T0321147

The Visible Woman

The Visible Woman

Imaging Technologies, Gender, and Science

Edited by

Paula A. Treichler,
Lisa Cartwright, and
Constance Penley

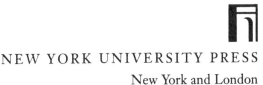

NEW YORK UNIVERSITY PRESS
New York and London

NEW YORK UNIVERSITY PRESS
New York and London

"Shooting the Mother: Fetal Photography and the Politics of Disappearance" by Carol Stabile originally appeared in *Camera Obscura* 28 (January 1992). *"The End of the Road*: Gender, the Dissemination of Knowledge, and the American Campaign against Venereal Disease during World War I" by Stacie A. Colwell, "Fetal Exposures: Abortion Politics and the Optics of Allusion" by Valerie Hartouni, "'Lasers for Ladies': Endo Discourse and the Inscription of Science" by Ella Shohat, and "The *Empire* Strikes Back: A Posttransexual Manifesto" by Sandy Stone originally appeared in *Camera Obscura* 29 (May 1992). "Mothers and Authors: *Johnson v. Calvert* and the New Children of Our Imaginations" by Mark Rose originally appeared in *Critical Inquiry* 22 (1996). "Beating the Meat/Surviving the Text, or How to Get Out of This Century Alive" by Vivian Sobchack originally appeared in *Body and Society*, vol. 1. Reprinted by permission of Sage Publications, Ltd. "Maybe Next Year: Feminist Silence and the AIDS Epidemic" by Paula A. Treichler and Catherine A. Warren originally appeared in *The Gendered Epidemic*, edited by Nancy L. Roth and Katie Hogan (New York: Routledge, 1998). Reprinted with permission.

Library of Congress Cataloging-in-Publication Data
The visible woman: imaging technologies, gender, and science / edited by Paula Treichler, Lisa Cartwright, and Constance Penley.
p.   cm.
Includes index.
ISBN 0-8147-1556-7 (clothbound: alk. paper). — ISBN 0-8147-1568-0 (pbk.: alk. paper)
1. Women—Health and hygiene—Social aspects.   2. Health services accessibility.   3. Imaging systems in medicine.   4. Feminist theory.
I. Treichler, Paula.   II. Cartwright, Lisa.   III. Penley, Constance.
RA778.V53   1998
362.1'082—dc21   97-45325
                    CIP

New York University Press books are printed on acid-free paper, and their binding materials are chosen for strength and durability.

Manufactured in the United States of America

10 9 8 7 6 5 4 3 2 1

Contents

Acknowledgments

The Visible Woman's birth is the product of a collective and not entirely uncomplicated labor, and as editors we would like to thank the major participants in this process. Eric Zinner, of New York University Press, has from the beginning supported this project with spirit and vision. The journal *Camera Obscura* and the *Camera Obscura* editors, Constance Penley in particular, made possible the two journal issues we published earlier on this topic and supported their transformation into the present (very different) book. Rachel Adams, *Camera Obscura*'s managing editor, coordinated all aspects of *The Visible Woman*'s pre-publication existence and, indeed, took the final manuscript to Federal Express at about the same moment that she took herself to Columbia University as a new assistant professor. Russ Coon, *Camera Obscura*'s succeeding managing editor, helped us complete our remaining tasks as editors. Finally, we thank the peerless Janet Lyon for giving *The Visible Woman* her name.

Paula A. Treichler, Lisa Cartwright, and Constance Penley

Introduction

Paradoxes of Visibility

The Visible Woman traces the development of several key medical and scientific technologies and examines their claims to make the human body—especially the female body—newly visible. These technologies have emerged as U.S. medicine and health care struggle with a series of largely unanticipated crises. The HIV/AIDS epidemic is foremost among these, yet other problems claim time and resources as well: the resurgence of tuberculosis and other infectious diseases, mounting evidence of enduring assaults on the human immune system, rising breast cancer rates, threats to reproductive choice and decreasing reproductive options, the rise of such occupational and environmental illnesses as repetitive stress injury and chronic fatigue syndrome, an expanding population without access to adequate health care, and the rapid restructuring of health care delivery in ways that are fragmented and poorly understood. One could add to this inventory the deeply divisive social questions that health and medical crises raise: concerns over civil rights and civil liberties, over "equality" and its attainment through federal policy initiatives, over the state of the global ecosystem, over the definition of what is "normal" and "natural" and how it is to be determined, and over the objective and value-free nature of scientific and biomedical research and practice.

During roughly this same period, visual technologies have emerged as a pivotal agent in the representation of diverse phenomena, ranging in scale from the computerized imaging systems that Western military forces used to chart and destroy vast territories in the Gulf War to the minute optical exploration of the body's interior made possible through techniques like video endoscopy, a fiber optics process used both to image (on a video monitor) and to treat (with laser surgery) such conditions as endometriosis. Images derived from MRI (magnetic resonance imaging), computerized tomography (computer-digitized X-ray imaging), and DNA sampling, colorized and sharpened to enhance their aesthetic appeal, regularly illustrate specialized journals like *Cell* and *Science* as well as popular magazines like *Scientific American* and *Life*. Given the power of these new technologies and their claims of unprecedented access to the natural world, it is not surprising that we acknowledge and think about the nation's health crises—whether biological, social, or environmental—through the visual images most readily available. To take just one example, HIV, "the AIDS virus," has achieved unequivocal superstar status among late-twentieth-century biomedical images. Schematic models of HIV regularly adorn book and magazine covers, electron micrographs document a range of HIV's daily activities, an enormous 3-D glass sculpture of HIV draws crowds and media coverage at international AIDS conferences, and, as the signature graphic for ABC's news magazine the *AIDS Quarterly*, a bright green image of HIV emerges out of the darkness to fill the screen over a throbbing *Jaws*-like soundtrack. Even if we cannot name the parts of the virus or identify their functions, we are members of an industrialized, technologized, highly literate society. We have lived our lives with the knowledge that invisible microbes cause disease, that "viruses" are an especially troublesome category of microbe, and that scientists who study these things can show us what they look like. Well acquainted with the conventions of scientific representation these viral images embody, we recognize them as what viruses are supposed to look like; the idea and the image have come to seem natural to us.[1]

Close scrutiny and analysis of images of HIV, however, reveal questions, even paradoxes. Like the products of other medical and scientific imaging systems, including X-ray, ultrasound, and MRI, they claim to make "the natural" newly visible, yet they simultaneously reinforce what we have already learned to see. Certainly a new technology, theoretical perspective, or scientific initiative may make material phenomena visible in ways that are exciting, useful, or more humane. Yet visibility is not transparency. Rather, we argue here, visibility is itself a claim that must be carefully examined: in acknowledging what is seen, and newly seen, we need to be equally vigilant about what is not seen, or no longer seen. To illuminate unseen connections, one of feminism's longstanding commitments, is an important goal of this volume.

Drawing upon and elaborating intersections among feminism, film theory, imaging technologies, and cultural accounts of science and medicine, *The Visible Woman* examines scientific and medical technologies that claim to newly clarify "the natural" in the light of parallel research that seeks to monitor, reinterpret, or contest those claims. Employing imaging technologies outside official medicine and science, or approaching imaging critically and self-consciously, the authors included here exemplify a much larger and heterogeneous group of patients, consumer advocates, activists, academics, and artists who are exploring ways to communicate their own understandings of current health and medical crises and to articulate their own experiences of health and disease. Across many populations and cultural domains, they are claiming knowledge, recognition, and rights for diverse kinds of bodies—among them, bodies that are gendered and transgendered, aging, racially and ethnically diverse, and physically and mentally disabled. Working with numerous electronic technologies (video, cable, computer networks) as well as sophisticated scientific and medical knowledge, these commentators are working to extend the range and vocabulary of patient knowledge and agency.

The Visible Woman also explores the symbiosis between scientific and popular imaging technologies. The culture and technological history of film and television repeatedly overlap and intersect with the culture and history of scientific and biomedical imaging. As we have noted in the case of HIV, there is crossover as well in the deployment of images and imaging technologies. Science and medicine furnish the raw material and the technological apparatus for narratives and spectacles in virtually all venues of popular culture. At the same time, science and medicine, in turn, regularly employ the representational conventions of popular entertainment. Yet while articles on scientific and medical imaging technologies in both specialized and general media certify that scientists, physicians, and imaging technicians cheerfully harness their technical images to popular vehicles, these same articles simultaneously declare themselves aloof from popular culture. To take just one example, the authors of a 1987 medical textbook on magnetic resonance imaging (MRI) open their discussion as follows: "I don't know about you, but when I turn on my television to watch the football game, electromagnetic waves, transistors, and picture tubes are the farthest thing from my mind. I have no trouble applauding a well-executed touchdown pass without understanding the operation of the television set." The authors establish electronic imaging as the shared foundation for both MRI and TV, but they quickly proceed to distinguish them: "Unlike in the case of the 'boob tube,'" the authors warn, "some understanding of the rudiments of MR image making is absolutely necessary in order to even vaguely understand the image. Without this knowledge one runs a serious risk of ineffective or even erroneous interpretation."[2] The magnetic resonance image, in other words, is not like television and other forms of entertainment media culture. MRI is addressed to a specialized audience of trained technicians who alone are able to produce and interpret accurately its highly abstract images. And the medical student audience is cautioned against viewing the diagnostic image as they would a televised football game.

Popular images, in this view, can be understood with no specialized knowledge of production and interpretation, but understanding scientific images requires highly expert technical training. Even among experts, however, new imaging technologies are taken up as though they will resolve questions definitively. Despite growing recognition of complexity and ambiguity in production and interpretation across cultural domains— that is, complexity in both technical and popular imaging processes—the notion of transparent representation and correct interpretation persists as a dominant theme in the imaging literature.[3] Long-standing and current controversies are being rewritten and reread through the lenses of new imaging technologies, and these inscriptions, in turn, will help determine how our medical futures are written. Reiterating our argument that visibility is not transparency, we want to look closely at the cultural and political filtering these "lenses" perform.

The Visible Woman, accordingly, explores three interrelated paradoxes of visibility. The first paradox is that today's scientific initiatives and imaging technologies enable us as never before to see the brain and body at work, their interior connections, and their complex relationships to widely divergent exterior phenomena. Yet the knowledge and insights about health and disease that these technologies make possible are shaped and constrained by existing networks of power, cultural values, institutional practices, and economic priorities.[4] In the process, systemic and structural issues related to, for example, the environment, access to health care, and patterns of reproduction are often transformed into the problems of individuals to be solved individually and privately, using guidelines produced from within the discrete domains of established disciplines and professional blocs. The second paradox—a paradigmatic exemplar of the first—concerns the new visibility of gender and women's health in science and medicine. This new women's health agenda is founded upon a well-documented history of feminist politics and women's health activism; yet it achieved its present prominence only by obscuring or obliterating its problematic political roots in struggles over abortion, reproductive choice, patient autonomy, and egalitarian ideals of health access for women across class, race, and employment status. In consequence, science and medicine, newly readied to take on "women's health" and solve "women's health problems," do so in an environment largely stripped of historical and political significance and of bodies deemed too problematic to be seen. The third paradox is that science and medicine, having defined the health problems of the late twentieth century in terms they are uniquely authorized and equipped to address, must ensure that new imaging technologies, too, remain within the domain of their expertise. Arguments ostensibly about the knowledge and training required to accurately read these new imaging narratives are also arguments about professional authority. Hence whatever our practical, personal responses to and experiences of these sophisticated new imaging technologies, it is crucial that we understand their performative character, that is, their role as a staging ground for struggles over agency and control. The urgency of this drama for women accounts, in part, for our emphasis in *The Visible Woman* on medicine and medical representation as a central focus of analysis. While "science" may offer a more philosophically satisfying site for speculation about the social and cultural construction of reality, medicine is easily as institutionally entrenched in its claims to scientific truth, as powerful in its account of the human body, and as skillful in its use of the visual as a significant resource in debate. In the rest of this introduction, we will more fully articulate these points and their paradoxical dimensions.

I

In March 1992, the venerable *New England Journal of Medicine* instituted a regular feature on medical imaging designed to display for its readers (primarily academic physicians) "a broad representation of useful and clinically important visual images." To emphasize that "imaging" extends an

existing tradition in medicine, *Journal* editor Jerome P. Kassirer introduced the new feature by listing images physicians routinely encounter:

> skin lesions, funduscopic views, blood smears, bone marrow smears, urine
> sediments, microbiologic specimens, joint aspirates, x-ray studies (chest,
> abdomen, pelvis, limbs, skull), recordings of electrical potentials (electrocar-
> diograms, electroencephalograms, and electromyograms), gross pathology
> specimens, histologic sections (routine, immunofluorescent, electron
> microscopy, special stains), endoscopic views, scans (CT, magnetic reso-
> nance imaging, radionuclide), sonograms, arteriograms, and venograms.[5]

Nonetheless, Kassirer continued, the whole notion of "imaging" poses
problems for medical scientists:

> To interpret an image, we use information from experience and memory to
> create a model of reality. The layers of imagery go even deeper; many of the
> images we use in medicine are already models. Microscopical slides are not
> living cells; CT scans of adrenal tumors are only representations of the
> actual tumor; ultrasound representations of a septal defect are sound waves
> converted into a film or video image, not the defect itself. Often, therefore,
> we are creating mental models of physical models, a process somewhat
> removed from classical hands-on auscultation, percussion and palpation.

"Images," Kassirer argues, unlike "classical hands-on" contact with the
patient's physical body, are multiply mediated through experience, memory, and diverse modes of representation; despite their apparent close correspondence to material reality, they may introduce new problems and
ambiguities into the diagnostic process. Kassirer does not pursue this line
of argument, however. Having carefully identified many of the complex
problems associated with interpreting medical images, he concludes with
a straightforward assertion about their value: "such models, whether once
or even twice removed from reality, are invaluable aids to perception and
interpretation, functions critical to the performance of doctors"; moreover, imaging, appropriately used, leads ultimately to "appropriate patient
care" (Kassirer, 829, 830). We need not quarrel with the pragmatic claims
of Kassirer's argument to note that its presumption of continuity with
existing medical practices also presumes the continuity of existing medical
networks and cultures, including the traditional one-to-one doctor-
patient relationship.

The reduction of important structural and interpretive complexities to
the provider-consumer relationship is accomplished with even greater dis-
patch in the *Journal of Reproductive Medicine*, which in January 1992 pub-

lished a symposium on imaging techniques for practicing obstetricians, gynecologists, and reproductive endocrinologists. Here (in contrast to the *New England Journal* argument), the representational value of imaging was taken absolutely for granted: the only pitfalls for physicians in using these new imaging techniques are competitive, not interpretive. Introducing the papers, guest editor Alan H. DeCherney emphasized that imaging technologies are therapeutic as well as diagnostic, noting as further evidence of imaging's popularity that many medical school radiology departments are changing their names to departments of medical imaging.[6] But "we are newcomers to this technology," he continued, warning physicians in reproductive medicine of the need for continuing mastery of new imaging techniques. Even ultrasound is no longer confined to obstetrics: there "is more than a fair possibility that in the future, every woman will undergo ultrasonography as part of her gynecological examination"; indeed, the "need for ultrasonography in postmenopausal women is beginning to emerge."[7]

II

The Visible Woman appears at a time when women's health has achieved particular visibility. Clearly, as the *Journal of Reproductive Medicine* suggests, a powerful economic narrative is emerging that targets many imaging technologies specifically to women and, simultaneously, constructs new markets for imaging. At the same time, a research initiative under the auspices of the National Institutes of Health (NIH) is inserting women's health into research agendas, academic curricula, and policy mandates. Established in 1990, the NIH initiative was provoked in part by a series of long-standing public claims about rising rates among women of breast cancer, HIV/AIDS, and other diseases and conditions; about differential biomedical research and clinical treatment according to gender, race, class, and age; about possibilities and problems associated with new reproductive technologies; about challenges to traditional understandings and enactments of sex, gender, and bodies; and about women's labor in a changing workforce. As this list goes on, it is clear that positions on health and gender are closely linked to a number of ongoing historical controversies and structural concerns.

It is this larger context that illuminates the paradoxical nature of the new visibility of gender and women's health in science and medicine and, with it, the targeting of many imaging technologies to women. Certainly for seasoned women consumers of health care, it is a new experience to

find women's needs so explicitly acknowledged. Whether we are undergoing routine gynecological care, neurological assessment of carpal tunnel
syndrome, or diagnosis and treatment of breast cancer, we rarely
encounter the mainstream health care system today without also encountering a specialized imaging process intended to be diagnostic, therapeutic, or both. Nor is it altogether surprising, given women's economic
importance as consumers in general, that our health needs have, in fact,
been efficiently reconstituted as a "market." We may welcome these technologies as less invasive and painful, with fewer side effects—or we may
resist them as further attempts to medicalize and market women's images.
In either case, feminist analysis is needed to identify precisely what kind of
narrative we want this to be.

One strategy for making private, unseen experiences available for visible public scrutiny marks the case of Cecil B. Jacobson, M.D., the "fertility doctor" who was charged in 1992 with multiple counts of criminal
fraud and perjury. Many of his women patients were undergoing artificial
insemination from anonymous sperm donors; if the procedures were
unsuccessful, Dr. Jacobson convinced women patients they were pregnant by prescribing hormones that would simulate positive urine tests,
then showed them ultrasound images of their nonexistent fetuses. He
went so far as to identify heartbeats, thumb-sucking, and other fetal
movements, and even suggested that these embryonic "visualizations"
already demonstrated desired traits. The notorious Dr. Jacobson went
beyond these practices (evidently not rare in the "fertility business") and
inseminated many of his unknowing patients with his own semen. By
producing a collection of offspring who resembled their doctor, this procedure (ironically, if not coincidentally) made it possible to transform the
private exploitation of isolated couples into a collective, and visible, prosecution of criminal fraud.[8]

Activist projects suggest other strategies for linking the private and
personal to the collective and political. Examples include AIDS/HIV
actions by groups like ACT UP; breast cancer activism; medical media
interventions like Kathy High's video *Underexposed: Temple of the Fetus* and
Carl George's *DHPG Mon Amour*, a film that documents the choice and
home administration of an experimental AIDS drug; interactive programs
like Ann Satterfield's *Treatment* and Kathy Shapiro and Richard Steen's *No
MisConception*, an interactive hypercard stack designed to introduce
women to a wide range of birth control methods; and the AIDS bulletin
boards and software packages that provide up-to-the-minute information
and commentary on a vast range of AIDS issues, theories, and treatments.

And as activist groups such as ACT UP (AIDS Coalition to Unleash Power), WHAM (Women's Health Action Mobilization), the National Black Women's Health Project, and NBCC (National Breast Cancer Coalition) are making clear, the identities of medical professional, consumer, and activist are not always discrete; transformation of medicine and science can and must take place from within, as well as on the margins of, institutional discourses and practices.

III

This brings us to the third paradox we identified above. The imaging technologies developed and popularized over the past decade or two are marked by continuing struggles over cultural authority and cultural inscription—over who will have the authority to define the role and meaning of these technologies and determine how they will be institutionalized. Such struggles call attention to what, precisely, is and is not seen. Just as a scientific fact at once designates something that is made and something that is not made (i.e., fabricated yet simultaneously certified as *not* fabricated), an image may at once count for what is seen and what is not seen. Such a tension marks recent medical debates. Two papers in the *New England Journal of Medicine* of January 7, 1993, on the problem of diagnosing thoracic aortic dissection (a tear in the wall of the aorta—a dangerous condition with a high mortality rate), describe the difficulties of evaluating the findings of rapidly evolving imaging technologies; among other problems, studies may be incommensurate over time.[9] Implicit in these discussions are problems of representation, interpretation, and the culture and conventions of reading images. Researchers responding in subsequent issues, however, focused exclusively on technique as the locus of the problem.[10] This shifts questions about medical representation to the representational capacities, merits, and deficiencies of specific kinds of technology, and shifts questions about meaning and interpretation to statistical concepts, for example, the specificity and sensitivity with which a given technique can represent a given property of the body.

Perhaps it is inevitable that meaning and interpretation within the practice of medicine be subordinated to the technical nuts and bolts of praxis. There is nothing wrong with discussing the pros and cons of various technological advances, but these concerns may preempt and displace more fundamental discussion of the cultural work that imaging systems accomplish and how they accomplish it. In a 1991 essay on medical imaging, Sarah Kember succinctly explains the cultural place of the physician in new imaging systems. Her analysis illuminates the contradictory professional response to imaging technologies described by Kassirer: physicians' discomfort with imaging systems follows in part from the fact that these new optical technologies emphasize the declining status of their own sensory expertise. Kember suggests that the locus of power is no longer the physician's observing body; it is the self-correcting perceptual machine in which the observer is now incorporated—and monitored. In medical imaging systems, she explains,

> the observer becomes part of the observed. Attempts to include the observer in analysis have yielded various methods in the study of image perception, notably the construction of relative operating characteristic curves and concepts of sensitivity and specificity. The observer is incorporated into the computational system, as a design fault, or design limitation. The study of image cognition joins that of image perception and attempts to reveal the process by which the observer of a radiological image arrives at a correct diagnosis. Medical skill is completely conflated with visual literacy and diagnosis is redefined in the field of the computer and/as the clinic.[11]

Ultimately, Kember argues, taking a position with which many experienced clinicians would undoubtedly agree, modern imaging systems produce a series of visual and cognitive analogies that successively correct for the deficiencies of the real and for physicians' own limited powers of observation (e.g., their inability to visualize invisible interior processes), forsaking the analysis of sameness and difference on which such clinical operations as autopsy depend. Kember concludes that it "is the widespread cultural desire for analogy which totals the totaled machine of postmodernism (analogy does for postmodernism what the eye does for empiricism) and medicine's progress is thereby part of a significant cultural and historical regression" (Kember, 56).

Despite problems of theory, technological anxiety, and postmodern hype, imaging technologies are widely—even when grudgingly—perceived to provide accurate and noninvasive diagnosis and treatment. But another paper in the *New England Journal of Medicine* indicates that the widespread acceptance of medical imaging may, in fact, be an inverse indicator of its real clinical value. William C. Black and H. Gilbert Welch, physicians based at the Center for the Evaluative Clinical Sciences at Dartmouth Medical School, argue that technological advances in diagnostic imaging "create confusion in two crucial areas of medical decision making: establishing how much disease there is and defining how well treatment works." Advancing what is essentially a technical argument about the statistical representation of disease and mortality, Black and Welch start from the fact that increased detection of any disease increases its estimated prevalence; when prevalence appears to increase, the perceived probability that a given patient will actually die from it inevitably decreases.[12] Thus, although nothing has actually changed, it can appear that early detection and whatever treatment is given (which will rarely be carefully controlled through clinical trials) improve chances of survival, leading to overestimation of both disease prevalence and therapeutic effectiveness. Not only do these "consequences of modern imaging increasingly pervade everyday medicine," write Black and Welch, "the increasing use of sophisticated diagnostic imaging promotes a cycle of increasing intervention that often confers little or no benefit" (Black and Welch, 1237).

There are important lessons here for those researching the culture of medical imaging, as well as for imaging specialists. As Welch and Black argue, imaging can be shown in some cases to offer little or no benefit. And as we have suggested, diagnostic imaging presents complex yet widely underestimated interpretive challenges. But imaging is given largely uncritical media attention, assumed to be self-evident and nonproblematic in hundreds of research proposals and published papers, and enthusiastically promoted as a profitable medical specialty with little concern for interpretive practice.

The Visible Woman seeks to avoid both the technophilia that characterizes much of medical imaging and related scientific inscription and the technophobia sometimes embraced by science and medicine's critics. The authors in this volume, tracing the broader culture in which imaging and inscriptions are used and appropriated, acknowledge the specific and often conflicting needs and desires of the diverse communities and audiences, within and beyond medicine and science, in which these images and narratives circulate. By bringing to these questions a variety of perspectives and identities, we hope to generate productive alliances and debates that can more adequately comprehend and document the cultural work that science and medicine perform.

IV

The book is in three parts, loosely paralleling the three "paradoxes of visibility" just described. The opening essays profile four key crises faced by U.S. biomedicine and public health in the twentieth century and identify the changing historical, sociocultural, and political contexts in which these crises have been represented and managed. Setting the stage for the rest of the book, these four essays also demonstrate that the work of science and medicine cannot readily be separated from the discourses and representations through which that work is conceptualized, executed, and given public life.

In chapter 1, Lisa Cartwright examines the elaborate medical dissection and imaging process through which a series of "cyber-cadavers" for use in medical education and elsewhere are being created from selected corpses of real human beings. Invoking the theme and paradox of visibility itself, Cartwright interrogates the complicated discourse through which the abstract contract between science and society is worked out in one specific arena and traces some of its differential consequences for particular individuals and groups. She also compares and contrasts the rhetoric surrounding the "Visible Man" and the "Visible Woman."

In chapter 2, Stacie A. Colwell brings together feminist, historical, and public health perspectives to examine the U.S. War Department's campaign against venereal disease during World War I. She specifically analyzes the ideological, organizational, and cinematic commitments and compromises that produced *The End of the Road*, a film warning women about syphilis and rightly celebrated, despite its moralistic good girl/bad girl narrative, as a groundbreaking effort to offer a program of education about sexuality and health to a wide female audience.

In chapter 3, Paula A. Treichler and Catherine A. Warren use quantitative and qualitative measures of AIDS coverage in feminist and nonfeminist print media to track and analyze U.S. feminism's problematic stance toward the AIDS epidemic. Even as women with AIDS and HIV infection grew more visible during the 1980s and heterosexual intercourse emerged as a significant mode of transmission, U.S. mainstream feminism remained largely invisible in the struggle against the epidemic. One result is that straight men, the major source of HIV infection and other STDs in women, remain largely invisible as well.

To conclude this section, Anne K. Eckman's essay in chapter 4 takes up the science-society contract in another arena, examining the recent initiative of the National Institutes of Health to improve U.S. women's health research. Launched after a stinging government critique of women's health research, the NIH initiative is designed to overcome the "Yentl syndrome," a metaphor for the tendency in biomedical science and clinical medicine to assume the male body as the normative standard. Acknowledging the progress signaled by the initiative, Eckman also asks at what scientific and political price this progress in women's health is to be won. One price, she suggests, is that now this new body of "women's health" had to be cleansed of controversial issues like abortion, midwifery, and hormone replacement therapy. Only then, made over into the study of heart attacks and bone loss, could women's health be lauded and widely publicized.

The second part of *The Visible Woman* concerns, precisely, the domain of controversy expunged from mainstreamed "women's health." These essays constitute a series of case studies on reproductive choice and new reproductive technologies, including the uses of imaging in obstetrics and gynecology. In chapter 5, an essay on fetal photography going back to *Life*'s 1965 display of Lennart Nilsson's celebrated fetal images, Carol Stabile examines the place in popular media of scientific and medical imaging of the "unborn child," and the ways in which these images function to assert fetal personhood and autonomy at the expense of pregnant women's identity and rights.

Valerie Hartouni examines in chapter 6 the ways in which "the grammar and culture of abortion have been profoundly refigured" over the last decade, attributing this change in large part to the increased public presence of the "free-floating fetal form" (in photographs, in videos, and in fetal medicine and other subspecialties of obstetrics and gynecology that rely on such imaging techniques as ultrasound). The focus of her critique, however, is not the medical or popular media texts in which fetal images are so often featured, but Aline Mare's 1991 *S'Aline's Solution*, an experimental videotape distributed through art and alternative media venues. Drawing on a strategy commonly used in prolife media, such as the notorious television documentary *The Silent Scream*, Mare's video uses images of the interior of the body to grant a reality to the fetus, setting it up as a character with whom viewers may identify, then purporting to represent the fetus's perspective as it experiences a saline abortion.

Both Stabile and Hartouni explore conventions of visual and textual representation in a range of contemporary reproductive narratives and specifically the growing public celebrity in U.S. culture of the fetal subject. The further evolution of representational strategies to resolve reproductive disputes is examined by Mark Rose in chapter 7. In *Johnson v. Calvert*, a landmark "surrogate mother" case in which one woman furnished ovum for fertilization and another carried the fetus to term, the question asked was, "Who is the mother?" Faced with conflicting biological claims, the California court used the paradigm of intellectual property law and asked, "Who first originated the concept of the child, intended to bring it into being?" The court's extension of copyright law to the determination of motherhood, Rose argues, constitutes a remarkable moment not only in surrogacy law but also in the history of authorship.

In chapter 8, Ella Shohat also takes up the ways in which disease is seen, defined, and managed through optical technologies. Her focus is endometriosis, a disease characterized by the adherence of the tissue from the uterine lining to all the "wrong" anatomical sites (the ovaries, fallopian tubes, or even the stomach). A disease traditionally associated in the medical literature with "career women" who choose not to bear children, endometriosis is currently managed by laparoscopy, a surgical procedure in which a laser and minute camera are inserted into the narrow passages of the reproductive system. Shohat critiques the scientific narrative of conquest and desire that informs this medical procedure, but also considers the ways in which women have organized around "endo discourse" to challenge and restructure the definition, diagnosis, and treatment of this disease.

The essays in the final part explore links between microlevel and macrolevel domains, between individual agency and the structural arrangements and institutional systems in which agency is enacted. These essays ask where space for agency exists and at what levels social and political change can occur. In doing so, they address the dual drama of medical imaging and inscription as a representational system and as a staging ground for professional authority, agency, and control.

In chapter 9, Michael Bérubé and Janet Lyon survey the highlights of mental retardation's cultural evolution in the United States. Elements of this history (in which mentally retarded children only recently became visible) readily lend themselves to a quasi-Foucauldian analysis of faceless, agentless programs of social control in which "all institutions mirror the culture's worst repressive fantasies as they inexorably strive for internal order and homogeneity." As parents of a child with Down syndrome, however, they ask a different question: Can you be Foucauldian about the past and yet retain hope for the present, for your own children?

In chapter 10, an essay whose title, "The *Empire* Strikes Back," was occasioned by *The Transsexual Empire*, Janice Raymond's 1979 book-length discussion of male-to-female transsexuals, Sandy Stone takes as a starting point documented accounts of transsexuals who have undergone male-to-female surgery. This manifesto makes a powerful case for the cultural importance of a transsexual identity that breaks with the gender binarism so stubbornly maintained not only in medicine and social science, but also in the women's movement and broader culture. It is a critical reminder both of the limits of medical discourse where gender identity is concerned and of the potential for radical retooling of institutional technologies of imaging, cultural inscription, and body reconfiguration.

Like other essays in *The Visible Woman*, Vivian Sobchack's essay in chapter 11 shows great respect for the "lived body"—how it inhabits concrete spaces and how the researcher's work can preserve this respect. Reflecting upon the body as it is taken up by such celebratory postmodernists as Baudrillard—that is, as a technobody primarily *"thought* always as an object and never *lived* as a subject"—Sobchack offers a witty commentary on her life after cancer with a bionic leg made of titanium and fiberglass. The paradoxes of visibility we address in this introduction are evident in Sobchack's contrast between the hypervisibility of new technologies with their intimations of transcendence and the vanishing material and mortal body that gives that transcendence reality and meaning.

In chapter 12, Richard A. Cone, a biologist, and Emily Martin, a cultural anthropologist, offer a collaborative interpretation of the body, the globe, and what it means to be healthy. The essay examines and seeks to link phenomena at very different levels: the operation of the mucosal immune system, the rising global rate of allergy and autoimmunity, and changes on a global scale in the ways we produce and consume food. Their interpretation postulates connections among domains that ordinarily belong to separate disciplines and suggests that gender is relevant at all points in the system. The unconventional format of the essay reveals the different ways that science and culture think and talk about these issues, at the same time demonstrating the fruitful possibilities of a cooperative, collaborative, analytic dialogue.

Like Colwell's essay on *The End of the Road* in this book's opening section, Gaye Naismith's concluding essay in chapter 13 examines the representation of gender and disease in film. Todd Haynes's *[Safe]* explores different approaches to the diagnosis and treatment—indeed, the existence—of environmental illness by following one woman's bleak quest for health in late-twentieth-century southern California. Where *The End of the Road* ultimately reached the screen as a compromise among the several warring organizations involved in its creation, Naismith reads *[Safe]* as a series of totalizing, mutually exclusive accounts of reality, each of which, by intensifying the visibility and responsibility of "the individual," obscures real responsibility for structural problems of the environment and U.S. society and thus renders genuine individual choice and political intervention invisible. Only outside the film—for example, along the lines of inquiry suggested by Cone and Martin and by models presented elsewhere in the book—can current cultural crises be made sufficiently visible to be effectively addressed.

Notes

1. Other examples that deploy the medical-scientific image as popular media spectacle for validation and support include the Human Genome Project's effort to construct a human record of genetic codes, the popular imaging conventions that accompany NASA's past and present initiatives, the ubiquitous ultrasound images put forward to shore up and naturalize claims about fetal development and fetal medicine, and the jumble of technical images and science fiction scenarios used to illustrate the breakthrough cloning experiment of spring 1997.

2. Jeffrey C. Weinreb and Helen C. Redman, *Magnetic Resonance Imaging of the Body* (Philadelphia: W.B. Saunders, 1987) 4.

3. A less prominent theme in the imaging literature concerns the ongoing problems of the field, such as its lack of standardized codes, across both laboratories (e.g., the same color coding may signify two different things in two different laboratories) and technologies (e.g., MR and PET [positron emission tomography] images are computed differently, hence their data cannot easily be correlated).

4. Nelly Oudshoorn, describing the results of her study of the medicalization of the female body, comments as follows:

> One of the reasons why science succeeds in convincing us that it reveals the truth about nature is that the social contexts in which knowledge claims are transformed into scientific facts and artifacts are made invisible. Science makes us believe that its knowledge claims are not dependent on social context. During the development of science and technology the established links with the worlds outside the laboratory are naturalized.

"A Natural Order of Things? Reproductive Science and the Politics of Othering," 122–132 in *FutureNatural: Nature/Science/Culture*, ed. George Robertson et al. (London and New York: Routledge, 1996) 124.

5. Jerome P. Kassirer, "Images in Clinical Medicine," *New England Journal of Medicine* 326 (March 19, 1992): 829–830.

6. The name change may also represent the determination by radiologists to steal the march on other specialties that might lay claim to expertise in interpreting new imaging systems—neurologists, for example.

7. Alan H. DeCherney, guest editor, "Imaging Techniques in Reproductive Medicine: A Symposium," *Journal of Reproductive Medicine*, 37.1 (January 1992): 1–2. A decade before, DeCherney authored an editorial in the *New England Journal of Medicine* (February 18, 1982) applauding a study that claimed to show a sharp drop in fertility among women over age 30; both the article and the editorial—as well as the wave of uncritical media coverage of the "infertility epidemic"—blamed women for choosing careers over reproduction. Researchers who disputed the existence of this "epidemic" made no headway in the media. When results from a longitudinal nationwide study published in 1985 definitively

invalidated the 1982 finding, reporter Susan Faludi asked DeCherney whether he now had second thoughts about his sermonizing editorial. "No, none at all," he told her; "the editorial was meant to be provocative. I got a great response. I was on the *Today* show." Susan Faludi, *Backlash: The Undeclared War Against American Women* (New York: Crown, 1991) 2.

8. It should be noted in the Jacobson case that the New York district attorney made efforts to protect the actual identities of the couples who agreed to join the prosecution's case. See Diane M. Gianelli, "Fertility Doctor Charged with Fraud over Methods," *American Medical News* February 24, 1992: 1.

Another poignant example of the deployment of imaging emerged in journalist Ellen Hopkins's interviews with couples undergoing in vitro fertilization; here, one woman interviewed suggests how an image can come to stand not only for the "unborn child" but for a host of failed reproductive technologies:

> Before transfer, they give you a Polaroid of your embryo. . . . You look at this greenish picture of a few dividing cells, and you will that photo to assume life, you will that photo to become your baby. And when it doesn't, all you can do is put that photo in a drawer.

"Tales from the Baby Factory," *New York Times Magazine*, March 15, 1992: 80.

9. Christoph A. Nienaber, M.D., et al., "The Diagnosis of Thoracic Aortic Dissection by Noninvasive Imaging Procedures," *New England Journal of Medicine* 328.1 (January 7, 1993): 1–9; and Cigarroa et al., "Diagnostic Imaging in the Evaluation of Suspected Aortic Dissection—Old Standards and New Directions," *New England Journal of Medicine* 328.1 (January 7, 1993): 35–43.

10. For example, see the responses to Nienaber and Cigarroa in the correspondences section of the *New England Journal of Medicine* 328.22 (June 3, 1993): 1637–1638.

11. Sarah Kember, "Medical Imaging: The Geometry of Chaos," *New Formations* 15 (Winter 1991): 55–66. Citation from 64.

12. William C. Black and H. Gilbert Welch, "Advances in Diagnostic Imaging and Overestimations of Disease Prevalence and the Benefits of Therapy," *New England Journal of Medicine* 328.17 (April 29, 1993): 1237–1243. The logic is as follows: If in a given year 100,000 people have a disease and 1,000 people die from it, the mortality rate is represented as 1,000/100,000 = .01 percent. If detection increases estimated prevalence of the disease to 120,000 while the same 1,000 people die from it, nothing changes except the denominator, but it will appear that the mortality rate has fallen to 1,000/120,000, or .008 percent.

Lisa Cartwright

1

A Cultural Anatomy of the Visible Human Project

In 1986, a long-range planning committee of the National Library of Medicine, a division of the National Institutes of Health, speculated about a coming era when the library's widely used bibliographic and factual database services would be complemented by libraries of digital images, distributed over high-speed computer networks and by high-capacity media. The committee encouraged the library to investigate the feasibility of producing a biomedical images library of its own. The Planning Panel on Electronic Image Libraries was formed and in 1990 proposed the ground plan for

a first project: building a digital image library of volumetric data representing a complete, normal adult male and female. This Visible Human Project will include digitized photographic images for cryosectioning, digital images derived from computerized tomography, and digital magnetic resonance images of cadavers.[1]

The library's speculation about the future flow of digital biomedical images was remarkably prescient. In 1986 the application of digital imaging in clinical settings was largely limited to specialized areas, and a computer interface that could link text, graphics, video, and audio on computers around the world was still just the fantasy of a few computer entrepreneurs. By 1994, the year the Visible Human Project's first completed database, dubbed the Visible Man, was unveiled to a global audience of World Wide Web users, digital imaging had become ubiquitous in U.S. medicine, and digital anatomical programs were available in relative abundance on the Web and elsewhere. The National Library of Medicine already provided access to a searchable database of nearly 60,000 images. The Web site titled "Anatomical Imaging Sites on the World Wide Web" now lists over 100 destinations, and a single company, A.D.A.M. Software, Inc., whose acronym stands for Animated Dissection of Anatomy for Medicine, advertises over 15 anatomical multimedia programs tailored to users ranging from physicians and scientists to schoolchildren and families. Why, among these images, was press coverage of the Visible Man so extensive? Why the fanfare surrounding its completion in 1994 and the Visible Woman's in 1995? What makes the Visible Man and Woman so different from previous anatomical models and previous ways of organizing biomedical knowledge?

This essay takes up these questions about the project's reception and its difference through an analysis of its various images, texts, and techniques. My central concern is sex difference and other aspects of cultural difference as they are (or are not) represented in the project. In their study of representations of male and female anatomy in texts for U.S. medical students, Susan C. Lawrence and Kate Bendixen show that in the century from 1890 to 1989, anatomy texts remained consistent in their disproportionate use of male figures or male-specific structures to illustrate or describe human anatomy. In these texts, the normal human body is pervasively presented as male, making it impossible to learn female anatomy without first learning male anatomy (e.g., "the clitoris is commonly described as 'homologous with the penis in the male' ").[2] By presenting the female body as a variation on the male, or by presenting the male body as a standard for gender-neutral medical information (as was sometimes the case), these texts contributed to the neglect of health conditions specific to women and the tacit perception of female-specific aspects of anatomy as innately abnormal. Adriane Fugh-Berman, a physician who attended Georgetown Medical School in the mid-1980s, writes about the place of female-specific anatomy in medical teaching: "The prevailing attitude toward women was demonstrated on the first day of classes by my anatomy instructor, who remarked that our elderly cadaver 'must have been a Playboy bunny' before instructing us to cut off her large breasts and toss them into the thirty-gallon trash can marked 'cadaver waste.' "[3]

The salient point here is not that the instructor has a prurient interest in sexualized body parts, but that he views with professional contempt and dismissal parts of the female body precisely because they bear sexual meanings not tied to reproduction. Fugh-Berman's anecdote suggests that anatomy's treatment of the female body may be seen, in this case at least, as the repressive side of a broader cultural tendency to privilege women's bodies as objects of visual pleasure. Terri Kapsalis's recent analysis of gynecology texts cogently demonstrates how such popular conventions of representing sexuality as pornography can serve to make visible that which medicine refuses to image. Kapsalis quotes a female gynecologist: "When I was in medical school, a fellow student had never seen a naked woman and would start sweating anytime anybody mentioned a pelvic exam. . . . A bunch of us bought him a copy of *Penthouse* so he would know what he was going to be looking at."[4]

In light of these accounts, the National Library of Medicine's decision to make the female body visible rather than opting to create a singular Visible Human on the basis of a male body sounds progressive. As a branch of the National Institutes of Health, the Library had reason to ensure representation of female anatomy. As Anne Eckman explains in her contribution to this volume, the NIH was taken to task in a 1990 Government Accounting Office report to Congress for failing to meet a research protocols policy stipulating that biomedical research should emphasize conditions and diseases unique to, or more prevalent in, women. In the wake of the publicity that surrounded this report, women became the focus of new initiatives by the NIH and other medical entities, with one result that in 1991 the term *women's health* entered the *Index Medicus*, the National Library of Medicine's widely used bibliographic index of medical knowledge, signaling among other changes a pervasive recognition of the need to endow women "with a fully visible and complete set of organs."[5] The Visible Woman may be seen as one example of this initiative to make women's bodies visible.

The act of making women visible, however, does not in itself address the complex question of how gender difference is constructed and given value in medicine.[6] Lisa Jean Moore and Adele E. Clarke document historical changes in what (if anything) counts as "the clitoris" in twentieth-century anatomy texts, demonstrating among other things the heterogeneity of representations of, and the contests of definition over, this body part where it is made visible.[7] Thus, it becomes necessary to analyze the ways that difference is assigned to bodies and their parts, and is encoded in medical images. My analysis focuses on the cultural and technical conventions used to produce the Visible Man and Visible Woman. A $1.4 million government-sponsored project that aims to foster the creation of a universally acknowledged set of anatomical images of designated normal male and female bodies, the Visible Human Project promises, in the words of one journalist, to make it possible for scientists to "study human bodies in ways never before possible."[8] According to the Center for Human Simulation at the University of Colorado, the team that contracted with the library to produce the project database, the images were created "to provide a universally-accessible, national resource for anatomical information for researchers, educators, medical professionals, as well as the general public."[9] How will universal concepts about what is normal anatomy—and which bodies may serve as a standard in medicine—hold up against the specific physicality and history of the citizens on whose bodies the Visible Human Project is based? Moreover, how does this new standard compare to anatomy's past representational practices? My angle on these broad questions is to retrace the acquisition and presence of these images in their current incarnations on the Web and in various commercial productions. My goal is to demonstrate that this massive and universalizing project replicates certain well-known characteristics of older anatomical paradigms, notably the taking of a male body as the standard in medical research and the use of the cadavers of criminals for anatomical dissections, but with an ironic twist: against earlier anatomical practices that identified the criminal body as innately pathological, the body of the Visible Man, based on the cadaver of a convicted felon, is now the basis for a medical norm. A second example of this return to earlier anatomical paradigms is the project's use of older and more broadly familiar conventions of photography and surface modeling in conjunction with more abstract image processes to produce this new anatomical standard. As I demonstrate below, this combination of strategies results in a unique kind of realism[10] that is difficult to reconcile with the range of applications imagined for the project. My overall aim is to show that the Visible Human Project, promoted through the rhetoric of new technologies and advanced scientific knowledge, ultimately is confounded in its goals of creating a new standard for medical research and education.

The Visible Human Project's Difference

A number of factors set the Visible Human Project apart from the plethora of digital anatomical resources on the market. Most important is its paradoxical status as the last word in virtual-body imaging and the closest thing to an actual living body. The most striking example of the latter is the project's use of "corpses" (a term used to refer specifically to bodies in the early period after death) rather than "cadavers" (a term generally applied to bodies preserved for anatomical study).[11] As Paula Treichler notes,

> Traditional anatomy texts and classes are based on photographs or illustrations or (more recently) computer-generated images of dissections of cadavers in various stages of preservation and decomposition—and most often cadavers are old people, sick people, or people with lots of pathology. So the Visible Man represents for the first time a young, healthy, "normal" guy whose tissues and organs are the closest thing possible to a living body. Medical students often describe the shock of seeing living tissues and organs in surgery that look nothing like what they saw dissecting cadavers. The Visible Man and Visible Woman will change that.[12]

The Visible Man and Visible Woman are the closest thing possible to fresh, healthy living tissue and organs because the people used to produce them died in states of relative health and their bodies were immediately frozen rather than chemically preserved. The Visible Man consists of 24-bit digitized computed tomography, magnetic resonance, and photographic images of over 1,800 1.0-millimeter cross-sectional slices of a male corpse, and the Visible Woman is composed of 5,000 images of .33-millimeter slices of a female corpse.

The Visible Man and Visible Woman are regarded as realistic not only because they are based on the closest thing to a living body, but because they are the closest medicine has come to creating accurate and detailed virtual bodies using advanced biomedical imaging techniques. Writing about anatomical representations published between 1900 and 1991, Moore and Clarke note that "precisely because anatomy is *not* cutting edge biomedical science and has supposedly been comparatively stable, we can see its (re)constructions more vividly."[13] The Visible Human Project is a watershed in anatomy because it uses advanced biomedical imaging techniques, and in doing so it dramatically breaks away from the relatively stable view of bodily structure presented in prior anatomical constructions. The corpses used to produce the Visible Man and Visible Woman

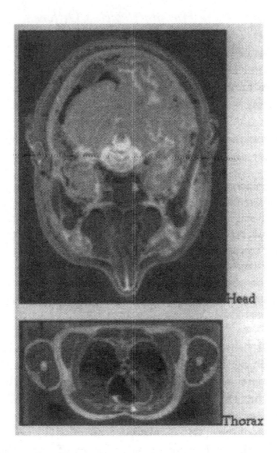

Figure 1.1   Photographic cryosections of head and thorax of the Visible Man.

were subjected to computerized tomography and magnetic resonance imaging. It is widely reported (in project literature and press accounts) that the research team that produced the data sets embedded in gelatin and deep-froze the two corpses, then sawed them each into four large chunks and passed these through a cryogenic macrotome—a kind of high-tech meat slicer. Then, as they milled away[14] each body from head to toe in ultrathin increments, a color photograph was taken of each of the flat cross-sectional planes exposed on the face of the remaining frozen block (figure 1.1).[15] These thousands of cryographs were then numbered in series and scanned into a computer animation program, which would eventually allow users to stack, disassemble, and volume-render discrete parts or whole bodies. Programs based on the data sets allow users to move optically through these highly detailed images of body sections via hypermedia links, three-dimensional reconstructions, and fly-through animations in which one can construct and travel through the minute spaces of various systems from a range of vantage points.

The image of slicing fresh bodies evokes earlier anatomical techniques—the messy practice of physically unlayering bodies through hands-on dissection, for example. For users of the project database, however, actual contact with the viscera of corpse, cadaver, or living body is conveniently replaced by virtual contact. Participants in the many interactive and virtual reality programs designed using Visible Human data are able to see and manipulate fresh organs and tissue carefully simulated to approximate living structures so closely that surgical techniques may be practiced upon them with great precision. As one project program advertisement suggests, users may "explore an entire human body with the click of a mouse!"[16]

The rhetoric of the virtually real appears frequently throughout discussions about the project. The Center for Human Simulation states that its goal is to enable the user to interact with the Visible Human imagery "in very real ways," asserting in a caption beneath one Visible Man rendering that "the tattoo [visible in the image] and all of the colors are real" and "this is not a photograph!!" but a computer-generated view created directly from Visible Man body slices.[17] Ben Schneiderman, head of the Human-Computer Interaction Laboratory at the University of Maryland at College Park, also emphasizes the realism of the Visible Man as compared to other anatomical renderings: "Medical textbooks give us a highly interpreted view of the human body, emphasizing key organs. This [the Visible Man database] was a raw and fresh perspective that told me things about my own body that I never knew before."[18] A Women's Wire news story reiterates the premium placed on realism in the nonscientific press, revealing details about the woman whose body was used to make the Visible Woman data set in order to support the assertion that "the images are not artificially created forms."[19] The combination of raw, fresh (unpreserved) flesh and virtual imaging thus confers on the Visible Man and Visible Woman a level of authenticity well beyond that conferred on the photograph of the cadaver, the digital image, or most any other mode of anatomical documentation prior to the Visible Human Project's inception.

What further sets the project apart from other contemporary anatomical programs is its pervasive presence in both public as well as professional settings. The stated goal of the Center for Human Simulation is to "enable the user, from the 12-year-old science student to the practicing surgeon," to use the database.[20] Although the images are not in the public domain, a sampling of them can be downloaded from the Web by anyone without revealing one's identity, and the entire data sets can be downloaded, for a fee, through a licensing agreement.[21] The Visible Man's 400-plus licensees include physicians in the U.S. Army, who are using the Visible Man to simulate the passage of shrapnel through flesh and bone; an interdisciplinary team at the State University of New York at Stony Brook, which has created an interactive fly-through animation of the Man's colon as a step toward developing a scanning test for colon cancer; the publishing company Mosby, Inc., which is creating a commercial CD-ROM and printed atlas in conjunction with a computer animation company; and teachers and students at Smoky Hill High School, who are creating their own Visible Human Digital Anatomy Project. The project's global scope is indicated by the presence on the Web of its Far East site, based at the University of Singapore.[22] The National Library of Medicine is working on imaging transmission technologies that would broaden this already wide base of licensees in much the same way it now makes accessible to countless medical professionals 8.6 million text-based records dating back to 1966 and an index of articles from over 3,800 biomedical journals (through database services such as Medline). As a featured project of the federal entity that brings us Medline, the self-proclaimed "premier bibliographic database covering the fields of medicine, nursing, dentistry, veterinary medicine, the health care system, and the preclinical sciences,"[23] the Visible Human Project stands a strong chance of becoming the international gold standard for human anatomy in coming years.

The current high profile of the Visible Man goes beyond medicine proper. His appearances in 1995 through 1996 included a gallery exhibition in Japan, where Visible Man images were displayed alongside body renderings by Leonardo Da Vinci, as if to suggest that this model is the new paradigm of human anatomy. The Man also served as a model for ergonomic furniture: designers studied the range of his motion to design more comfortable seating.[24] Each month new videos, interactive videodisks, and CD-ROMs based on both the male and female data sets are introduced through Web sites and advertisements placed in journals ranging from *Science* to *Wired*. Stories about the Man have been featured in venues ranging from international news wires and National Public Radio to local newspapers and the *Chronicle of Higher Education*.

The Visible Man's public profile is high in part because his was the first data set to be completed (because an appropriate male cadaver became available first, not because a male body was deemed more necessary to the database). A more significant source of his celebrity, though, is the fact that the press revealed information about the identity of the man whose corpse was used to make the male data set. The story behind this breach of donor privacy is significant to my consideration of sexual and cultural difference in at least two ways. First, whereas medical accounts of the actual and potential uses of the Visible Man represent him as a universal anatomical norm, medical accounts of the Visible Woman highlight factors about her body and identity that potentially limit her data set's applicability to research that is not universal, and not even universally female. While the recognition of the specificity of bodies is not a bad thing, this discrepancy of treatment raises several questions: Why are the attributes of sex made prevalent only in the case of the female body? And how do researchers justify elevating the Visible Man to a universal standard while specifying the need (as we shall see) for more than one female model? Second, while the Visible Man has attained an honorable public profile, whether as modern-day hero or martyr to science, the Visible Woman has been much less glamorously received.

The Visible Couple: Internet Angel and Postmenopausal Housewife

It seems only natural that a project that so strongly foregrounds the real of the bodies involved would invite cultural narratives about those bodies. This tendency has extended to the ascription to the project of conventional heterosexual family models, not only by the press but by project personnel. "The Visible Man has been an incredibly big success," states Donald Lundberg, director of the National Library of Medicine. "But you have to have a female body to go with the male."[25] The prevalence of this view that the female body is necessary only after, "to go with," the male is evident in accounts of the project that refer to the Visible Woman as a "mate" (as in *Science*'s news story, "Visible Man Gets High Resolution Mate") or to the data sets collectively as "the Visible Couple" or a "digital Adam and Eve."[26] The implication, of course, is that female anatomical information is necessary for the analysis of reproductive anatomy. Accordingly, the Visible Woman is the basis for such projects as a grant proposal to the Women's Health Research Program of the Department of Defense involving use of the images for virtual reality training in gynecologic and reproductive health care.[27]

In at least one respect, however, this particular configuration of the Visible Couple doesn't quite mesh with the larger family picture imagined by the Center for Human Simulation. The discrepancy hinges on the age-appropriateness of the Visible Woman for her role as partner to the Man. Whereas the Visible Man is based on the corpse of a 39-year-old, the Visible Woman's source was 59 when she died. How age is deemed medically relevant has bearing on the construction of cultural norms and standards in the project. Where the Visible Man's age is mentioned, it is cited as evidence of his status as an exemplar of normal (healthy and fit) male anatomy. Victor Spitzer, head of the Center for Human Simulation, describes the middle-aged 39-year-old corpse in terms of youth and fitness: "In a younger body," he explains, there is good muscle tone, and you can see the anatomy. In an older body things get smaller."[28] Press coverage also tends to overstate the Man's youth (39 is hardly young) and fitness, suggesting that these characteristics are central to collective mythologies about the normal male body. Wheeler notes that Ben Schneiderman, the person who learned about his own body from the Man data, "was surprised . . . by the way the images revealed the strength of the thighs."[29] Even the Man's weight (199 lbs.) is referenced only in passing, not as a factor in assessing whether his body does, in fact, constitute a norm.

The project's presentation of the Visible Woman suggests different criteria for normal female anatomy. The Visible Woman is represented as older, her age is linked to her sex and reproductive function, and specifically it is implied that she is postmenopausal. Victor Spitzer, a member of the team that produced the data sets, states the team's intention to seek further subjects—identified as "a fetus and a premenopausal woman"—to complete the data bank, implying that unlike the Man the current Visible Woman is not an adequate standard because she is postmenopausal and presumably therefore unsuited to demonstrating processes of reproduction.[30] The Visible Woman comes into being not only as a counterpart to the male model, but as an incomplete one at that. A premenopausal woman and a fetus are needed to make the Visible Family a viable reproductive unit. In their study of gender and sex bias in anatomy and physical diagnosis text illustrations, Kathleen Mendelsohn and colleagues found that women are dramatically underrepresented in illustrations of normal, nonreproductive anatomy, with one outcome that students may develop an incomplete knowledge of normal female anatomy except with respect to the reproductive system, which is not underrepresented; because "society has traditionally valued women most for their reproductive function and their role as mothers, it is not surprising that scientists and physicians would share this bias."[31] Similarly, women become visible in the Visible Human Project primarily on the basis of their reproductive function. The current and future Visible Women exist in relationship to menopause, a term that does the double duty of inscribing age and reproductive ability as essential aspects of normal women's anatomy.

Perhaps ironically, women probably stand to benefit from the availability of more specific models for medical research and teaching. As Lawrence and Bendixen note, the neglect of representations of women's anatomy leads to a lack of training in health conditions specific to women. They conclude that more images are better. The project's treatment of difference, however, is clearly problematic because the difference at issue, in concept at least, primarily seems to be reproductive anatomy. The prospect of gender-neutral uses of images (i.e., illustrations in which gender is not made obvious by the image or the caption) is worth considering since the Man data set in particular has been used for a number of projects, such as the colon fly-through, in which gender is not apparently a central issue. As by far the more detailed of the two image sets, however, the Visible Woman is likely to become the more useful model for programs requiring detailed data (virtual reality renderings for surgical simulations, for example). Mendelsohn and colleagues note that the use of apparently neutral illustrations poses an interesting dilemma: "Although neutral illustrations avoid bias by portraying neither sex," they explain, "they do not address the known physical and functional differences between the sexes" beyond those of the reproductive system. They conclude that "neutral illustrations should be avoided in favor of equal representations of both sexes."[32] It remains to be seen whether the existing Woman data set will also be used to support sex-specific research on subjects other than reproduction, and whether the Man data set will be identified as sex-specific in research that is not about the reproductive system. The outcome of these questions will be determined not by the producers of the database alone, of course, but collectively by the vast range of federal and commercial entities using the image sets for discrete research and educational programs.

The dilemma of neutrality posed by Mendelsohn and colleagues is indeed an interesting one with reference to the Visible Human Project since professional and popular accounts rarely fail to identify not only the gender but other aspects of the cultural identity of the respective bodies. At this point, each data set bears a considerable amount of cultural baggage, so that even in the most scientific of applications it would be difficult for those involved to overlook the identities inscribed in the images. Shortly after the Visible Man's Web debut, the press identified him as

John Paul Jernigan, a 39-year-old convicted felon executed by the State of Texas who had willed his body to science. In 1981, Jernigan was caught by surprise in the midst of a home burglary in which he stabbed and fatally shot the homeowner. Texas courts found Jernigan guilty of murder and sentenced him to death by lethal injection. Twelve years after the crime, prison workers attached an IV catheter to Jernigan's left hand and administered a drug that effectively suppressed the brain functions that regulate breathing. As journalist David Ellison has put it, the drug made Jernigan forget how to breathe.[33]

Jernigan may have led a life of crime, but on at least one count, he was a model citizen: he had signed a donor consent authorizing scientific use of his body upon death. Jernigan's generous intentions might have been thwarted by the fact that the cause of his death was lethal injection, a process that left his organs contaminated and hence useless for transplant into another (living) body. However, his age, body type, and health condition suited perfectly the needs of the researchers from the University of Colorado at Boulder who had won a contract from the National Library of Medicine to produce the Visible Human database.[34] A relatively healthy corpse in such fine condition is hard to get. The team, which had been searching for over a year, seized the chance to acquire Jernigan's corpse for the part of the Visible Man.

Neither the library nor the Center for Human Simulation meant for Jernigan's identity to become public knowledge. Michael Ackerman, library head of the Visible Human Project, explains that "the cadavers which the project receives are anonymous donations. In the case of the male cadaver, he died of court-ordered lethal injection in Texas on August 3, 1994. From this information the press tracked down his life story."[35] The Visible Man raised the historical specter of anatomy's use of the cadavers of charges of the state—principally criminals and the insane—for autopsy.[36] Some of the press broached this issue (minus the historical perspective) as an ethical question, ironically overlooking the questionable ethics of their own decision to broadcast Jernigan's name and life history. National Public Radio delicately posed the question of using a prisoner's body while noting the project's technological achievements. David L. Wheeler's article in the *Chronicle of Higher Education* recounts minor details of Jernigan's story (such as the contents of his last meal), dubbing him an "Internet angel" and even proposing a narrative of divine retribution through service to science. "In his life, he took a life," Wheeler writes. "In his death, he may end up saving a few."[37] (Though the article was published a few months after the release of the Visible Woman, she is mentioned only in passing.) That the story's appeal is Jernigan is made clear from the lead pull quote, the ethical implications of which are never pursued in the article text: "From the cadaver of an executed murderer, scientists produce digital anatomical images."[38]

If Jernigan's public persona is Internet angel, the Visible Woman might be said to have the less stellar title of Internet housewife. Although the donor whose body became the Visible Woman remains anonymous as per her legal instructions, certain facts about her identity and health have become public knowledge: she was a 59-year-old Maryland housewife; she had "never been sick a day in her life"; she died in her sleep of a myocardial infarction. According to one account, her husband, who had read a news story about the project, specifically requested that her body, which she had left to science, be donated for the part of the Visible Woman. Gender is thus at issue in the public construction of the Visible Woman's persona as well, with her husband acting as broker, not only volunteering her body for the job but providing the information he deemed suitable to the press.[39]

The project's highly touted realism poses another interesting dilemma vis-à-vis neutrality versus specificity: that of markers of racial identity (or their absence) in the data sets. Surprisingly, Jernigan's racial identity has not been discussed alongside his other vital statistics in descriptive accounts. Given the disproportionately high percentage of black men in prison populations, it is surprising that Jernigan's racial identity has not come up along with his other vital statistics in descriptive accounts. His mug shot, which has been published (in monochrome not color), would suggest that he is white; however, a determination based on appearances can only be speculation. This guess is reinforced by some of the imagery associated with the project. One of the options of a volume-rendering program based on the Visible Man and Visible Woman is to allow the user not only to reassemble the form of the body, but to reconstitute its containing organ, the skin. The Visible Man and Woman's optically and physically decomposed bodies are uncannily reconstituted quite literally in the flesh, using a high-resolution 3-D surface-construction algorithm called Marching Cubes.[40] These full-body surface models include dimensional renderings of the face, a part typically concealed in medical images in order to maintain the anonymity of the subject (figures 1.2 and 1.3). The conventional photographic clarity of these images differs dramatically from the kind of realism and clarity associated with the photographic cross-sections. Here we see body images that eerily resemble conventional full-body photographs of living bodies. The fact that these images are

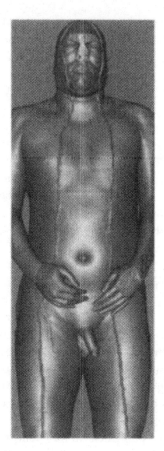

Figure 1.2 From the Marching through the Visible Man Web site by Bill Lorensen.

accessible on the Web poses obvious problems for the maintenance of subject anonymity and, moreover, raises questions about the encoding of racial difference that have been entirely unaddressed. In its colorized appearance on screen, this rendering has a uniform pinkish beige tone, matching precisely the old Crayola crayon whose label "flesh" implied that whiteness is the norm and this particular hue is the standard skin tone. Certainly this almost comical cliché of flesh tone is not an example of the program's highly touted realism; the computer rendering can't possibly match the corpses' actual skin tone. Is it an example, then, of the project's idea of what constitutes viable standards and norms? The decorative tattoo on the Man's chest present and highlighted in the caption of the image described on page 27 has been erased from this rendering,

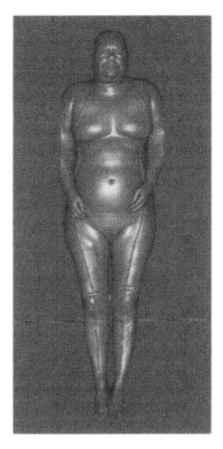

Figure 1.3   From the Marching through the Visible Woman Web site by Bill
Lorensen.

suggesting that it is not meant to replicate the specificity of Jernigan's
body. Regarding the project's quest for a detailed anatomical model, we
must ask which aspects of the body matter and which aspects are permitted to remain in the realm of crude stereotype.

A Universal Standard or a "Cataloger's Nightmare"?

The project's rhetoric of realism merits closer examination with respect to
its agenda of facilitating anatomical knowledge. A Center for Human Simulation document notes that "the current knowledge explosion in biomed-

ical sciences necessitates greater efficiency in training, data search, and testing for all health care professionals" in the area of anatomy, which "provides much of the fundamental vocabulary of the health care professional" but poses difficulties in dimensional visualization.[41] While the Center sees the Visible Human database as a means to greater efficiency in the organization and dissemination of anatomical knowledge, there is evidence that the project may be introducing unanticipated degrees of complexity to the field. Spitzer has remarked, "The Visible Man is useful if you already know anatomy. It's difficult to learn any anatomy from him."[42] This is a rather startling statement, given that the aim of the project is precisely to teach and to clarify anatomy. It appears that the project's emphasis on detailed realism has paradoxically confounded its goal of furthering anatomical knowledge. Wheeler writes that "as scientists moved beyond their initial aesthetic reactions to the images . . . they were quickly confronted with the Visible Man's most important failing," that is, the absence of labels showing which organs are where among the thousands of images in the data set. As Ackerman puts it, "For a librarian, this is very unsettling. It's like having books lying all over the place not indexed or cataloged."[43] This disarray is exacerbated by the incommensurability of written and visual data in computer programs and by the fact that the photographic cross-sections were not shot at uniform intervals and with consistent magnification levels, adding to the difficulty of correlating information from one body slice to the next. These problems of organizing the data and standardizing the images are certain to be addressed as programs fostering image-text compatibility are developed and as the data continue to be processed by program licensees. However, it is unclear whether these problems will be resolved or exacerbated as hundreds of project users bring their respective organizing principles, needs, and esthetics to the job. The following Web posting by radiation oncologists at the University of North Carolina at Chapel Hill indicates how far the project might be from its goal of standardization and efficiency:

> We (the Radiation Oncology department at UNC, not NLM) are dealing with the frozen Male CT scans and have found many errors. We think that the information we have gathered about the images is important and so are sharing it. We are also sharing the corrected images at this time (cf. license agreement) but do not have sufficient resources to spend much time doing this!

> . . . [W]e needed to strip the arms from the body because they are not in normal scanning position for a pelvic study. We also needed all of the scans

in the head & neck area to be of identical zoom (magnification factor). We will make some of these reworked scans available to other institutions, free of charge over a network connection, after the recipient signs a license agreement with the NLM. Of course, this depends on our current work-load.[44]

Problems of image standardization and organization suggest that anatomical knowledge is not always commensurable across fields, and hence a universal anatomical model is not viable. The problem of commensurability is undoubtedly aggravated by the proliferation of medical subspecialties, which include a multitude of imaging modalities, each with its own conventions for rendering and interpreting data and its own idea of what constitutes realism. The range of images (computed tomography, magnetic resonance, and photographic) that comprise the Visible Human Project suggests that the disarray of the database goes beyond lack of unity within each body set to include (potential) lack of translation or correspondence across modalities. The Center for Human Simulation sets as its general goal facilitation of collaboration among an impressive list of specialists, but the length of this list in itself indicates the potential for problems of commensurability of knowledge and goals. It includes anatomists, radiologists, computer scientists, bioengineers, physicians, educators, mathematicians, pathologists, anthropologists, medical information specialists, and library scientists.[45] Ironically, the very proliferation of new technologies that has made the Visible Human Project so appealing has also created needs so specific that a universal database, much less universal bodies, cannot adequately serve them.

   This crisis of commensurability can be characterized in terms of a paradox of visibility: the Visible Human Project was devised in part in answer to a demand for anatomical images providing greater and more detailed information about the human body. In filling this demand, the project has generated a level of quantity and detail beyond that which its users are equipped to process. Moreover, as the UNC case above demonstrates, the very specificity of the data precludes its universality. This paradox suggests that it would be fruitful to consider more closely the techniques used to produce and interpret the Visible Man and Visible Woman.

   In their analysis of anatomical representations of the clitoris, Moore and Clarke note that two kinds of images were predominant in texts published between 1981 and 1991: photography of cadavers—a technique whose introduction they describe as resulting in "a new vivid realism"—and the newer techniques of computer-generated imaging—which, they argue, "delete the range of variation" among bodies and, moreover, "delete the body itself" insofar as computer-generated images are more difficult to translate than conventional photographs.[46] Moore and Clarke express concern that computer images' deletion of specific characteristics of gender, race, class, and culture along with their general dematerialization of the body may ultimately eliminate women from the anatomical picture, much as they have been disappearing in reproductive discourses.[47] The Visible Human images fit and exceed the categories described by Moore and Clarke, suggesting a new paradigm for the 1990s. I have cited numerous sources suggesting that the project's color photographs of corpses introduce a new realism even more vivid—and certainly more vivified—than cadaver photography. And the computed tomography scans, magnetic resonance images, and cryographs all involve computer imaging techniques that make it difficult even for trained researchers to visualize the whole body on the basis of these images (the "nightmare" of uncataloged cryographs). The computer-generated graphics noted by Moore and Clarke, however, are essentially line drawings. They do not share the Visible Human images' detailed correspondence with actual bodies. Whereas the graphics Moore and Clarke describe fail to evoke a body because they are schematic and abstract, the Visible Human images fail to evoke a body because they detail "parts" so minute and so arbitrarily segmented that they preclude ready recognition and categorization. For instance, a single .33 cross-section of the Visible Woman's torso might provide a bit of data about any number of structures including the breasts, the lungs, the heart, the skeletal system. Though the data are highly detailed, they may be hard to place in context of an entire body because (a) the slice does not correspond to conventional ways of dividing the body for anatomical study (according to systems or organs, for example); and (b) the wealth of minute detail makes it difficult to determine which aspects of the data field matter and which do not. The very aspect of the project lauded by Schneiderman—the fact that its computer renderings are not highly interpreted like other anatomical images—becomes a factor in its lack of "face recognition." Ironically, close attention to anatomical detail—to differences right down to the cellular level—is a factor in the apparent failure of individual images in isolation from the set to evoke the material body. At this point in time, the images may take on embodied life for some after significant modification (as in the various interactive and virtual reality programs that give the Visible Man and Visible Woman attributes such as dimensionality, wholeness, and flesh color). But, of course, it is only a matter of time until those working with the project in their laboratories, secondary school classrooms, and home computer workstations encode and enliven the discrete images with new cultural meanings. What those meanings will be vis-à-vis gender, race, and other differentials remains to be seen.

Conclusion

It is striking that the Visible Human Project, a federal initiative to generate a universal set of anatomical norms, was launched at a moment when the government also began to subsidize the Human Genome Project, an even broader-based (and more heavily funded) international search for a detailed universal encoding of life. The projects share the paradox of seeking to create a universal archive through which to represent and to know human biology, while rendering their respective body models with a level of specificity that may ultimately confound goals such as the establishment of a norm. Both projects are beset with the difficulty of determining what data are relevant from among the surfeit of information represented. However, while genome research is largely the province of official science, the Visible Human Project exists in a somewhat more ambiguous zone between medicine, media, and science. Available on the Web and through a relatively inexpensive licensing fee, the Visible Human database approximates shareware (computer programs distributed widely and for free) when compared to the findings of genome research. As such, the Visible Man and Woman may be viewed, used, and altered in ways neither anticipated nor approved by the National Library of Medicine and the Center for Human Simulation. This factor suggests that there is no singular Visible Human Project, but rather a heterogeneous range of project applications and, moreover, that the possibility exists for using the data in unexpected ways.

How will this potential play out with regard to the representation of sexual difference? I noted above that women may benefit from the availability of more specific models for medical research and teaching. But one could easily argue from either perspective: that an army of Visible Women would better support research on diseases with manifestations particular to age, genetic makeup, or any other set of characteristics and conditions; or that such research might foster wrongful designations of sex-based pathology. The relevant question, however, is not whether more or fewer images of women will aid or offset the inadequate regard of women in medicine, but what agendas the current and future Visible Women will serve, and how anatomical difference will be constructed through the various imaging techniques used to render these models. Will the highly touted realism of the simulations based on the Visible Human data sets always replicate conventional views of the gendered body, or will they introduce new ways of seeing, ultimately shaking anatomy's static paradigms of binary sexual difference? Are anatomy's visible women likely to be biomedical Stepford wives, supporting research that reinforces historical views of women as exceptions to (male) anatomical norms and creating new needs for women on the basis of iatrogenic anxieties about their difference being pathological (e.g., the need for hormone therapy)? Or will more detailed and diversified anatomical models support inquiry into sex-specific factors of health and disease including and beyond conditions linked to reproduction? Moreover, will the project eventually recognize the limits of its current familial model and generate a range of male and transgendered as well as female anatomical specimens? The current disarray of the images, the mix of project licensees and Web-site image poachers, and the range of potential applications of the data make it difficult to place a bet on any one answer. For the moment, the heterogeneity and confusion of this "universal" database makes these questions remain promisingly open.

Notes

1. National Library of Medicine (U.S.) Board of Regents, "Electronic Imaging, Report of the Board of Regents," U.S. Department of Health and Human Services, Public Health Service, National Institutes of Health, 1990. NIH Publication 90–2197.

2. Susan C. Lawrence and Kate Bendixen, "His and Hers: Male and Female Anatomy in Anatomy Texts for US Medical Students," *Social Science and Medicine* 35.7 (October 1992): 925–33. Citation from 925.

3. Adriane Fugh-Berman, "Man to Man at Georgetown: Tales Out of Medical School," *Nation* (January 20, 1992): 1, 54.

4. See Chapter 4 of Terri Kapsalis, *Public Privates: Performing Gynecology from Both Ends of the Speculum* (Durham, NC: Duke UP, 1997) 81–111. Quotation from 81. This is not to imply that women's sexual organs are not represented in medical textbooks. On this point see Lisa Jean Moore and Adele E. Clarke, "Clitoral Conventions and Transgressions: Graphic Representations in Anatomy Texts, c. 1900–1991," *Feminist Studies* 21.2 (Summer 1995): 255–301.

5. Anne K. Eckman, "Beyond 'The Yentl Syndrome': Making Women Visible in Post-1990 Women's Health Discourse," chapter 4 in this volume.

6. Evidence that making women visible will not in itself address this larger issue can be found in the numerous critical studies of scientific and medical representations of the body which have shown that historically where bodies and their parts are identified as sex- or race-specific these models have often been used to support arguments about the biological bases of pathology to the exclusion of environmental and social factors. The literature on the construction of sexual and racial difference in anatomy, science, and medicine is extensive. It includes: Nancy Leys Stepan, *The Idea of Race in Science: Great Britain, 1800–1960* (Hamden, CT: Archon Books, 1982); Ludmilla Jordanova, *Sexual Visions: Images of Gender in Science and Medicine between the Eighteenth and Twentieth Centuries* (Madison: U of Wisconsin P, 1989); Thomas Laqueur, *Making Sex: Body and Gender from the Greeks to Freud* (Cambridge: Harvard UP, 1990); Cynthia Eagle Russett, *Sexual Science: The Victorian Construction of Womanhood* (Cambridge: Harvard UP, 1989); Londa Schiebinger, *The Mind Has No Sex? Women in the Origins of Modern Science* (Cambridge: Harvard UP, 1989); Sander Gilman, *Pathology and Difference: Stereotypes of Sexuality, Race, and Madness* (Ithaca: Cornell UP, 1985); Elizabeth Fee, "Nineteenth-Century Craniology: The Study of the Female Skull," *Bulletin of the History of Medicine* 53 (1979): 415–433; David Horn, "This Norm Which Is Not One: Reading the Female Body in Lombroso's Anthropology," in *Deviant Bodies*, Jennifer Terry and Jacqueline Urla, eds. (Bloomington: Indiana UP, 1995) 109–128; Allan Sekula, "The Body and the Archive," *October* 39 (1986): 3–64; Thomas Forbes, "To Be Dissected and Anatomised," *Journal of the History of Medicine and Allied Sciences* 36 (1981): 490–492; Giuliana Bruno, "Spectatorial Embodiments: Anatomies of the Visible and the Female Bodyscape," *Camera Obscura* 28 (1992): 239–261. For opposing discussions of more recent findings regarding biological difference, see Simon LeVay, *The Sexual Brain* (Cambridge: MIT Press, 1993); and Jennifer Terry, "Anxious Slippages Between 'Them' and 'Us': A Brief History of the Scientific Search for Homosexual Bodies," in *Deviant Bodies*, Urla and Terry, eds.

7. Moore and Clarke 255–301.

8. Jacqueline Stenson, " 'Visible Woman' Makes Debut on the Internet," *Medical Tribune News Service*, November 28, 1995.

9. From the Web site of the Center for Human Simulation, February 2, 1996.

10. I'd like to clarify my use of the term "realism" since much of this essay takes issue with its use. In their classic introductory film studies textbook, David Bordwell and Kristin Thompson argue against using the term realism as a standard of value in judging films because the conventions associated with realism vary according to historical period, genre, and other aspects of context (*Film Art*, 5th ed. [New York: McGraw Hill, 1996]). The same argument can be made about realism in science and medicine. It is worth asking whether conventions of realism are in fact the most useful means of "learning more" about, or "better representing" the body in anatomy. Catherine Waldby provides a more extended discussion of the Visible Human Project in terms of conventions of realism and representation

in "Revenants: The Visible Human Project and the Digital Uncanny," *Body and Society* 3. 1 (March 1997): 1–160.

11. My definitions of "corpse" and "cadaver" are drawn from *Dorland's Illustrated Medical Dictionary*, 27th ed. (Philadelphia: W.B. Saunders, 1988), 383 and 251.

12. Paula Treichler, in a personal note.

13. Moore and Clarke 257.

14. I use the term "mill away" rather than "slice" because the latter implies that the material cut away is intact, whereas I believe the material cut away is so thin that it probably could not be maintained as an intact slice.

15. Accounts of the process appear in numerous sources. See the Visible Human Project Web site, Project Overview, http://www.nlh.nih.gov/research/visible_human.html

16. From the Web site of Micron BioSystems' Visible Productions, advertising the Visible Human Male Videodisc.

17. From the Web site of the Center for Human Simulation, February 2, 1996: http://www.uchsc.edu/sm/chs. The image has since been replaced by another rendering of the visible man. A 1996 Web advertisement for the first CD-ROM to be based on Visible Human Project data emphasizes the Visible Man's unique wholeness and accessibility, inviting potential clients to "[i]magine exploring an entire body with the click of a mouse!" (Micron BioSystems' Visible Productions advertising the Visible Human Male CD-ROM).

18. Quoted in David L. Wheeler, "Creating a Body of Knowledge," *Chronicle of Higher Education*, February 2, 1996: A6, A7, A14. Quotation from A7, A14.

19. Web archive of the Women's Wire News for November 28, 1995.

20. From the Web site of the Center for Human Simulation.

21. The cost is $1,000 in the United States, Canada, and Mexico, and $2,000 elsewhere.

22. Visible Human Project Far East site at the University of Singapore, http://medweb.nus.sg/vhp/vhp.html

23. From the Medline homepage, http://www.nlm.nih.gov/databases/databases.html

24. Wheeler A14.

25. Donald Lundberg quoted by Jacqueline Stenson, " 'Visible Woman' Makes Debut on the Internet," MEDTRIB, the *Medical Tribune* News Service, November 1995.

26. See Constance Holden, " 'Visible Man' Gets High Resolution Mate," *Science* 270 (1995): 1927; Gary Stix, "Habeas Corpus: Seeking Subjects to be a Digital Adam and Eve," *Scientific American* 268.1 (1993): 122–123.

27. From the Center for Human Simulation Web site.

28. Quoted in Wheeler A7.

29. Wheeler A14.

30. Quoted in *Women's Wire* news for November 28, 1995. This report also notes that the Visible Woman may at some point be used to demonstrate processes of aging.

31. Kathleen Mendelsohn, Linda Z. Nieman, PhD, Krista Isaacs, Sophia Lee, and Sandra Levison, MD, *Journal of the American Medical Association* 272.16 (October 26, 1996): 1267–1270, citation from 1269.

32. Mendelsohn et al. 1270.

33. David Ellison, "Anatomy of a Murderer," *21–C* (March 1995): 20–25.

34. From the Web site of the Center for Human Simulation.

35. Quoted by Amy Friedlander, editor of *D-Lib Magazine*, in response to online queries about Ackerman's "Accessing the Visible Human Project," *D-Lib Magazine*, October 1995. (The magazine's byline is "the magazine of digital library research.")

36. See, for example, Ruth Richardson, "A Dissection of the Anatomy Act," *Studies in Labor History* 1 (1976): 1–13.

37. Wheeler A14.

38. Wheeler A6.

39. See Stenson, " 'Visible Woman' Makes Debut on the Internet"; brief from the National Library of Medicine, *Gratefully Yours* (a newsletter published by the NLM), September/October 1995; and Bill Lorensen, "Marching Through the Visible Woman" Web site (http://www.graphics.stanford.edu/~lorensen/vw/vw.html). Lorensen works for the GE Imaging and Visualization Laboratory.

40. See Lorensen, "Marching Through the Visible Woman" and "Marching Through the Visible Man"; and W. E. Lorensen and H. E. Cline, "Marching Cubes: A High Resolution 3D Surface Construction Algorithm," *Computer Graphics* 21.3 (July 1987): 163–169.

41. From the Web site of the Center for Human Simulation.

42. Quoted in Wheeler A14.

43. Wheeler A14.

44. Gregg Tracton, Web posting of August 16, 1996, http://www.radonc.unc.edu/visiman/whatishere.html

45. From the Web site of the Center for Human Simulation.

46. Moore and Clarke 289.

47. Moore and Clarke 289. On the disappearance of women in reproductive discourses, see Valerie Hartouni, *Cultural Conceptions: On Reproductive Technolgies and the Remaking of Life* (Minneapolis: University of Minnesota Press, 1997) and Carole Stabile, "Shooting the Mother: Fetal Photography and the Politics of Disappearance," chapter 5 in this volume.

Stacie A. Colwell

2

The End of the Road

Gender, the Dissemination of Knowledge, and
the American Campaign against Venereal
Disease during World War I

"Two roads there are in life," states the prologue to the
1918 American Social Hygiene Association Film, *The End of the Road*.[1]
Instructed by her mother "in the 'good' of sex," Mary Lee, the film's heroine, follows one road "upward towards the Land of Perfect Love," by
becoming an army nurse and marrying the film's hero, Dr. Philip Bell.
Vera Wagner, Mary's childhood friend, follows the other, "wrong road,"
down "into the Dark Valley of Despair where the sun never shines." Vera,
whose mother refused to educate her in "the 'good' of sex," learns for herself "the 'bad' of sex." Coming of age in a time when "wild oats" were
being "sown to the luring medley of 'Jazz,' 'Gin,' and 'Jalapies,'" Vera
contracts syphilis from a nonmarital relationship but is saved by Mary and
Dr. Bell, who convince her to accept treatment and instill in her a "holier
regard for courtship" and a "better understanding of marriage."

Alarmed by reports of high rates of venereal disease among the draftees
to the First World War, the American Social Hygiene Association

44

(ASHA), in collaboration with various federal agencies, conceived of *The End of the Road* as a companion feature for women to *Fit to Fight*, the Association's venereal disease education film for enlisted men. *Fit to Fight*, the first such picture ever produced with government support, was essentially an army lecture film bracketed by two reels of dramatic material.[2] Believing that the educational component of *Fit to Fight* was made more effective by the added narrative, the Association opted to make their second film, *The End of the Road*, as a feature film. "Much information and counsel for conduct" could be better imparted by the lecture "being interwoven with the plot," the producers concluded, and "the excellent portrayal of character" would make "a strong appeal to youth's best impulses."[3] Moreover, wrote the screenplay author, Katherine Bement Davis, a "love story" was "necessary to hold the interest of the young women who see the film."[4]

Intended for a noncommercial audience of women and girls over the age of sixteen, this didactic feature-length "women's film" was to be shown by a trained lecturer as part of a larger venereal disease instruction program. However, shortly after the film's production, due to the enormous "demand for the motion picture method of educating civilian groups," ASHA and the U.S. Public Health Service (USPHS) contracted with the Public Health Film Company for the film's additional use in commercial theaters. In order "to protect the films from misuse," ASHA copyrighted them and the USPHS stipulated screening conditions "to safeguard the films from sensational exploitation."[5]

Believing all precautions had been taken, the various producers and promoters anticipated that the film would be as favorably received as were the two other films of the same genre released in the preceding months.[6] Undoubtedly, they were unpleasantly surprised by the public debate that followed the film's commercial opening in February, 1919. Within months of its release, ASHA was compelled to withdraw *The End of the Road* from all commercial screenings and eventually to discontinue the film entirely.

The film and its reception clearly reflect the peculiar conditions of its production. Written by Katherine Bement Davis, a sociologist and Director of the War Department's Committee on Protective Work for Girls; directed by Army Lieutenant Edward H. Griffith of the War Department's Committee on Training Camp Activities; performed by a supporting cast of enlisted men; filmed by cameramen from the Medical Department of the Army; and distributed jointly by ASHA and the USPHS, the film was, not surprisingly, an amateur project even by the standards of the time. This amateurism and the didactic story line combine to create a film whose intent and text are unusually transparent.

Herein, I will trace the genealogy of the production and text of *The End of the Road*; contextualize the film's postwar censorship and discontinuation; and examine the broader consequences for women's lives of the antivenereal campaign of which it was a part.

The American Social Hygiene Association (ASHA)

Produced by ASHA on behalf of the U.S. War Department Commission on Training Camp Activity, *The End of the Road* is a visual record of the unique confluence of events that led to its production almost three-quarters of a century ago.[7] As such, *The End of the Road* begins with the establishment of ASHA, its nominal parent organization. Organized in 1913 as a hybrid of the social purity and sex education movements, ASHA was incorporated in March, 1914, as the legal union of the American Vigilance Association (AVA) and the American Federation for Sex Hygiene (AFSH). The union of these two groups was, in fact, the last in a series of recent mergers undertaken in the Progressive Era zeitgeist of efficiency.[8]

Although the social purity groups united by the AVA and the sex education societies brought together by the AFSH shared the common ambition to counter the perceived epidemic of venereal diseases, the two movements had previously resisted unification because of deep-seated differences in ideology, agenda, and composition. A social purity organization, the AVA had its deepest roots in the nineteenth-century abolition and women's movements and sought social reform through moral uplift. For the AVA social purist, the eradication of venereal diseases was best achieved by "rescuing" prostitutes from their "depraved" occupation.[9] Most of the organizers and charter members of AFSH, on the other hand, were physicians who eschewed moral arguments and sought instead to reduce the incidence of venereal disease by such preventative measures as sex education and medical intervention.

Despite their overlapping purpose and the more recent duplication of their efforts, the two groups were consolidated only after the death in 1913 of AFSH founder and leader, Dr. Prince Morrow, and even then only after pressure from the philanthropist John D. Rockefeller, Jr.[10] Rockefeller, who became an ardent foe of prostitution and venereal diseases after chairing a grand jury on white slavery, pledged future financial support and exerted considerable political pressure to induce the two groups to unite. At a meeting in October, 1913, engineered by Rockefeller, the leaders of the two groups accepted his financial pledge and established the union organization, ASHA, whose "distinctive objects" were "sex education, the suppression of prostitution and the reduction of venereal diseases."[11]

ASHA's Incorporation into the Government

Having secured considerable financial support as well as political hegemony over earlier movements and agencies, the newly organized union of social purists and physicians sought to translate their "distinctive objects" into national policy. Their next step was to build a partnership between the Association and the government. For the first few years following the Association's founding, however, the federal and state governments took little notice of ASHA's work; this situation changed with the coming of the war.[12]

After three years of lobbying for government involvement in their campaign against venereal disease, ASHA, working in conjunction with the Young Men's Christian Association (YMCA), secured its foothold in the government following their joint complaint to Secretary of War Newton Baker about the swollen ranks of prostitutes accompanying General Furston's army in their 1916 pursuit of Pancho Villa. Concerned not by the immorality of this caravan, but by the implied increase in venereal disabilities, Baker agreed to mount an investigation. Raymond Fosdick, ASHA's lawyer, was selected to conduct the inquiry and submitted a confidential report to Baker that carefully couched the perceived consequences of this situation in terms of diminished military efficiency and weakened troop morale.

In the months following that August 1916 report, as the possibility of American involvement in the First World War increased along with the threat of an impending draft, the "problem" that Fosdick described gained larger significance.[13] Government officials had become convinced of the need to develop a campaign against venereal disease, first, to preserve military efficiency and, second, to assuage the citizens who were writing Washington to urge the government to protect the spiritual and physical health of draftees. "I understand that the moral conditions in our military camps . . . are anything but good," wrote one mother to the Secretary of the Navy, "the parents must have some guarantee that the moral atmosphere will be . . . high."[14] Letters such as this, together with the public alarm at the reports of high national rates of venereal disease, induced the federal government to incorporate wholesale into its structure the venereal disease campaign of an Association with known roots in both the

social purity movement and the medical community. Meanwhile, in antic-
ipation of subsequent events, and at the suggestion of William F. Snow,
ASHA's General Director, the entire male staff of the Association volunteered for active military duty, angling for the commission to lead the
nation's battle against the venereal enemy.[15]

Apprised by Secretary of War Baker of the conditions in the training
camps, President Woodrow Wilson accepted a proposal by Fosdick to create a clearing house of voluntary social agencies to oversee programs in
the camps and to keep the areas around the camps "decent and
respectable."[16] On 17 April 1917, Baker created the Commission for
Training Camp Activities (CTCA) within the War Department to coordinate this work and named Fosdick as its chair. With the Association in
uniform, Fosdick chose a group of prominent Progressive leaders and fellow ASHA members to serve with him.[17] Thus began the national campaign against venereal disease, a campaign whose concern was the health
of men and whose impetus and agenda came originally from outside government, channeled inward by the incorporation of the tenuously aligned
social reformers. The distinctive agendas of the different reform factions
within ASHA/CTCA are discernable within the text of the film that the
group produced.

The Film

Writing in October, 1918, Katherine Bement Davis describes the project as
having "been most carefully worked out in consultation with physicians on
the side of fidelity to medical fact, and with teachers as to the psychological
effect." "The stories in the film are all taken from life," continues Davis:

> Two girls grow up side by side in a small town. One girl has the right kind of
> mother [Mrs. Lee], who has met her child's inquiries as to the beginning of
> life with the truth, and all through the years of the girl's adolescence has
> been her confidante and friend. The other girl's mother [Mrs. Wagner] is a
> different type. She is a woman who has had ambitions she has never been
> able to gratify, and whose one idea for her daughter is that she shall make a
> rich match and be placed in a position where she need not work and may
> gratify her fancies. The prologue shows the difference in training of the two
> girls. The story begins with the day the two girls graduate from the local
> high school. Later, both come to New York. Mary [Lee], actuated by a
> desire to be of service to the world, enters a hospital to take a nurse's train-
> ing. Her friend Vera [Wagner] comes, hoping to have wider opportunities

for matrimonial choice. She has taken a position in a department store. The two girls' stories develop in line with their early training. Mary, strengthened by principles and high ideals, resists temptation, while Vera, making advances which have as their purpose no real desire to do wrong, but only to attract, is led to accept the attentions of a man [Howard Lord] who has no thought of marrying her, and step by step goes along the road that leads in the end to disease, desertion and disgrace. Mary, in her hospital work, comes in contact with girls and women whose careers are the direct outcomes of the paths they have chosen to follow. The war comes. Mary becomes an army nurse. . . . The love story . . . is skillfully interwoven and leads to the climax in the last scene overseas, where . . . Mary and her lover [Dr. Bell] discover each other.[18]

There are, within this narrative, elements that can be clearly identified with the constituent groups within ASHA. The social purity faction previously represented by the AVA contributed to the film their ideological perspective on sexuality and their environmental determinism. The members originally comprising AFSH promoted an ideology they billed as "scientific" sex education, a frank and candid sexual discourse, and the positive role of the physician. The film's author added a third perspective. As a sociologist Ph.D. who ran the Laboratory of Social Hygiene, an institution that was part research, part female reformatory, Davis was uniquely situated to synthesize the perspectives of both the social purists and the physicians, as well as to inject her own contrary opinions.

The American Vigilance Association Agenda

Construction of Sexuality

The agenda of the social purity reformers within ASHA, that is to say those members who were represented by the American Vigilance Association before the groups' merger, is evident in the script's ideation of sexuality and its depiction of the factors that precipitate Vera's "fall." The film's portrayal of sexuality is one of inherent danger that is best met by the continence of both parties. Indeed, the only sexual act alluded to in *The End of the Road* that does not lead to catastrophe is the story of Mary's mother, describing her planned, or at least desired, pregnancy. The danger of intercourse for purposes other than procreative is revealed in a brief tangent that aptly precedes all discussions of venereal disease. Embarking on her career in nursing "at a New York hospital," Mary, the heroine, meets "the most brilliant surgeon of the visiting staff, Dr. Philip Bell." "I want you to take a case of mine," Dr. Bell informs Mary, introducing her to a young immigrant parlormaid who has been "transferred to the hospital from the reformatory so she might die free." The maid, Mary's first patient, confides that she was seduced by the household's chauffeur who, despite earlier promises to the contrary, refused to marry her when she became pregnant. "I was not myself," the deflowered "wild rose" concludes, "I killed him."[19] The patient then falls back on the pillow, either exhausted or dead. There is no infection in this scenario, but emphasized is the social purity message that sexual activity alone is dangerous, driving one to insanity and criminal behavior.

This social purity ideation of sexuality has as its correlate the understanding that sexual continence was the only safe route for both sexes. This correlate is rooted in the nineteenth-century "voluntary motherhood" movement that sought to increase married women's sexual control but that also promoted male sexual continence.[20] It is important to note here, however, that although the rhetoric of the continence proponents claimed to do away with a double standard by applying to men the standard women had been measured against, the aim was not equality in sexual freedom or pleasure but in shared abstinence. This "single standard" is also promoted in *The End of the Road*. When Paul Horton, Mary's childhood sweetheart, is informed of his imminent deployment to Europe, he begs Mary to "give me a memory I can never lose." Mary recoils at the suggestion: "Paul, how could you suggest such a thing! You who said you loved me—why you don't know what love means!" In the following sequence, Paul's brashness is contrasted with Dr. Bell's proper courtship. Mary then breaks with Paul and becomes engaged to Dr. Bell, for whose patience "a fine comradeship with Mary is [his] reward."[21]

The inclusion of this ideal of sexual continence within the film illustrates one of the unresolved discrepancies amongst the film's producers and promoters: the ASHA constituent groups, the federal government, and the film's author. ASHA's constituent group, the American Vigilance Association, actively promoted this ideal of sexual continence. Additionally, the General Medical Board of the U.S. Council on National Defense officially rejected the doctrine of "sexual necessity," declaring that "continence is not incompatible with health and is the best preventive of VD." Congress, too, moved by the above-mentioned public appeals, formally endorsed the continence prescription; included in their Draft Act was a provision forbidding prostitution within five miles of a military post and granting the Association funding to inculcate the men in the ways of sexual continence.[22]

Many leaders of the armed forces, however, were not convinced that sexual continence was necessary, or even beneficial, to the health of the fighting man. These leaders linked their dissent to those within the medical community, many of whom were represented by the other ASHA constituent, the American Federation for Sex Education, and with whom Davis sympathized.[23] Together, they lobbied successfully for the establishment of chemical prophylaxis stations and the distributions of the "prophylaxis packets." Despite the efforts of the social purity constituents and the challenges to prophylaxis from the popular press, all attempts to limit the use of prophylaxis stations or to reprimand morally the errant servicemen were overruled.[24] The contradiction posed by the ASHA's and the CTCA's demand for sexual continence while handing out prophylaxis packets was allowed to stand for the duration of the war in the interest of military efficiency.

Regulating the Environment

In addition to the social purity conception of sexuality, a second ideology of the American Vigilance Association illustrated by the film was their conception of regulating the environment to eliminate vice. The social purity movement had initially sought to reduce the prevalence of venereal disease by reducing the prevalence of prostitution. Along with their number one goal of "abolishing the red light district," the purity movement sought to provide an environment that would "distract" men from prostitutes and prevent women from entering that occupation.[25] Described below are the various influences detailed in the film that the social purity movement identified as catalysts of immorality.

Alcohol

There was considerable overlap between Prohibitionist organizations such as the Women's Christian Temperance Union and the social reformers within ASHA. As a result, ASHA and others working through the CTCA immediately banned alcohol within a five-mile radius of the camps. "Alcohol," the reasoning went, "rendered the subject not only less fit for military duty, but even more definitely exposed to the ravages of venereal disease."[26] As stated by ASHA members, alcohol's "depressing effect is first evident on the higher cerebral centers with a resulting loss of the normal moral tone and consequent exposure to venereal disease."[27] In *The*

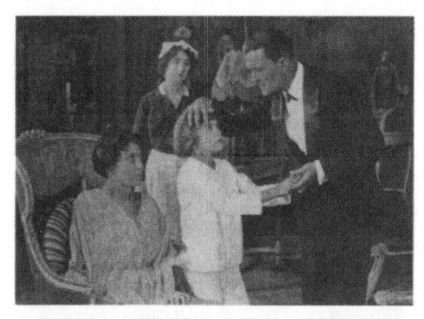

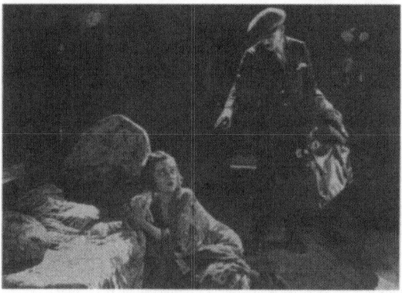

Figure 2.1   "Blind from Birth" and "Deserted." Stills from *The End of the Road*. Published in Katherine Bement Davis, "Social Hygiene and the War, Part II: Woman's Part in Social Hygiene," Social Hygiene, vol. IV (October, 1918): 549.

End of the Road, this supposed correlation is repeatedly emphasized. For instance, Mary and Dr. Bell, chaperoned by his mother, go on an outing to a country club where "between dances . . . the Cocktail Consumer's League and the Local Order of Highball Hounds hold a joint session." Scanning the crowd, wide-eyed at the heavy drinking, Mary witnesses "the champion catch-as-can flirt of his social clique, Russell Ellbridge," lure away "Marian Sinclair, a debutante fascinated by his reputation," for a walk—literally and figuratively—down the primrose path. Ellbridge, we learn, is a married man whose wife Dr. Bell treats for gonorrheal arthritis and whose son is blind because of "the sins of his father" (figure 2.1).[28] To hammer the point home, Dr. Bell and Mary are called away from the club to treat an accident victim at "a notorious roadhouse nearby" where Mary spots Vera, her foil in the drama, seated with a man at a nearby table, decidedly drunk. A drawn-out scenario ensues that temporarily rescues Vera from her drunken, diseased companion, Howard. Referring to both illicit sex and alcohol, Mary cautions Vera to "think of the consequences now . . . [or you] sha'n't find happiness at the end of the road."

Tobacco

The advice books for mothers invariably disapproved of tobacco, as smoking by women signified a loosened morality. In fact, at the time of the film's release, it was a contested issue whether scenes of women smoking were grounds for censorship.[29] Supporting that censorship, ASHA acknowledged "the recognized safeguards against sexual perversions" to be "abstinence from alcohol, tobacco . . . and all other drugs which impair self-control, even momentarily."[30] In the film, the only woman to smoke is Vera, a habit she assumes only after her seduction and one she quits following her rehabilitation.

"Unwholesome" Home and Work Environment

Certainly the film belabors the differences in Mary and Vera's home lives as the fundamental determinant of their later actions. In a series of juxtaposed shots that also illustrate class-bound codes for women's recreation, Mary's mother is shown reading to Mary from Dr. Jane S. Parker's book, *Ideals of Social Relationships Written for Girls in their Teens* (figure 2.2), while, seated in an identical composition, Vera's mother is shown perusing a magazine as Vera reads from an illustrated novel, the open page of which depicts a rakish man.[31] Where Mary and her suitor Paul are always

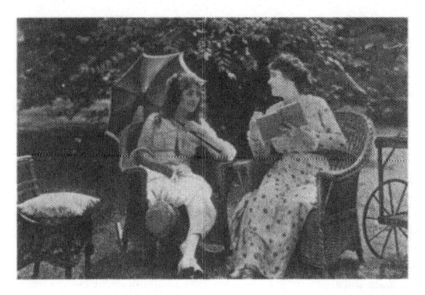

Figure 2.2   "Mary at 17." Still from *The End of the Road*. Published in Davis, "Social Hygiene and the War, Part II," 550.

carefully chaperoned by her mother, Vera is caught by her mother "spooning" with her beau Arthur in a dark corner of the garden. Where Mary is shown to have a friend in her mother, Vera is reprimanded by her mother in every shot in which the two appear—an interaction, we are shown by the mother's letters, that continues even after Vera moves to New York. Lastly, following that "thrill that comes once in a lifetime— Commencement Day," Mary, with her mother's support, chooses to move to New York to pursue the socially acceptable career of nursing and, presumably, to live in the nurses' dormitory. Vera, on the other hand, moves to New York at her mother's insistence. "You'll never be able to marry a rich man if you work for a living here," Mrs. Wagner tells Vera. "It's different in a place like New York—if you had a position there you might meet some wealthy young fellow." In New York, Vera lives in a dingy cramped room in a rundown area and is employed "at a New York Bargain counter."[32]

The choice of Vera's employment was not accidental. From the 1880s to the 1920s, numerous investigations of department store life were undertaken by women's reform associations, such as the National Consumers' League, the Women's Trade Union League, and the Young Women's Christian Association, all of which had overlapping membership with the social purity movement led by the AVA. Their highly publicized investigations stressed the ill health, exhaustion, and impoverished social lives of the department store "girls." The most sensational charge, however, was that department store saleswomen were in special peril of prostitution, whether professional or occasional. The public nature of the stores, their sumptuous atmosphere, and the low wages paid combined, so the argument went, to grease the transition from bargain counter to counterpane.[33] Hence, Vera's near-seduction, as mentioned above, occurred when she was unchaperoned and drunk in an almost deserted roadhouse. Vera's actual seduction takes place across the counter where Howard tells her, "Better quit this job. I'll give you a real one."[34]

Diet, Dress, and 'Do

The fourth and last catalyst of vice, which pertains to women's personal appearance, drew on the beliefs of other women's reform organizations that overlapped with the social purity movement. Echoing the contemporary interest in the effects of diet on physical and moral health, the preface to the inaugural issue of ASHA's *Social Hygiene* recommended "moderation in eating" and "abstinence in youth from hot spices" as two of their "recognized safeguards against sexual perversions."[35] Food of "miserable quality," states another *Social Hygiene* article entitled "The Unadjusted Girl," "has direct bearing on physical degeneracy and consequent delinquency."[36] Contrasting the moral health of the women's high school relationships, Vera's beau is shown presenting her with a box of chocolates, which she rapidly consumes while seated too close to him on the bench. The film then cuts to Mary, properly chaperoned, receiving a hat from her admirer, who is then seated in an armchair across from her. Later, when Vera is shown in her dressing gown, despondently draped over the loveseat in Howard's flat, we are informed that she "eat[s] too much candy."[37]

Closely related to the efforts for diet reform was the nineteenth-century health reform movement's attention to styles of dress. The resurrection of this ideology during wartime, however, was not for the health of the woman caught in binding clothing but for the sake of her male company (figure 2.3). "The too transparent waists, showing plainly all the underclothes beneath, the dresses cut too low in the neck, the gowns that cling too closely to the figure," explains Mrs. Woodallen Chapman, "stimulate the lower desires and passions if one is not careful both by dress and behavior to avoid everything physically suggestive."[38] ASHA's goal, then, said Lecturer Rachelle S. Yarros, was to teach the young woman

IMPROPER DRESS MAY DO HARM BY AROUSING EMOTIONS HARD TO CONTROL.

Such a dress is both inappropriate and improper at a party for Soldiers

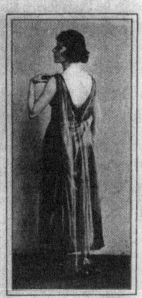

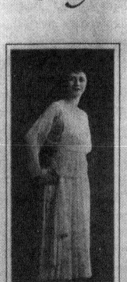

This party gown is modest, pretty, simple and inexpensive.

It has been adopted by the Junior League in New York City.

Figure 2.3 "Improper Dress . . ." Wall poster for the Social Hygiene Campaign, 1918. Published in Davis, "Social Hygiene and the War, Part II," 527.

to realize that she cannot play with love; that indecent manner of dress, dancing and behavior, flirting and coquetting and leading on, while not directly injurious to herself, and as a matter of fact giving her a good deal of the kind of satisfaction for which she longs, are unfair, because the boy is overstimulated by such manifestations.[39]

And, of course, in the film, Mary's hems are lower and her necklines higher than Vera's.

The hairstyles, too, have significance. Elsewhere in ASHA's journal, Ruth Kimball Gardiner warns mothers of daughters to "be especially careful what you say about the way in which [they wear their] hair." "A girl who will take her mother's advice about all other points of personal appearance," Ms. Gardiner continues, "will resent bitterly any interference with the way she wears her hair."[40] Vera's mother failed to heed this advice when she tells Vera, "I think you should put your hair up—no man wants to rob the cradle."[41] In the next sequence, high school commencement, Vera is shown tentatively touching her chignon and fixing her skirts while Mary, sporting a long braid fastened with a large, girlish bow, listens attentively to the speaker.

The American Federation of Sex Hygiene Agenda

The second constituent group of ASHA, the American Federation for Sex Hygiene (AFSH), also inserted its agenda into *The End of the Road*. Naturally, this group sought to promote "biological and not moral" sex education, and, composed primarily of medical workers, to endorse the use of scientific terminology and present a favorable portrayal of the physician.[42] However, while the ambitions of the AFSH certainly appear more unified and directed than those of the AVA constituents, they are also problematic in that their agenda, promoted as objective and scientific, is as ideologically bound as that of the AVA.

Sex Education

As evidence of education's centrality to AFSH's agenda, the first third of *The End of the Road* is devoted to the promotion of sex education. The question, then, is educate whom, what, where? According to the ASHA platform, the "who" of sex education is everyone, boys as well as girls, servicemen as well as housewives. The "what" of sex education is "the study of the whole process of reproduction and the nurture of children, the meaning of marriage, prostitution, venereal diseases, illegitimacy, and the hygiene of sound recreation."[43] And the "where" is everywhere: "the home, the church, the school and the community."[44] This definition of sex education reflects ASHA's ideal of "dispersing old prejudices and inhibitions" and providing "purely scientific" instruction, an ideal that proved largely rhetorical.[45] In its articles of incorporation, ASHA claimed that its objective was "to acquire and diffuse knowledge of the established principles and practices and of any new methods, which promote or give assurance of promoting social health."[46] ASHA, however, departed from the "purely scientific" by using a nonscientific, socially constructed, interpretation of "social health."

Despite their insistence that everyone should receive sex education, ASHA invoked its discretionary interpretation of "social health" to determine what parts of the "whole process of reproduction and . . . the meaning of . . . venereal diseases" different groups should, in fact, be taught.[47] Not surprising, given ASHA's affiliation with the CTCA, the men in the armed forces were to receive the most complete education. The film that ASHA produced for the enlisted men, *Fit to Fight*, was also its most educationally complete, for it includes images of prostitution, instruction in venereal prophylaxis, and language appropriate to discussions of these social problems, that is "harlot," "streetwalker," "venereal disease," and "clap." Men in industry were not so privileged. In addition to avoiding street language (perhaps at the expense of comprehension), the "Men's Lecture Series" prepared for civilians did not include descriptions of venereal disease prophylaxis, a serious omission given that these men would have to bear the treatment costs as they were denied access to the free venereal disease clinics established for the enlisted men.

Moreover, boys in industry, an estimated 5 million between the ages of 14 and 20, did not get the "square deal" that the title of their lecturer's instruction book promised. The sex education prepared for this group was to be limited to the "Keeping Fit" program that emphasized general health instruction. As with the program for civilian men, the boys' program did not include information on the treatment or prophylaxis of venereal diseases nor did it discuss the early signs and symptoms of the diseases. The instruction manual for hygienists working with boys emphatically warns in bold face type that "lectures on venereal diseases and sex hygiene should not be given . . . [as the] introductory remarks as outlined on general health are sufficient."[48]

Finally, the ASHA produced a fourth series, "Keeping Fit Exhibit for Negroes, an adaption for colored boys and men," by introducing unspecified "suitable changes in reading materials."[49] When preparing *Fit to Fight* for the collective group of civilian male audiences over the age of 16, ASHA pooled its restrictions and edited out much of the street language, most of the scenes with prostitutes, and all descriptions of prophylaxis and the acute stages of venereal diseases.

The sex education that girls and women actually received was an even paler approximation of the ideal of complete instruction in reproductive physiology and venereal disease. The primary tenets of ASHA's education program provided that "instruction in sex subjects should never be given to the two sexes together"; that "none but obviously high-minded teachers" with "suitable training" should provide instruction; and that only women teachers should instruct female audiences.[50] Such proscriptions, not based on any pedagogic or psychological study but on Victorian social convention, severely limited the number of instructors who would be both eligible and willing to lead female sex education classes. One of the motivations for ASHA to produce *The End of the Road* was to create a self-explanatory, standardized educational vehicle to circumvent their self-constructed bottleneck.

Another moral dilemma was what to include in girl's and women's sex education. Regarding instruction about venereal diseases, Prince Morrow, the founder and long-term leader of AFSH, had averred that the catastrophic consequences of venereal disease "will continue until women know, as they have a perfect right to know, the facts which so vitally concern their own health and the health and lives of their children."[51] This viewpoint, however, was widely challenged, even within ASHA. As Ruth K. Gardiner warned in the pages of *Social Hygiene*, "Too much talk of venereal disease to a girl whose experience of life is perforce small, usually leads to morbidity and ugly fear."[52] Such worries were also raised concerning the girl's instruction in normal sexual physiology. As a popular child psychologist warned, "a large portion of those in our nerve sanitariums are there because of unconscious fear of sex."[53] Although the prominent ASHA lecturer Dr. Rachelle S. Yarros, together with Katherine Davis, convincingly countered that they had universally positive response from their lectures to women, this wariness of sex education crept into *The End of the Road*.[54] This ASHA film, for instance, contains none of the images or language describing venereal disease transmission that were allowed to remain even in their civilian men's education film, *Fit to Win*. Instead, Mary Lee receives a euphemistic explanation of "where babies come from" related in a decorous mix of third and first person and including the reassurance that Mrs. Lee "forgot the pain of your coming into the world when nurse put you into her arms."[55] Mary receives equally euphemistic instruction regarding courtship: "You must keep intimacy for the one you love" since "flirting and what young people call spooning—playing at love—is cheapening the greatest emotion of life."[56] What is not included in this venereal education film for women is Mary's home education in venereal disease. In fact, the viewer is uncertain whether Mary ever discussed venereal diseases with her mother, as she did childbirth and courtship, or whether she received instruction during her nurses' training, or whether she was as ignorant as Vera in this matter. Lastly, although the intertitles reveal an obvious attempt to dispel any "ugly fear of sexuality," the film never mentions the contemporary discussions on the nonreproductive pleasures of sexuality for women.

Just as the "who" and the "what" of sex education were more complicated than the universalism that the AFSH members within ASHA aspired to, the "where" of such instruction was also more limited than "everywhere." The instruction of girls by their mothers in sexual matters had long been the chief vehicle of female sex education. Beginning in the 1890s and a regular feature in the 1910s, the popular press, especially women's magazines, began running features on exactly how to impart this knowledge. Reformers perceived two problems with this method of girl's sex education. First, the mothers themselves were often ignorant about such matters and thus could not adequately instruct their daughters. Second, the dissemination of Freudian principles in the popular press precipitated anxieties that, "just as the thoroughbred setter dog may be rendered forever 'gun shy' and useless . . . by an explosion too near his ear," a young girl may be permanently damaged if exposed "to the wrong way of obtaining such knowledge" of sex.[57] This "wrong way" of sex education was also enacted in The End of the Road. In a sequence set up as an explicit contrast to Mary's forthright home education, we are told: "Vera's natural curiosity leads her to a source of information distorted and obscene." Pictured is Vera, seated beside a gangly, decidedly lower-class woman in her late teens who prefaces her explanation of reproductive physiology with "it's turrible bad an' you mustn't tell I told you but Gladys Hicks' gotta fella fifteen an' he told her how babies are made."[58]

While ideally, sex education was to be provided at home, by the parents, the ASHA and other organizations recognized that this was not always the case. As the CTCA described the situation for young men:

It is one of the great failures of society . . . that on the subjects of rational sex hygiene, prostitution, and venereal diseases, the very great majority of young men have no background whatsoever, excepting one supplied by the streets and by obscene stories. . . . It is up to the government to supply this background not given by their civilian life . . . to educate these boys on the vital subjects of reproduction, sex hygiene, and venereal diseases, etc., in the teaching of which their parents and home communities have been so woefully negligent.[59]

The AFSH reformers within ASHA had long supported sex education in the public schools as a safety net and had lobbied the federal government to support this effort. Yet, as discussed earlier, the government's interest in sex education was limited to whatever was needed to maintain a fit army. The government was concerned with women's health only inasmuch as women threatened (that is, slept with) military personnel. In the film, however, the social reformers promoted a larger role for the government. Vera's "fall" was the result of the "noneducation" she received from her mother, but her "salvation" is the attention and education she receives from the uniformed Army doctor, Philip Bell.

In sum, for better or worse, women's duty to educate their children was usurped by health reformers who intervened on behalf of the federal government to gain authority over this instruction. The means of instruction employed by the reformers were multiple, private dialogues with subgroups, imparting limited and unequal information. As a film specifically for middle-class white women, and which presents an edited body of information, *The End of the Road* itself demonstrates the divorce of the ASHA's reformist ideal of a complete and scientific education from the subjective programs they (ASHA) actually developed.[60]

Proper Terminology and Candor

The second element of the AFSA agenda that the ASHA sought to promote in *The End of the Road* was the replacement of euphemism in discussions of venereal disease with proper terminology. "Stress the importance of a decent vocabulary," ASHA tells parents; "only the terminology of science is free from obscene association."[61] As Davis points out: "In a vague way, many women knew . . . [about] venereal diseases, but almost never by name."[62] Seeking to correct this ignorance, *The End of the Road* intertitles display the word "gonorrhea" once and "syphilis" twice. This was somewhat of a bold gesture: six years before, Margaret Sanger's pamphlet "What Every Girl Should Know" had been confiscated by the U.S. Post Office because the references to syphilis and gonorrhea were considered "obscene" under the Comstock Law.[63] (The successful challenge to this act was led in part by the AFSH.) The tentative public acceptance of such vocabulary is exemplified in the *New York Times* review of *The End of the Road*: "The picture is not pleasant nor euphemistic. Neither is the subject with which it deals. It is unpleasant, however, only to the degree necessary for force, and plain spoken only to the extent necessary for clearness. It is never morbid; one feels clean after seeing it."[64]

As indicated by the review's reference to "unpleasantness," ASHA's use of what it called "good Anglo-Saxon words" did not, however, mean that the ASHA had rejected the Victorian sensibility it displayed elsewhere.[65] ASHA's insistence on proper medical terminology reflected the physician constituency of ASHA's AFSH faction and that subunit's attempts to codify a specific scientific discourse that would legitimate their aspirations toward professionalism. There is, for instance, much inconsistency in the application of this linguistic reformation elsewhere in the film. Mrs. Ellbridge's hysterectomy, for example, is described, but the words "prostitute," "venereal disease," and mention of the sexual activity that transmitted the infections do not appear in the intertitles. Indeed, the graphic pictures of women disabled and deformed by syphilis and a child blinded by gonorrhea are described as resulting from "criminal folly" and "the sowing of wild oats."[66]

Ideal of the Physician

The third and final ambition of the AFSH constituents of ASHA was to insert into *The End of the Road* an ideal of physicians. Prince Morrow, the founder and leader of AFSH, had been a regular participant in nineteenth-century struggles to define medical confidentiality. Morrow was a resolute opponent of the "medical secret," the collusion between physicians and venereally infected male patients that resulted in the infection of their unsuspecting female partners.[67] Writing about this conspiracy, Dr. Davis states:

> Physicians who have known the true facts concerning the complaints with which their women patients were afflicted have observed a conspiracy of silence. We have talked about "female weaknesses," "female diseases," "the

complaints of women," when, as a matter of fact, women have been infected with one or the other of the venereal diseases.

On two separate occasions in the film, Dr. Bell violates the unwritten compact of the "medical secret" by discussing with Mrs. Ellbridge the gonorrhea she contracted from her husband.[68] Moreover, to illustrate his true progressive stripes, Dr. Bell consoles her with the observation, "The ignorance, prudery, and false standards of our fathers are more to blame than your husband."[69]

Davis as Auteur

In addition to AVA and AFSH, the constituent organizations of ASHA that produced the film, there was one other influence on the script of *The End of the Road*, namely, its author, Katherine Bement Davis. There are two incidents wherein Davis subordinated the ASHA agenda to her own. First, the ASHA implicitly endorsed women's role as mother and home-maker. Davis, however, has Mary pursue a career in nursing, while Vera, working in a munitions factory at the end, is "happy in the conscious of doing her part in the world struggle."[70] Second, ASHA explicitly endorsed the "promotion of laws and conventions favoring early marriage," believing that it would limit premarital sexual experimentation and thus reduce venereal disease.[71] Davis, however, has Mary reject Paul's proposal twice. First, Mary contended, "We're too young to think about marrying Paul—we must wait a while." Later, Mary refuses him a second time on account of her career, a bold explanation given eugenic alarm at bourgeois women's employment. "I have work to do, too, Paul, I've volunteered for overseas service—I can't marry you."[72]

The Film's Reception

Despite the conflicting agendas of Davis's and ASHA's constituent groups, *The End of the Road* is a coherent film, starring well-known thespians, Richard Bennett and Claire Adams, and was shot at the Rockefeller's scenic estate at Pocantico Hills. The film's promoters, commercial and otherwise, were not unreasonable in hoping that the film would prove popular and profitable like other films of the genre.[73] They were undoubtedly surprised by the events of *The End of the Road*'s official opening in Syracuse, New York.

After booking the film's opening run at the Empire Theater for February, 1919, the Syracuse manager staged a private screening for "a semi-censoring committee composed of leading Syracuse clergymen, medical men, dramatic editors and city officials."[74] After the showing, all but one of the committee gave *The End of the Road* their unconditional approval. After thinking on it overnight, the holdout, Assistant Public Safety Commissioner S. T. Fredricks, "at length branded the picture as unfit to be exhibited here publicly." Called in as a representative of the War Department to ameliorate the situation, Captain (then Lieutenant) Edward H. Griffith, the film's director, helped arrange another screening, this time for society and club women. Following the news of this special women's screening, a Syracuse news correspondent reports that "there was a near riot as a result, but the picture came through with one hundred percent approval, including a hearty endorsement of the wife of the Commissioner for Public Safety"—and Fredricks's boss. The strategy worked. Fredricks withdrew his objections and the picture opened, on schedule, before a house of 1,500 moviegoers.[75]

The following month, March, 1919, proved reassuring to the film's promoters and producers, as telegram requests for the film from state and local health boards outstripped availability, and negotiations began between the CTCA and the YMCA for the printing of additional copies.[76] April, however, brought the disquieting news that the National Association of the Moving Picture Industry (NAMPI), highly vocal in the public dialogue on censorship, was organizing opposition to the film.[77] In May, the NAMPI declared *The End of the Road* to be "morally unfit," and it formally petitioned U.S. District Attorney Clyne "to bar the film from the mails, express and railroad."[78] That same month the Illinois counsel for NAMPI initiated proceedings in that state to block further showings of the film and to prosecute any theater owner who continued to run the film. Then, in July, ASHA preemptively withdrew the film from New York City theaters following the decision of the U.S. Circuit Court of Appeals that upheld Licensing Commissioner Gilchrest's ban on *Fit to Win*.[79] That same month ASHA was challenged by the Executive Committee of State and Provincial Boards of Health of North America and agreed to withdraw *Fit to Win* from all commercial showings, and to restrict the audiences of *The End of the Road* until "a careful study of this film" could be made.[80] By August, only six months after the film's opening, ASHA executive officer William Snow broached the subject with distributor Ira Silverman of dismantling their contract for the film's commercial showings.[81]

The Controversy

It has been proposed that this abrupt reversal in the film's reception represented a backlash against some elements in the genre of social hygiene films.[82] Certainly this reaction involved, in part, a rejection of certain discussions and subtexts within the films. But the full explanation is more complex, encompassing changes affecting the film's promotion and audience, as well as factors relating to the postwar return to normalcy.

Producers and Promoters

The government, representing the CTCA, the Medical Division of the Army, and the USPHS, together with ASHA was responsible for the production and promotion of *The End of the Road*. This complex voluntary-federal relationship that spawned the film broke down at the war's end. One explanation for the spurning of *The End of the Road* was the film's effective orphanage by its promoters and producers in the face of the rising public censorship.

With the war in Europe won, the two factors that had prompted the government's alliance with ASHA, public opinion about the camp's morality and military concern for efficiency, were moot. As for the specific participants within the government, from Armistice Day to the end of that federal fiscal year, the same seven-month period during which the film was released and its withdrawal initiated, the picture's nominal parent organizations regrouped and renegotiated their wartime alliances. As the demobilization camps emptied, the CTCA, the film's main promoter, was disbanded and its members absorbed piecemeal into the U.S. Interdepartmental Social Hygiene Board (ISHB), the U.S. Public Health Service (USPHS), and civilian life.

With the CTCA eviscerated, the only other government bodies represented in the film's production left to intervene were the Medical Division of the Army and the USPHS. The former, the Medical Division of the Army, lacked a mandate to intervene in civilian women's education, though, as I mentioned, Lieutenant E. H. Griffith, the film's director, did orchestrate the resolution in Syracuse. In contrast, the USPHS did have a mandate and, moreover, its Division on Venereal Disease owned 34 copies of *The End of the Road*, for loan to state and local health boards. Instead of intervening on behalf of the film, however, the USPHS Surgeon General, Rupert Blue, ran a notice in the September 20, 1919, issue of *Moving Picture World* that announced: "This is to inform you that the Public Health Service has withdrawn its indorsement [*sic*] of the films, 'Fit To Win,' 'End of the Road,' and 'Open Your Eyes,' and all other pictures dealing with venereal disease that have been shown or are being shown commercially."[83] Yet, in light of the above discussion of the sex education promoted by the AFSH physicians within ASHA, it is not so surprising that their counterparts, the physicians within the USPHS, would reject the commercial motion picture as a sex education vehicle: it was public, presented uniform information regardless of audience composition, and was not interpreted through a "trained lecturer."

Who was left to oppose the film's commercial discontinuation? ASHA, like the government, was in a state of flux. As one of the six members on the ISHB, William J. Snow, the ASHA Executive Officer, was compelled to concur with fellow ISHB members that *Fit to Win* was "not a useful after-the-war film for general circulation outside of the army."[84] But *The End of the Road*, he felt, "should continue until a clear opinion has developed concerning the desirability or undesirability of its being shown through commercial channels."[85] Other AVA and AFSH constituents of ASHA not absorbed into the ISHB or USPHS did, in fact, continue to use the film in educational programs but, with the demise of the CTCA, they lacked a spokesperson to defend its commercial showings. That left only Davis to defend her film. However, in February, 1919, when the censorship juggernaut got its first push in Syracuse, Davis set sail for Europe on the "Ship of Service" to investigate the postwar condition of the social hygiene movement.[86] For the record, though, actress Claire Adams, who played Mary Lee, did travel to both Syracuse and Pittsburgh to defend the film she had starred in.

Audience

The film's promoters and producers may have failed to defend the film, but *The End of the Road*'s viewer numbers and box office receipts indicate that the theatergoing public accepted it. Club women, women within social reform movements, and nonaffiliated bourgeois women, collectively the film's targeted audience of middle-class women, clearly supported the film, as evidenced by their defense of its opening in Syracuse. Indeed, in the months between the film's release and the dissolution of the Committee, an Illinois women's voluntary umbrella organization, Women's Committee of the Council of National Defense, reported that their Social

Hygiene Department managed to show *The End of the Road* to as many as fifty-four thousand women. The commercial shows, too, appeared to be at least as popular. Even after the NAMPI began its campaign against VD films, *Variety* reported in May, 1919, that *The End of the Road* was still "playing to capacity in the fifth week" of its run in Brooklyn.[87] And, as the bottom line, the film was making money, drawing almost $9,000 in one week at a Philadelphia theater and commanding "top dollar price" in Syracuse.[88]

In addition to these traditional measures of reception, the film engendered sufficient controversy that two separate studies were undertaken to determine its effect upon its audience. The first study, conducted during the summer of 1919 by Professor Maurice A. Bigelow using Columbia University summer students, supported the film unequivocally. Bigelow reported that an "overwhelming majority of these students were of the opinion that *The End of The Road* should be continued in public showings." Bigelow, confident of his results, said he "believ[ed] this evidence is most important."

ISHB was apparently unconvinced and, that same summer, made a grant of $6,600 to the Psychological Laboratory of Johns Hopkins University for a second study of "the informational and educative effect upon the public of certain motion-picture films used in the various campaigns [against] . . . venereal disease."[89] In cooperation with ASHA and Johns Hopkins, eminent psychology researchers Karl Lashley and John Watson investigated the educational value and emotional appeal of both *Fit to Win* and *The End of the Road* in a variety of experiments on different populations. Their research revealed that women, both white and African American, were by far the least knowledgeable in all categories of information concerning VD.[90] Moreover, the study demonstrated that women gained more technical knowledge than men from the film and suffered no demonstrable emotional reactions, though the researchers carefully probed for such responses. When specifically questioned about the more graphic details virtually all stated "that all parts of the picture" should be shown, and all insisted that young women should be shown the film, at least before marriage, but preferably around ages of 14 to 16.[91] In contrast to this, "the majority of men objected to the showing of the film to women" of any age.[92] In sum, the investigators reported that the women

were glad to have seen the picture and to have been aroused to many facts of which they were ignorant before, and they thought the picture should be shown more widely in that community. . . . No one in this group appears to have been shocked by the picture or to have felt any ill effects from it. On the contrary, all seem favorably impressed both during and after the performance.[93]

But these carefully obtained results were only indirectly translated into concrete suggestions to ISHB about the film's screenings. Although the investigators found the film had little effect on the sexual behavior or use of prophylaxis by men (and they tellingly did not investigate this outcome in women), they concluded that the films should be shown only to male, or at least gender-segregated adult audiences; that the material should be greatly simplified; and that the subject should be "handled with great skill and shown only under careful regulation."[94]

There is no obvious reason why Lashley and Watson disregarded their own data and why their results, together with those of Bigelow, were not used to reintroduce the films as educational tools and to extend VD instruction programs for women. The difficulty for the Hopkins's researchers and the members of ASHA and ISHB to put aside their concern about the propriety of educating women on sexual matters—a concern heightened, perhaps, by the recent social dislocations of suffrage and women's wartime employment—may have contributed in part to their odd research conclusions. Indeed, among their recommendations, Lashley and Watson suggested that ASHA's policy of segregating the audiences by gender be extended to all of the film's showings. This suggestion was clearly a response to general anxieties over showing previously restricted sexually suggestive material to women in a darkened, permissive, and coed public space.[95] By segregating the audiences by gender, the Hopkins's researchers and the ASHA and ISHB members privatized public displays and discussions of women's sexuality in accordance with their residual notions of separate spheres of influence. The conflict of this notion of male/public and female/private with the format of the cinema was, in fact, recognized and debated within the contemporary press.[96]

Finally, the postwar reorganization of the CTCA had specific significance for women's ability to participate in the debate and affect the policies that would regulate their lives. For women as a group, the CTCA had, as a clearinghouse for voluntary organizations, directly incorporated a large number of women's organizations into the government per se. Following the immediate postwar reorganization, the women's groups "cooperated with" but were not a part of ISHB, and when ISHB was absorbed by the USPHS after July 30, 1922, even this "cooperation" ceased. Most women within the CTCA returned to civilian life as those individuals transferred to ISHB or USPHS were nearly exclusively degreed professionals, overwhelmingly male and disproportionately from the AFSH faction within ASHA.[97] The net result of the reorganization was twofold. First, the disbanding of the CTCA marginalized or even eliminated women and AVA faction members from the debates surrounding the policy on "the women's film" and the propriety of women's sexual education. Second, by removing women from the decision-making arena, those women at the grassroots level who supported the film, predominantly bourgeois women within the clubs and social reform movements, had no conduit to voice their demand for the film and the education it provided. In short, evidence suggests that many women, the film's intended audience, saw the film, approved of it, and believed it "should be shown more widely in that community," but their vehicle to voice this opinion had been disbanded and prominent members of their community marginalized.

Content

The film's content also shaped its reception and subsequent commercial withdrawal. The aspects of the film identified above as elements of the broader agendas of AVA and AFSH may have affected the film's reception by audiences beyond its above-described supporters. Second, the film's departure from some of the genre's conventions surrounding the etiology of VD may explain, in part, the difference in reception between *The End of the Road* and the earlier, more stereotypical pictures. In a period characterized contradictorily by normalcy and social revolution, the film's departures had specific references to wartime phenomena that may have offended or alienated postwar viewers.

Outdated Agendas

"I want my girl to do as she pleases, be what she pleases regardless of Mrs. Grundy," wrote Zelda Fitzgerald of her daughter Scottie, using "Mrs. Grundy" as a shorthand for prudery and opposition to the postwar standards of pleasure and consumption.[98] "Mrs. Grundy" was also a shorthand for the social purists, like those represented by AVA within ASHA. Although Fitzgerald was writing in 1924 when she proclaimed that she wanted her daughter "to be a flapper," the Flapper, so identified with the 1920s, was already a powerful public image in 1913 when, as *Current Opinion* declared, "sex o' clock" had struck in America.[99] By late

1919, the AVA's "Mrs. Grundy" and the agenda of the AFSH faction of
ASHA had become outdated for many Americans.

ASHA's AVA construction of sexuality as dangerous, their promotion of
sexual continence, and the implicit suggestion that VD was a retribution
for immorality, would have been ridiculed by a rising number of young
women like Scottie Fitzgerald and criticized by a burgeoning number of
proponents of Freud, Free Love, and other such contemporary philosophies. During the war such social critiques were silenced by the zeitgeist
of patriotism. Moreover, women's sexuality itself was also constructed as
unpatriotic. As an ASHA/CTCA pamphlet explained:

> Girls must be made to realize that they bear a responsibility to the soldier
> and that their patriotic duty is to avoid weakening the soldiers devotion to
> his country's best interests by arousing his emotions to a pitch which will
> tend to divide that devotion.[100]

Other elements within *The End of the Road* identified above as part of
the AVA philosophy of environmental determinism would fail to resonate
beyond club women, conservatives, and older Americans. The vilification
of alcohol, for instance, would be viewed as either redundant or prudish in
this period around Prohibition. Tobacco use, too, was popularized during
the war by cigarette company campaigns and women's use was becoming
more commonplace. The enormous number of women who joined the
workforce during the war period, particularly in nontraditional occupa-
tions and who, as a consequence of their new economic independence,
became consumers in the leisure culture, made the AVA descriptions of
women's proper environment equally outdated. Last, the loose dresses and
long tresses ASHA's film and poster campaigns promoted were quickly
disappearing from women's fashion magazines.

The AFSH's agenda promoted in *The End of the Road* also appeared to
lose relevancy. AFSH's primary platform was sex education but the home
instruction so heavily stressed in the film appeared less urgent in the
immediate postwar period when a record 22 percent of all public schools
offered sex education and 85 percent of principals supported such curricu-
lums.[101] Language reform, AFSH's second objective, was so successful that
the film's one intertitle with "gonorrhea" and two with "syphilis" may
have seemed less shocking to many 1919 cinemagoers than their continued use of "wild oats" and "primrose path." Additionally, the objections to
the graphic photographs that accompanied the purportedly frank discussion appeared less gruesome alongside the concurrent rash of vampire
movies, an irony not lost on some of the film's defenders.[102] The final

AFSH ambition of popularizing their representation of the ideal physician who, among other attributes, rejected the "medical secret" was also dated. The state-by-state reform of marriage laws that required of the couple a physician's certification of health was believed by many to obviate that responsibility for the physician.

Conventions and Meanings

With the sole exception of *The End of the Road*, all of the ten or so other VD hygiene films present women as the initial source of infection.[103] This was in keeping with the dominant construction of venereal disease as one in which the loci of infection were prostitutes, usually conceptualized as immoral, lower-class, or immigrant women.[104] Departing from the proto-type VD hygiene film, however, *The End of the Road* is the only film to emphasize men as the source of infection and to present only intraclass disease transmission.

Unique in portraying only male-to-female transmission, *The End of the Road* shows only Vera's Howard and the "champion catch-as-can" Russell Ellbridge as the initial disease vector. At first, this seems to break with the traditional ideology and absolve women as plague carriers. However, in addition to presenting a male etiology of VD, this "woman's film" portrays these infectors as unreformable, thus breaking another of the genre's conventions. Whereas the other films almost invariably include the rescue and repentance of the infectious women, the unrepentant and unsympathetic Howard leaves Vera, presumably to repeat the experience, and Mrs. Ellbridge, in the hospital for a hysterectomy as a result of the gonorrhea she contracted from her husband, brushes aside his bedside promises as something she has heard before. Only the infected women, themselves, in this film, are in any sense rescued or repentant. Davis explains *The End of the Road* as "an effort to make girls see that . . . in the spiritual world as well as in the physical world, the law of cause and effect prevails . . . that sorrow and suffering . . . follow self-indulgence."[105] Hence, the breaks with convention actually suggest that even when infected, rather than infecting, women are still guilty of sexual activity and the venereal disease their punishment.

Another departure from the genre's conventions is the absence of the infecting prostitute or lower-class woman to introduce the initial infection, which would only then be passed, via the marriage bed, to middle-class women and children. Besides Ellbridge's wife, the infections in *The End of the Road* are from the playboy Ellbridge to socialite Marian Sinclair and from Howard Lord to his at least financial equal, Vera Wagner. This intrabourgeois model of venereal disease transmission in *The End of the Road* has two resonances with the contemporary society.

This transmission model played, first, on the widespread middle-class paranoia about "race suicide." The ASHA literature, replete with such propaganda, explains its eugenic fear as arising from situations where "those designed by nature to be the future fathers and mothers of the race are so incapacitated by venereal disease as to be either unproductive [of children] or else menacing to the welfare of their offspring."[106] The infections (and the implied possibility of sterility) of Vera and Marian and Mrs. Ellbridge's hysterectomy were all recognizable symbols from the contemporary eugenic discourse that equated the damaged reproductive capacity of white, bourgeois, women with the demise of civilization.

Just as women's infections and hysterectomy were signifiers of contemporary eugenic ideologies of "race suicide," sexual activity in this wartime production had as its special reference the "social murder" committed by sexually active women.[107] The absence of the infecting prostitute as a lower-class conduit for venereal disease in *The End of the Road* reflected recent research about the VD incidence pattern. "We found that venereal disease was not coming from prostitutes," Raymond Fosdick, CTCA chairman, told a congressional committee, "but from the type known in the military camps as the flapper—that is, the young girls who were not prostitutes, but who probably would be to-morrow, and who were diseased and promiscuous."[108] "Gonorrhea and syphilis are 'camp followers,' " announced one ASHA publication that was said to have reached eight million readers.[109] In sum, the bourgeois community was forced to accept that "sex o' clock" had indeed struck within their own social strata and that numbering among the "camp followers" (sexually active unmarried women, also known as charity girls, camouflage dames, camp runaways, patriotic prostitutes, army flappers, and khaki mad girls) were the daughters of their community.

The connection between *The End of the Road* and the phenomenon of the camp followers was not tenuous, but drawn by many Americans because of Davis's reputation. As the Commissioner of Corrections in New York City, Davis was frequently featured in the popular press, her fame renewed regularly by national awards and honorary degrees for her research on female offenders.[110] Her eventual appointment as director of the CTCA's Committee on Protective Work for Girls (CPWG) would also have been noted by many Americans, as would her billing as the film's author and director.

The CTCA had sought and received the responsibility to enforce the Draft Act's required ban on prostitution inside the training camps and within the "moral zones," the area in a five-mile radius of the camps. To meet this responsibility, the CTCA created the CPWG in September, 1917, "to promote law enforcement, sex education and activities for girls."[111] Seeking to counter the increasing number of nonprofessional, sexually active young women, Maude E. Miner, the CTCA's first chair, appointed 150 women as protective officers to patrol the nation's streets, amusement parks, dance halls, beaches, and other places "where darkness is a shield to conduct," looking for wayward young women and returning them home.[112]

As the CPWG's caseload grew exponentially over the following year, another unit, the Law Enforcement's Section on Women, joined the effort to resolve the "girl problem." The new plan, in conjunction with the Department of Justice, implemented a program of compulsory exams for arrested women and incarceration of infected repeaters. Outraged by these policies, Maude Miner resigned her position as chair of the CPWG. "I could not be satisfied to see the girl's interests entirely subordinated to the interests of the soldiers," wrote Miner, "and the only reason for caring for the girls in the detention homes and reformatories reduced to just that."[113] The work of the Section nevertheless was continued and extended by Miner's replacement in the CPWG chair, Katherine Davis.

The aim of Davis's research and the intention of the CPWG programs were to distinguish between and reform both "the khaki mad girl" and "the other girl who has already crossed the line" into prostitution.[114] Davis described the former as "lure[d] by the uniform":

Young girls, thrilled with patriotism, sometimes fail to realize that the uniform covers all the kinds of men there are in the world; men of high ideals . . . or, in the worst instances, men who feel that their own physical appeal must be gratified, no matter who suffers. And so, many girls, through ignorance, through emotion, take steps which will lead to bitter regret.[115]

These "charity girls," who "may become professionals in time" were arrested, investigated by CPWG caseworkers, examined, and, if uninfected, usually sent home "in the hope of diverting her from a life of prostitution."[116] "The other," the "Temptress" who was thought to have "already crossed the line, was deemed dangerous, not only to the young men whom she allures, but, earning money easily, dressing more showily, furnishes a dangerous example to girls of weak will and unsatisfied desires."[117] When arrested, she was likely to be examined and incarcerated without trial "in an institution located in the country where there is abundant opportunity for outdoor work," in order to insure "the protection of the military and naval forces of the United States against VD."[118] Under Davis, the CTCA arrested some thirty-five thousand "civilian persons"—all women. Of these women, the 15,520 found to be infected with VD or, as "prostitutes," at risk of contracting and spreading VD were held in detention homes for an average stay of ten weeks or, in reformatories, for an average stay of a year.

Like the other social critiques mentioned, the outcry against the abrogation of these women's civil rights and suspension of the writs of habeas corpus were silenced by wartime patriotism. Indeed, reports that socialist women, who were antiwar, were being arrested as a form of political harassment similarly failed to engender any policy review.[119] The end of the war brought a waning interest in venereal disease and a return to "normal life." Many Americans were uninterested in reviewing their wartime policies or reliving them on the screen. Normalcy held little room for panic over "race suicide" or "charity girls" and as such, orphaned by its producers and promoters, the film's outdated and potentially offensive content may have permitted its censors to override the support from among its intended audience of women and disenfranchised social reformers.

Epilogue

In addition to illustrating this unusual voluntary-federal collaboration and the magnitude of the wartime campaign against venereal diseases, the fate of *The End of the Road*, in particular, may be read as a bellwether of change in venereal control strategies and women's role in the public health. In March, 1921, the Sixty-Sixth Congress of the United States voted *not* to provide funds for the continuation of the Interdepartmental Social Hygiene Board after June 30, 1921. Convinced by the testimony of the American Medical Association and others that ISHB's services were redundant, the House Appropriations Committee transferred ISHB's responsibility for coordinating research and education on venereal diseases to the United States Public Health Service. The USPHS also assumed the Board's budget, a budget ten times that of the USPHS's Section on Venereal Diseases. The demise of the Board, the CTCA's postwar incarnation, signaled an end to all wartime ties, formal and cooperative, between voluntary agencies and federal government.[120] For the USPHS, Congress's actions were read as a mandate for the reform priorities of medical treatment, scientific research, and public school sex education. With an almost identical agenda and overlapping membership, the USPHS expounded on the programs developed by the AFSH faction within ASHA. Reflecting the supremacy of the AFSH disease-centered model of infection control (i.e., scientific research, the provision of prophylactic and treatment facilities, and scientific sex education) over the AVA environment-centered model (that is, prohibition, increased women's wages, detention facilities for prostitutes), the budget, which under the ISHB had invested three times as much in educational research as scientific, was gradually shifted to reflect the new priorities. With the demise of ISHB, the opportunity for dialogue between these two views disappeared and the programs were insulated within the government from public critique.[121] With this insulation of the USPHS educational programs, the strategy of imparting unequal information to different subpopulations was continued. The government's discretionary power to determine what knowledge people were to have in matters concerning their own health was the most disconcerting development and one that had particular significance for women.

For most of the nineteenth century, women had been the accepted leaders in movements for public and personal health reform and the expected educators of their children in matters of sexuality. With the impending war, various social reform organizations were taken into the government in alliance with nascent professional groups to coordinate the nation's war efforts. As part of the reform movements, women, as individuals and organizations, were also incorporated under this federal umbrella and were allotted considerable, albeit traditional, responsibilities for running the Hostess Houses at military camps, the women's and girl's reformatories and detention homes, and the civilian women's educational programs. With the war's end, women's organizations were gradually "demobilized" from the government and, as a result, women's avenues for influencing public health policy were dismantled. Though hidden by the "successes" of women's reform efforts, namely Prohibition and Suffrage, the demise of Interdepartmental Social Hygiene Board was significant for individual women committed to venereal disease control or sex education. Indeed, the disbanding of ISHB was even more significant for women collectively, as insulated officials with their private agendas took over the regulation of women's access to information about their own sexuality and reproduction. *The End of the Road* was, in this regard, a dead end.

Notes

I wish to thank the Museum of Modern Art and Dr. Byron Ruskin for access to *The End of the Road*; Lisa Cartwright for generously providing me with archival materials; Paula Treichler for her encouragement and advice; Sonya Michel, Evan Melhado, Leslie Reagan, and the Women of the Big Yellow for their many helpful comments and criticisms; and especially Rick Canning for his invaluable assistance and support throughout.

1. Prologue to *The End of the Road*, which appears as intertitles 4–14. For the film's discussion below, I have numbered the intertitles from 1 to 139, as they appear in the Metropolitan Museum of Art's Film Archives copy of *The End of the Road*, a postwar edited version. This film was copyrighted by the American Social Hygiene Association Inc., in March, 1919, six months after its completion in late September, 1918, and a month after its commercial opening in February, 1919. Letter from ASHA General Director, Major William F. Snow to Surgeon General Ireland, September 2, 1919, Records of the Office of the Surgeon General, Record Group 112, File Number 4.52, National Archives, Washington, DC; *American Film Institute Catalog of Motion Pictures Produced in the U.S., Feature Films, 1911–1920*, ed. Patricia King Hanson (Berkeley: University of California Press, 1988) 241.

2. Allan M. Brandt, *No Magic Bullet: A Social History of Venereal Disease in the United States Since 1880* (New York: Oxford University Press, 1987) 54. *Fit to Fight*, a training camp film shown to all recruits, was produced under arrangements similar to those described above for *The End of the Road*. After the war, in 1919, *Fit to Fight* was revised for use in civilian education, the discussions of venereal prophylaxis were omitted, an epilogue was added, and the picture was retitled *Fit to Win: Honor, Love, Success.*

3. Letter from Major Snow to Surgeon General William Crawford Gorgas, 4 January 1918, Records of the Office of the Surgeon General, Record Group 112, File Number 4.52, National Archives, Washington, DC; ASHA, *Catalogue of Social Hygiene Motion Pictures, Slides and Exhibits* (New York, n.d.) 4–5.

4. Katherine Bement Davis, "Social Hygiene and the War, Part II: Woman's Part in Social Hygiene," *Social Hygiene*, vol. IV (October, 1918): 525–560, 558.

5. Snow to Ireland, 2 September 1919.

6. *The Spreading Evil* (James Keane, 1918) and *The Scarlet Trail* (John S. Lawrence, 1918). "Jolo," *Variety* (22 November 1918): 46; Edward Weitzel, *Moving Picture World* (11 January 1919): 246.

7. For excellent analyses of the American and British campaigns against venereal disease, see Brandt, *No Magic Bullet*, and Annette Kuhn, *Cinema, Censorship, and Sexuality, 1909–1925* (London: Routledge, 1988).

8. ASHA, *The American Social Hygiene Association, 1914–1916*, no. 41 (New York: ASHA, 1916): 9.

9. David J. Pivar, "Cleansing the Nation: The War on Prostitution, 1917–1921," *Prologue*, vol. 12 (Spring, 1980): 29–40, 30. Note: herein the word "prostitute" is used to mean female sex workers. Although there were occasional oblique references to "both male and female prostitutes," all of the 35,000 "civilian persons" arrested and detained on suspicion of prostitution during the war by the CTCA were women. ISHB, *Manual for the Various Agents of the Interdepartmental Social Hygiene Board* (Washington, DC: GPO, 1920) 33.

10. Pivar, "Cleansing of the Nation," 30.

11. ASHA, *The American Social Hygiene Association, 1914–1916*, 3.

12. Michael Imber, "The First World War, Sex Education, and the American Social Hygiene Association's Campaign against Venereal Disease," *Journal of Education Administration and History*, vol. 16 (1984): 47–56, 47.

13. Imber, "The First World War," 225, footnote 17.

14. Mrs. R. G. Stone to Josephus Daniels, 25 April 1917, quoted in Brandt, *No Magic Bullet*, 57.

15. Imber, "The First World War," 49.

16. Imber 59.

17. Brandt, *No Magic Bullet*, 59.

18. Davis, "Social Hygiene and the War," 558.

19. Intertitles 62 through 70.

20. See Linda Gordon, *Woman's Body, Woman's Right: A Social History of Birth Control in America* (New York: Viking Press, 1976).

21. Intertitles 130, 131, and 74.

22. Brandt, *No Magic Bullet*, 61.

23. Although she advocated sexual continence, Davis also accepted prophylaxis as helpful in the fight against VD. Davis's report on ASHA in "Conferences," *Survey*, vol. 35 (20 November 1915): 193–194.

24. The only punishment to befall any sexually active serviceman was reserved solely for those who failed to report to the stations promptly after sexual exposure. For the Army, see USPHS, *The Attack on Venereal Diseases*, V.D. Bulletin No. 5 (Washington, DC, 1918): 9; for the Navy, see C. H. Lavinder, *Where Away: Some Things Worth Knowing About Venereal Diseases*, V.D. Bulletin No. 85 (Washington, DC, 1927): 13.

25. AVA, *The Social Evil in Syracuse, Being the Report of an Investigation of the Moral Condition of the City Conducted by the Committee of Eighteen Citizens* (Syracuse: AVA, 1913): endplate.

26. Lieutenant George Anderson, "Making the Camps Safe for the Army," *Annals of the American Academy of Political and Social Sciences*, vol. 79 (September, 1918): 143–151, 146.

27. J. E. Rush, "Critical Comment on Current Methods of Public Education in Venereal Disease," *American Journal of Sociology*, vol. 27 (November, 1921): 325–333, 329.

28. Intertitles 80, 82, 83, and 103.

29. Henry MacMahon, "Big Shears—or Common Sense? A Timely Discussion of the Problem of Moving Picture Censorship," *Independent and Harper's Weekly*, vol. 105 (25 June 1921): 662–680.

30. Charles Eliot, "The American Social Hygiene Association," *Social Hygiene*, vol. 1 (December, 1914): 1–5, 3.

31. Figure 2.2, a promotional still, shows Mrs. Lee reading aloud to Mary from *The Maid of Maiden Lane*. Though arranged in an identical tableau, in the film Mrs. Lee is shown reading to Mary from Parker's deportment manual.

32. Intertitles 45, 60–61, 76.

33. Susan Porter Benson, *Counter Cultures: Saleswomen, Managers, and Customers in American Department Stores, 1890–1940* (Urbana: University of Illinois Press, 1988) 134–135.

34. Intertitle 105.

35. Eliot, "The American Social Hygiene Association," 3.

36. Dr. Carrie Weaver Smith, "The Unadjusted Girl," *Social Hygiene*, vol. VI (July, 1920): 401–406, 402.

37. Intertitle 117.

38. Mrs. Woodallen Chapman, *A Nation's Call to Young Women* (Washington, DC: GPO, 1918).

39. Poster reprinted in Davis, "Social Hygiene and the War," 527.

40. Ruth Kimball Gardiner, *Your Daughter's Mother*, ASHA Publication No. 319 (New York, 1920) 552.

41. Intertitle 44.

42. John H. Stokes, *Today's World Problem in Disease Prevention: A Non–Technical Discussion of Syphilis and Gonorrhea* (Washington, DC: USPHS, 1919) 19.

43. New Jersey State Department of Health, *The Parent's Part* (Trenton: Bureau of Venereal Disease Control, 1918) 8.

44. ASHA, *Social Hygiene: The Home and the Community*, Publication No. 41 (New York, 1916) 20.

45. ASHA, *The Boy Problem*, Publication No. 284 (New York: ASHA, 1920) 1; Valerie H. Parker, *Social Hygiene and the Child*, ASHA Publication No. 542 (New York: ASHA, n.d.) 3.

46. "Articles of Incorporation" filed by ASHA in March, 1914, and reprinted on the flyleaf of Parker, *Social Hygiene: The Home and the Community*.

47. New Jersey State Department of Health, *The Parent's Part*, 8.

48. USPHS, *A Square Deal for the Boy in Industry for Those Interested in Work With Boys* (Washington, DC: GPO, 1920) 9.

49. ASHA, *Catalogue* 12.

50. Eliot, "The American Social Hygiene Association," 4.

51. Quoted in Brandt, *No Magic Bullet*, 29.

52. Gardiner, *Your Daughter's Mother*, 555.

53. Gardiner 542.

54. Dr. Rachelle S. Yarros, "Experiences of a Lecturer," *Social Hygiene*, vol. 5 (April, 1919): 205–222, 206–207; Katherine Bement Davis, "Women's Education in Social Hygiene," *Annals of the American Academy of Political and Social Science*, vol. 79 (September, 1918): 167–177.

55. Intertitles 16, 21–24.

56. Intertitle 38.

57. Gardiner, *Your Daughter's Mother*, 541.

58. Intertitles 35, 36.

59. William Zinsser, Director of the CTCA Section on Men's Work, "Working with Men Outside the Camps," *Annals of the American Academy of Political and Social Science*, vol. 79 (September, 1918): 194–203, 195–196.

60. Suzanne White, "*Mom and Dad* (1944): Venereal Disease 'Exploitation,'" *Bulletin of the History of Medicine*, vol. 62 (1988): 252–270, 266.

61. ASHA, *Social Hygiene: The Home and the Community*, 29. Also Eliot, "The American Social Hygiene Association," 2.

62. Davis, "Women's Education in Social Hygiene," 167.

63. Margaret Sanger, *What Every Girl Should Know* (New York, 1912); Brandt, *No Magic Bullet*, 24; Gordon, *Woman's Body, Woman's Right*, 214.

64. "Opening of *The End of The Road*," *New York Times* (2 March 1919): Section IV, 5: 2.

65. Stokes, *World Problem in Disease Prevention*, 14.

66. Intertitles 108 and 109.

67. This secret operated in either of two ways: a physician might treat an infected male without insisting that his female partner(s) be informed; or, if the female partner became infected and sought medical care, the physician might treat her without informing her of the proximate cause of her illness. Mark Connelly, "Prostitution, Venereal Disease, and American Medicine," in *Women and Health in America*, ed. Judith Walzer Leavitt (Madison: University of Wisconsin Press, 1984) 202.

68. Intertitles 101–104, 107.

69. Intertitle 104.

70. Intertitle 136.

71. ASHA, "Education to Combat Venereal Disease," *Survey*, vol. 45 (11 December 1920): 383.

72. Intertitle 129.

73. *Damaged Goods*, for example, the first film of the genre, was very favorably reviewed and, produced for less than $50,000, it was said to have grossed at least $2,000,000. Eric Schaefer, "Of Hygiene and Hollywood: Origins of the Exploitation Film," *The Velvet Light Trap*, vol. 30 (Fall, 1992): 34–47, 37.

74. News item, "Syracuse, February 19," *Variety* (21 February 1919): 71.

75. "Syracuse, February 19," 71.

76. Western Union Telegram, G. H. Sumner, Secretary, Iowa Board of Health to Surgeon General Gorgas, 1 March 1919; Letter, Max J. Exner, National War

Work Council of the YMCA, to Captain E. H. Griffith, CTCA, 6 March 1919; Letter, George R. Mott, National War Work Council of the YMCA, to E. H. Griffith, CTCA, 18 March 1919; Letter, E. H. Griffith to George R. Mott, 31 March 1919. Curatorial Records, Army Medical Museum housed in the Otis Historical Archives, Armed Forces Institute of Pathology, Washington, DC.

77. *"End of the Road* to be Stopped Showing Here," *Moving Picture World* (24 May 1919): 1167.

78. *"End of the Road* to be Stopped Showing Here," 1167.

79. News item, "United States Circuit Court of Appeals Bars *Fit to Win* Showing in New York City," *Exhibitor's Trade Review* (26 July 1919): 610.

80. Letter from Snow, "Copy of Letter sent to State Boards of Health," 3 September 1919, Records of the Office of the Surgeon General, Record Group 112, File No. 4.52, National Archives, Washington, DC.

81. Letter from Snow to Eugene B. Kelley, Commissioner of Health, Boston, MA, August 30, 1919, Records of the Office of the Surgeon General, Record Group 112, File No. 4.52, National Archives, Washington, DC.

82. See Schaefer, "Of Hygiene and Hollywood," 34. I question the extent to which increasingly graphic depictions helped precipitate the "backlash." *Damaged Goods*, the earlier, well-accepted, hygiene film included hospital footage very similar to that in *The End of the Road*. Moreover, none of the commercially released films contained footage of chemical prophylaxis. All mention of such procedures was carefully edited out from *Fit to Fight* while it was still being shown in the demobilization camps, long before its use before civilian audiences. See worksheet, "Titles: Copies for *Fit to Fight* for Mr. Zinsser's Department," sent to Major Snow, file date 12 September 1918, Records of the Office of the Surgeon General, Record Group 112, File Number 4.52, National Archives, Washington, DC.

83. Quoted in Schaefer, "Of Hygiene and Hollywood," 44.

84. The members of the ISHB were the Secretaries of the Treasury, War and Navy, plus three medical representatives, one each from the Army, Navy, and USPHS. *Report of the Interdepartmental Social Hygiene Board for the Fiscal Year Ending June 30, 1920* (Washington, DC: GPO, 1920): inside front cover.

85. Snow to Kelley, 30 August 1919.

86. Editorial Correspondence, "All Aboard the Ship of Service," *World Outlook*, vol. 5 (February, 1919): 18–20.

87. *"Fit to Win* Allowed to Run," *Variety* (2 May 1919): 66.

88. *"End of the Road* Barred," *Variety* (18 July 1919): 46; *Variety* (21 February 1919): 71.

89. Karl S. Lashley and John B. Watson, *A Psychological Study of Motion Pictures in Relation to Venereal Disease Campaigns* (Washington, DC: United States Interdepartmental Social Hygiene Board, 1922) 1.

90. Lashley and Watson, *A Psychological Study of Motion Pictures*, 23–25.

91. Lashley and Watson 50, 52.

92. Lashley and Watson 58.

93. Lashley and Watson 43.

94. Lashley and Watson 87.

95. Miriam Hansen, *Babel and Babylon: Spectatorship in American Silent Film* (Cambridge: Harvard University Press, 1991) 119; Kathy Peiss, *Cheap Amusements: Working Women and Leisure in Turn-of-the-Century New York* (Philadelphia: Temple University Press, 1986) 139–162.

96. White, "*Mom and Dad* (1944)," 253–254.

97. Neva R. Deardorff, "Throttling Social Hygiene," *Survey,* vol. 45 (19 March 1921): 883–884.

98. Quoted from Sara M. Evans, *Born for Liberty: A History of Women in America* (New York: The Free Press, 1989) 175.

99. Evans, *Born for Liberty,* 161; Brandt, *No Magic Bullet,* 49; "Sex o' Clock in America," *Current Opinion,* 55 (August, 1913): 113.

100. Chapman, *A Nation's Call,* 12.

101. "Report of the Committee on the Teaching of Hygiene in Public Schools. Part II—Domestic Science and Nature Study," *Bulletin of the American Academy of Medicine,* vol. 7 (April, 1906): 432; Imber, "The First World War," 52–54.

102. Rush, "Critical Comment on Current Methods of Public Education in Venereal Disease," 329.

103. Other films in the genre include *And the Children Pay* (Veritas Photoplay Co., Matrix Photo Plays, 1918, 7 reels); *Damaged Goods* (American Film Mfg. Co., Mutual Film Corp., 1914, 7 reels); *Fit to Fight* and *Fit to Win* (ASHA and CTCA, ASHA and USPHS, 1918/1919, 6 reels); *Open Your Eyes* (Warner Bros., State Health Films, 1919, 7 reels); *The Scarlet Trail* (G and L Features, 1918, 6 reels); *The Solitary Sin* (New Art Film Co, 1919, 6 reels); *Know Thy Husband, Wild Oats,* or *Some Wild Oats* (Samuel Cummins, Social Hygienic Films of America, 1919, 6 reels); *The Spreading Evil* (James Keane Feature Photo Plays, 1918, 7 reels). Also, for *Cleared For Action* (1918) and *Whatsoever a Man Soweth* (1919), no production or distribution information available.

104. William H. Zinsser, "Social Hygiene and the War, Pt. I: Fighting Venereal Diseases—A Public Trust," *Social Hygiene,* vol. 4 (October 1918): 497–514, 506.

105. Davis, "Women's Education in Social Hygiene," 176.

106. Poster reproduced in ASHA, *Social Hygiene: The Home and the Community,* 24.

107. Mary Macey Dietzler, *Detention Houses and Reformatories as Protective Social Agencies in the Campaign of the United States Government Against Venereal Diseases* (Washington, DC: GPO, 1922) 2.

108. Brandt, *No Magic Bullet,* 81 from U.S. House Committee on Military Affairs, Hearings on Training Camp Activities, 65th Congress, 2nd Session, 14 March 1918, 5.

109. Elizabeth Fee, "Sin vs. Science: Venereal Disease in Baltimore in the Twentieth Century," *Journal of the History of Medicine and Allied Sciences,* vol. 43 (1988): 141–164, 143–144.

110. Vern L. Bullough, "Katherine Bement Davis, Sex Research, and the Rockefeller Foundation," *Bulletin of the History of Medicine*, vol. 62 (1988): 74–89, 79.

111. Originally the responsibilities of the Committee on Protective Work for Girls fell to the Civilian Committee to Combat VD (CCCVD). Quickly, however, this "girl problem" was seen as too large for voluntary local organizations and was delegated to another CTCA committee, the CPWG. Brandt, *No Magic Bullet*, 78–79.

112. Miner, quoted in Brandt 83–84.

113. Brandt 85.

114. Jane Deeter Rippin, "Social Hygiene and the War: Work with Women and Girls," *Social Hygiene*, vol. 5, no. 1 (January, 1919): 125–136, 126.

115. Davis, "Social Hygiene and the War, Part II" 532.

116. Davis, "Social Hygiene and the War," 126, 128.

117. Davis, "Social Hygiene and the War, Part II" 533.

118. Mrs. Martha P. Falconer, "The Segregation of Delinquent Women and Girls as a War Problem," *Annals of the American Academy of Political and Social Science*, vol. 79 (September, 1918): 160–166, 162.

119. Pivar, "Cleansing the Nation," 34–35.

120. There was a woman's advisory Committee to the USPHS. However, as Pivar explains, "not only did [Surgeon General C. C. Pierce] permit the committee to do no more than advise, he asserted that it had no right to designate associations or persons with whom the service would work." Deardorff, "Throttling Social Hygiene," 883; Pivar, "Cleansing the Nation," 35.

121. Pivar, "Cleansing the Nation," 35.

Paula A. Treichler and Catherine A. Warren

3

Maybe Next Year

Feminist Silence and the AIDS Epidemic

> There is not one, but many silences, and they are an integral part
> of the strategies that underlie and permeate discourse.
> —Michel Foucault 1976, 27

In the first years of the HIV/AIDS epidemic, U.S. feminism largely accepted the stereotype of AIDS as a "gay man's disease" even though the stereotype relied upon assumptions about sex and gender that feminism had long challenged.[1] When heterosexual transmission was recognized as a growing source of HIV infection in women, mainstream feminists might at last have been expected to join the struggle against the epidemic—even relish this fresh opportunity to target straight men as a culprit and make more visible their continuing power over women. Yet silence and ambivalence remained standard operating procedure for mainstream U.S. feminism until the early 1990s and even now leaves much to be desired. As committed feminists, we believe feminism's indifference to the AIDS epidemic should not pass unexamined or unchallenged. In this essay, we use quantitative and qualitative measures of AIDS coverage in feminist and non-feminist print media to track and analyze feminism's problematic stance towards the AIDS epidemic. We conclude by propos-

ing a more activist and productive feminist media agenda for reporting
HIV/AIDS in particular and women's health in general.

Women and the "Gay Men's Disease"

Cases of AIDS and AIDS-like symptoms were reported in women as early
as 1982, only the second year of the AIDS epidemic's official existence.[2]
More than a decade later, in 1993, a woman named Beverly, recently diagnosed with AIDS, was interviewed for a prime-time news segment on the
growing epidemic among women. Beverly had gone to a series of physicians before one finally tested her and diagnosed HIV: "They never
looked for this disease in me," she told the reporter, "being as how they
thought it was a gay men's disease."[3]

How had Beverly and her physicians missed the news that HIV can be
transmitted to and from women? That AIDS was no longer "a gay men's
disease," if indeed it ever was? How had mainstream media themselves
missed the news? By 1988, HIV had been widely proclaimed "an equal
opportunity virus," transmitted through "what you do," not "who you
are." By 1993, several thousand women had been diagnosed with AIDS
and HIV infection in the United States—to say nothing of worldwide
estimates in the millions. Was Beverly unusually dense in failing to get the
message? Were her physicians unusually ignorant?

The short answer is no. The long answer is more complicated and contradictory. When a woman—any woman, indeed any person, in a rich,
technologically sophisticated, postindustrial democracy—can become
infected with a deadly virus years after the knowledge is available to prevent it, many sites of silence are implicated and many points of intervention have failed. What might have changed the broad cultural
understanding of women and AIDS? What might have enabled Beverly
and other women to identify and cope more effectively with the loaded
new risks the epidemic posed? What different representations, language,
educational approaches, spokespeople, or cultural models might have produced a different outcome? One way to begin to answer these questions is
to document the evolution of representation and understanding over the
course of the epidemic. In doing so, we can also look more closely at how
AIDS and HIV are presented by and to various U.S. constituencies—as
narrow personal risk, as urgent public health issue, as social phenomenon,
as cultural crisis. What meanings are articulated, to whom, and to what
are they linked?

This essay examines the failures, obstructions, and silences that have hindered our understanding of women's relation to HIV. It asks what we knew about HIV, when we knew it, and what lessons we can learn for the future. It also asks who is meant by "we." Who are the "we" with the knowledge to slow the spread of HIV to women? The "we" responsible for deploying that knowledge? The "we" who helped or impeded that deployment? In seeking answers, this essay is concerned not only with the conventional bad guys of AIDS scenarios—U.S. biomedical institutions, the media, Congress, the Christian right, and the rest of the usual suspects. It also explores the failures and silences of the "good guys"—the feminist movement and the field of women's studies, constituting a "we" closer to home. This "we" includes us, the authors.

Silence about AIDS was, of course, never total. Like most Americans, Beverly knew the basic AIDS 101 message: AIDS is caused by a virus. That virus can be transmitted through sexual behavior, sharing contaminated drug needles, or receiving contaminated blood or blood products. A fetus can become infected through its mother's infected blood. Finally, preventive behavior, such as the use of a condom, can reduce the likelihood of sexual transmission. But Beverly obviously still thought of AIDS as it had been initially and powerfully framed: a disease of the "4-H Club"—homosexuals, hemophiliacs, heroin users, and Haitians—with homosexuals leading the charge. Each of those four groups, though for somewhat different reasons, was presumed to be male. And where sexual transmission was concerned, AIDS was almost universally understood as "a gay men's disease."[4]

Numerous analysts have sought to explain the power of this early framing and to debate its immediate and long-term consequences. We do not intend to revisit these questions here.[5] Nor do we wish to argue that the linking of AIDS to the gay community is historically inaccurate. As Edward King eloquently emphasizes in his 1993 book *Safety in Numbers*, it was the gay population who first contracted AIDS and HIV in large numbers, who organized pioneering struggles against the disease, and who continue in many places to bear the brunt of the tragedy. (Despite these facts, many governments, including those in the United States and the United Kingdom, have still not launched significant public health education and intervention campaigns targeted specifically for gay men.) It is in the context of this framing that our examination of women and AIDS must necessarily occur. Additionally, key biomedical authorities on AIDS in the United States (C. Everett Koop, Mathilde Krim, and James Curran, among others) cautioned early and often that *no group* should feel complacent about this epidemic. The Centers for Disease Control (CDC) certainly never told women to relax. It should not be surprising, though, that in the numerous struggles to call attention to the epidemic and obtain funding, institutions long accustomed to overlooking women—medicine, the media, state and federal legislatures, and, to a degree, even gay men themselves—initially overlooked them in the case of AIDS as well. No one had time for a hypothetical future problem of women with AIDS in the face of federal indifference, CDC cutbacks, media passivity, and ambiguous data.[6]

As Beverly's case suggests, these early silences persisted and continued to affect what happened to women with AIDS. Only now, in the late 1990s, can we really begin to evaluate the costs for women worldwide. These include continued barriers to diagnosis and care, exclusion from treatment and support programs, lack of information about sexuality and reproduction, lack of preventive technologies designed for women, and lack of resources and support services for women, children, and families. Moreover, the HIV/ AIDS epidemic continues to fuel a relentless conservative agenda against women and amplifies already vocal calls for surveillance and punishment.[7] And finally, but not insignificantly, our theoretical models of AIDS are still based primarily on research studies of men with HIV. When the World Health Organization estimated in 1990 that three million women worldwide were infected with HIV, its chief of surveillance noted: "Whether the natural history of HIV infection in women differs to any significant degree from that outlined for men is not known, and the detailed studies needed to answer this question are very difficult to plan and put into effect" (Chin 1990, 4). By 1992, with the HIV "gender gap" steadily closing and estimates that global HIV infection among women would soon equal that of men, it was still the case that relatively little information existed specific to women.[8]

Yet some gender differences are clearly relevant to diagnosis, treatment, and the design and delivery of services. For example, preliminary findings from an ongoing international study offer striking evidence that women's risk of HIV infection worldwide is linked in complex ways to their gendered social and economic status: "In many settings, the cultural norms that demand sexual fidelity and docile and acquiescent sexual behavior among women permit—and sometimes even encourage—early sexual experimentation, multiple partnerships, and aggressive and dominating sexual behavior among men" (Gupta and Weiss 1993, 399). One might even say that women contract HIV infection not only because of "what they do" but also because of "who they are." As Beth Schneider has pointed out, the AIDS epidemic simply exacerbates the mundane inadequacies of existing women's health care:

> Women need more of what they needed before AIDS—drug treatment programs especially for those with children; sustained prenatal care; increased foster care services and childcare facilities; confidential counseling at family planning and prenatal clinics; continued access to abortion and state-funded abortions; sex education; national healthcare in some form; and basic survival provisions in food, clothing, and shelter (Schneider 1988, 104).

U.S. AIDS experts and opinion leaders interviewed in November 1994 for a study of AIDS stigma and discrimination emphasized that as women continue to become infected and ill, economic, social, and psychological costs will mount. The study's authors are pessimistic about the future: "Too often women are thought of as dispensable," they conclude, "and [their] dispensability as merely the natural order of things" (Public Media Center 1995, 16).

Such studies help document the effects of early silence about women and AIDS. Those familiar with the longer history of women's health might have predicted that when women with AIDS did turn up, little public concern would be expressed about them except as threats to others: to their innocent babies if they were known to be pregnant, to their innocent clients if they were believed to be prostitutes, to "the general population" if they were neither of the above. Indeed, the role assigned to women in AIDS at a 1987 conference, said physician Constance Wofsy, was "almost an invisible pass-through" (Gena Corea 1992, 82). Those familiar with the recent history of U.S. feminism, however, could not have predicted that feminists, too, would be largely silent on the subject of women and AIDS in those critical first years. While gay men fought against the disease, joined in their efforts by a core of health care professionals, community service providers, and a handful of activist lesbians and organized sex workers, most members of the mainstream feminist movement watched from the sidelines—or did not watch at all. Feminism did not take up the cause of AIDS even after heterosexual transmission became the fastest growing source of HIV infection in women. Here, feminism's special domain— straight men and their power over women—could, with some justification, have been evoked. Yet silence and ambivalence remained the operative status quo for mainstream feminism from 1981 until January of 1991, when *Ms.* magazine at last published a serious cover story on the scope and politics of the epidemic ("Women and AIDS" 1991). By then more had been done on behalf of women by individuals and groups *outside*

mainstream feminism, including, surprisingly, the slick women's magazines, as well as front-line health and service agencies, lesbians, predominantly male AIDS organizations like Gay Men's Health Crisis and ACT
UP, and academics in various eclectic coalitions.[9] Moreover, even though
the influence of the AIDS epidemic on policy, law, and health activism
continues to be profound, straight men remain largely invisible as a major
source of HIV and other STDs in women, and AIDS/HIV is still not a
firmly established item on the feminist or women's studies agenda.

Should it be? Yes. We believe that the AIDS epidemic encapsulates
many goals and issues fundamental to women's interests and women's
health: reproductive freedom, sexual equality, civil liberties, economic
self-sufficiency, the right to effective protection against conception and
disease, and the rest of a longstanding program. Even within the AIDS
establishment and AIDS activism, there remains the need for voices to
speak on behalf of women. A 1995 special issue of the PWA newsletter
Newsline on HIV and pregnancy makes clear that childbearing women
with HIV have few champions:

> For people with AIDS/HIV, the right to privacy and self-determination
> have been of paramount importance. Many battles have been fought over
> these issues and some have been won. Most people with AIDS and those
> affected are strong advocates for the right to make personal choices about
> everything from treatment to disclosure. Yet when people with AIDS are
> also female and pregnant, the discourse around privacy and individual
> rights often takes a huge shift (People with AIDS Coalition of New York,
> 1995, 7).

A Word about Method

Because we are interested in the evolution of AIDS awareness and concern
within various women's and feminist communities, we use media coverage
as an index of cultural knowledge. Because we are also interested in the
direction, flow, framing, and interpretation of information and thinking
about women and AIDS, we examine three specific domains of AIDS coverage in the print media: mainstream publications, glossy women's and
feminist magazines, and alternative (including academic) feminist publications. This provides a rough method of tracking contributions and challenges to the dominant reading of AIDS—that AIDS is a gay men's
disease and an epidemic that has little relevance for women. In asking who

speaks for women, we explore, in particular, the dynamic of feminist silence surrounding AIDS.

In the following sections, we present capsule chronologies of women and AIDS coverage during the critical period 1981–1988 for the three media domains just identified. We then discuss these findings in the light of several key theoretical issues: the problematic representations of women and gender that underlie the construction of conventional AIDS chronologies; the processes by which media, whether "dominant," "alternative," or "oppositional," frame issues for their readers and audiences; and the complex responsibilities inherent in silence as well as in communication. Even now, we argue, feminist attention to the HIV/AIDS epidemic remains inadequate; nevertheless, at a point in history when new HIV infections are in principle essentially preventable, although in practice far harder to prevent, feminist insights and resources are absolutely critical. The epidemic continues to offer opportunities for feminist voices to be heard and to have significant impact on the course of the epidemic and related decisions about women's health.

Chronological Overview of Media Coverage

In this section, we sketch how the HIV/AIDS epidemic—as disease, as disease affecting women, and as broad cultural crisis—was covered and constructed over time within three broad media categories or frames: the biomedical and mainstream press, the mainstream women's and feminist press, and the alternative women's press. The first category encompasses medical journals and leading media, where we find much of the key data through which accepted accounts of the epidemic and its epidemiology emerged; the second category encompasses media coverage in the glossy women's magazines, and in the glossy feminist magazines like *Ms.* and *New Woman*; the third category includes journals like *Spare Rib*, *Off Our Backs*, and *Gay Community News*, and academic feminist journals like *Signs* and *Hypatia*.[10]

Mainstream and Medical Coverage

1981–1982

On June 5, 1981, the *Morbidity and Mortality Weekly Report*, published by the Centers for Disease Control in Atlanta, described five cases of young, otherwise-healthy homosexual men with *Pneumocystis carnii* pneumonia in Los Angeles. Subsequent issues of the *MMWR* documented additional cases of unexpected illnesses in other cities. The mainstream media published three articles in 1981 on the new mystery disease plaguing gay men.

One year later, in July 1982, the CDC reported the first cases of the syndrome in men with hemophilia. At this point, the American Red Cross advised lesbians as well as gay men to voluntarily refrain from donating blood. In September 1982, an *MMWR* "AIDS Update" on the epidemic in the United States officially adopted the term *acquired immune deficiency syndrome*, or "AIDS." In this issue, it listed cases among women for the first time: of 593 total cases to date, 34, or 5.7 percent, were among women (*MMWR* 31 [Sept. 24, 1982]: 507–514). In December the CDC reported cases of immune deficiency and opportunistic infections in infants and posited the existence of "vertical transmission" from mothers to their infants in utero or shortly after birth (*MMWR* 31 [Dec. 17, 1982]: 665–667). By the end of December 1982, 57 adult women, or 6 percent of total cases, had been diagnosed with AIDS (*MMWR* 31 [Jan. 7, 1983]: 697–698).

The mainstream media were not immune to this medical news. By the end of 1982, the general mainstream media had published 10 articles on the baffling new "epidemic of immune deficiency." Several articles, including the first front-page story on AIDS in a major newspaper (*Los Angeles Times* May 31, 1982), focused on the appearance of AIDS not in gay men but in hemophiliacs and infants, the "innocent victims" of the epidemic.

1983–1984

By spring 1983, nearly two years into the epidemic, the CDC had found no evidence that "casual contact" contributed to the transmission of AIDS. In May 1983, however, a study in the *Journal of the American Medical Association* claimed to have identified cases of AIDS spread through "routine close contact" (Oleske et al. 1983). An accompanying editorial by Anthony Fauci noted the possibility of vertical transmission from mother to infant but emphasized the less likely but more sensational alternative of routine household contact. Predictably, the wave of national media coverage that followed underlined the dire implications of the household contact scenario. In response to intense pressure from the CDC and other AIDS authorities, the journal quickly downplayed the possibility of household contact in favor of vertical transmission—but this did little to contain the first round of "spread-of-AIDS" stories in the mainstream press. The ensuing "moral panic" (Watney 1996) was reinforced when reported AIDS cases reached 1,000—the kind of milestone the media rely on. By the end of 1983, two years into the epidemic, 77 articles had been published on AIDS in mainstream publications.

For 1984 the *Reader's Guide* listed a total of 70 articles on AIDS. Of those, 52 were medical in nature, a focus partially brought about by the news that researchers had isolated the virus said to be the agent responsible for AIDS. Although a few titles left open the possibility that both sexes might be affected by AIDS, for example, "AIDS Has Both Sexes Running Scared" (Cantarow 1984), no articles focused explicitly on women. Mainstream magazines mentioned and advocated safe sex for the first time in 1984. With the development of a test for antibodies to the virus, however, getting tested was pitted against safer sex and some articles urged anxious heterosexuals to get regularly tested as a solution to the problem of sex in the age of AIDS.

1985

In 1985, media coverage of AIDS in the United States increased dramatically. The *Reader's Guide* listed 176 AIDS articles, an exponential increase from 1984. In March, the first antibody test became available. In June, Hollywood great Rock Hudson acknowledged that he had been diagnosed with AIDS and was seeking experimental treatment at the Pasteur Institute in Paris. Between June and Hudson's death in October 1985, mainstream media coverage (print and electronic) climbed from an average of 18 stories to an average of 111 stories per month.[11] In July, *Life* ran a cover story on AIDS titled—in bold red letters—"Now No One Is Safe from AIDS" (Barnes and Hollister 1985). Cover photos showed a clean-cut white nuclear family, a black soldier in uniform, and a young white woman, all seemingly unlikely victims. All, in fact, had acquired HIV through familiar routes of transmission (respectively, blood products for hemophilia, transfusion, and sexual contact with a man with AIDS). The Burks, the wholesome nuclear family, were featured in many print and television stories, which typically cited the requisite elements that made them "innocent victims": they looked like "a typical U.S. family"; the father, Patrick, contracted HIV through contaminated blood products for treating his hemophilia; he then unknowingly passed the virus to his wife, Lauren, before he knew he was infected; and she, also unknowingly, passed it to their son, Dwight, during pregnancy or breastfeeding.

So it seems that despite erratic media coverage, "gay" had become the presumed norm. Only exceptions, non-gay AIDS cases, were news. The *Life* cover was widely reprinted (together with the infamous *New York Post* headline "Long Island Grandma Dead of AIDS"—see Shilts 1987, 320). Media images were now available as graphic icons for the disease and, inevitably, media coverage itself became a story. *Newsweek*'s bold red Hudson cover, for instance, appeared in the made-for-TV movie, "An Early Frost," broadcast on NBC in November 1985, to make the point that AIDS was an important public health crisis and information was widely available. While public attention was still riveted on the Rock Hudson case, which was interpreted by some to mean "regular guys" were at risk, *JAMA* reported (in October 1985) the possibility of female-to-male transmission of HIV [HTLV-III] among U.S. servicemen in Germany; investigator R. R. Redfield and colleagues suggested that "prostitutes could serve as a reservoir for HTLV-III infection for hetero-sexually active individuals" (*JAMA* [Oct. 18, 1985]: 2094–2096). Main-stream AIDS coverage for 1985 included only four stories explicitly about women and 10 about children.

Amid the consternation and confusion produced by these reports of seemingly "heterosexual" transmission, science writer John Langone's December 1985 article in the magazine *Discover* tried to set the record straight. In his view, AIDS posed no threat to the vast majority of hetero-sexuals because "AIDS is—and is likely to remain—the price paid for anal intercourse" (Langone 1985, 52). Though Langone's position departed from the thinking of a significant number of epidemiologists and biomedical authorities at the time, he argued with great clarity and few qualifications that a crucial physiological dichotomy between the rectum and the vagina protected women from HIV; unlike the "vulnerable rec-tum," the "rugged vagina" was built by nature to take abuse, and was therefore too tough for the virus to penetrate. Langone's assertion that AIDS was still, after all, a "gay men's disease" may not have been correct, but it was irresistibly clear and provided welcome relief from confusion and anxiety.

In the years to come, the media would often assert that women were as vulnerable to HIV as men and just as often categorically assert that they were not. (By the mid-1990s, when women began to account for more new infections and AIDS cases than men, they would assert that women were *more* vulnerable to HIV.) Meanwhile, the experts played their own version of is-she-or-isn't-she, with some espousing the Langone view, oth-ers disputing it, others voting don't know. Redfield et al.'s reports in

JAMA suggesting female-to-male transmission, for example, provoked intense debate, in *JAMA* and elsewhere, over whether it was possible for women to be infected with HIV and in turn infect men through sexual contact. One proposed alternative was that apparent transmission via female prostitutes was actually "quasi-homosexual" (Client B contracting HIV from the reservoir of infected semen from Client A)—a view that preserved the "gay men's disease" conception of AIDS.

1986–1987

In April 1986, the Association for Women's AIDS Research and Education (Project AWARE) in San Francisco launched a study to begin to assess HIV antibody seroprevalence in high-risk women in California; "high-risk" was defined as women reporting five or more sexual partners in the previous five years, and/or sexual contact with a high-risk male, and the study encompassed both prostitutes and non-prostitutes. The findings, published subsequently in the *MMWR* (36 [March 27, 1987]: 157–161), reported the same rate of seroprevalence in both populations— 4 percent. The prostitutes who tested positive reported a history of IV drug use. How was this interpreted? Poorly. A multi-center study of female prostitutes, entitled "Project 72," was initiated by the CDC to clarify the issues. Of the 1,396 women enrolled, seroprevalence among those with no reported IV drug use was 4.8 percent; but this was perhaps high because many women in the study were from the Miami area, with its higher migration from the Caribbean, where heterosexual transmission was more common. Other news compounded the confusion. A possible case of female-to-female transmission was reported in a letter to the *Annals of Internal Medicine* (Marmor et al. 1986). In March 1986, the Nevada Board of Health required prostitutes to be tested for HIV antibody as a condition of employment and, once employed, tested monthly thereafter (Campbell 1991); prostitutes themselves asked that clients be required to use condoms. In June, the CDC reported that IV drug use still accounted for the largest number of AIDS cases among women, at 20 percent; but the next highest category of transmission was "other," leaving a mysterious hole in the statistics. In November 1986, the *New York Times* spelled out AIDS's lessons to date: women are "obliged to take on a new kind of responsibility for their sexuality and to reassess their roles as health professionals, relatives, lovers and friends of people with AIDS." (No lesson was offered to men, straight or otherwise.) By the end of December 1986, the CDC reported a total of 2,062 adult women with

AIDS in the United States, compared to 27,627 men, or 6.9 percent of the total.

The problem was that only a small number of researchers were focusing specifically on women and how they were represented (see Corea 1992). The rest of the AIDS literature of this period tended to finesse the question of AIDS and HIV infection in women: in one review article on psychological issues in AIDS, for instance, women were mentioned only under such headings as "pediatric AIDS"; authors simply did not discuss the fact that most cases of "pediatric AIDS" presuppose a case of "maternal AIDS" acquired somewhere. The scenario was a familiar one: women with HIV/ AIDS were bracketed as individual exceptions or special populations, or as so pathologically diseased as to be uninteresting, or as mere medical surrogates for their male partners or children. Randy Shilts, in his best-selling *And the Band Played On* (1987), devoted only 10 pages to "heterosexuals," and used most of that space to concentrate on the story of a female prostitute. His only index entry for "women" mentioned that Larry Kramer wrote the homoerotic screenplay for the film *Women in Love*.

An effort to dispel this silence was made by researchers Mary Guinan and Ann Hardy, whose paper "Epidemiology of AIDS in Women in the United States: 1981 through 1986" appeared in the *Journal of the American Medical Association* (256 [May 17, 1987]: 2039–2042). Findings to date, they contended, confirmed predictions that HIV/AIDS was being transmitted heterosexually, to and from both women and men. Guinan and Hardy's article was one of the first medical accounts to focus on women as a broad population—rather than singling out prostitutes. While statistical increases among women were less dramatic than those encountered previously among gay men, they argued, vigilance and educational intervention were critical, especially in several identifiable sub-groups including female sexual partners of IV drug users. They challenged the "rugged vagina" hypothesis: in fact, they argued, we know very little about how much protection the vaginal mucus membrane affords, but epidemiological and clinical experience with other STDs suggested it might be quite permeable. Calling for prudence, they advocated risk-reduction behavior for women, including "celibacy and having only one lifetime sexual partner." In an accompanying editorial in *JAMA*, Constance Wofsy called attention to some of the misleading ways in which AIDS was represented visually (Wofsy 1987). People with AIDS were usually still pictured as gay males, she noted, and when images of women appeared, they were white and healthy. While such atypical images avoided stigmatizing or stereotyping women who *did* have AIDS and sent the important message that despite stereotypes about the epidemic, many kinds of people are potentially at risk, they also reinforced the incorrect message to women of color and others that they were *not* at risk.[12] Perhaps the one consistent message was that infected or not, the burden was on women themselves to prove they mattered. In a special AIDS issue in October 1988, *Scientific American* recapitulated the story of the Burk family, who had been featured in the big 1985 *Life* cover story (Barnes and Hollister 1985) as a typical American nuclear family who just happened to have AIDS (Patrick Burk's hemophilia was not evident in the photos). Reproducing a *Life* photo, *Scientific American* updated the Burks' story (p. 91): "When the photograph was made, Patrick and Dwight already had AIDS; they have since died. The daughter, Nicole, is not infected." The pattern of reporting on the condition of the husband and children, but not the wife, mother, or woman is not atypical. In these accounts, women remain primarily characters in other people's stories. Indeed, even in Guinan and Hardy's admirable article, they (or perhaps their journal editor) felt obliged to argue that women with HIV and AIDS were of "special interest" to medicine for several reasons—none because women themselves were worthy medical subjects:

> Women with AIDS or [HIV] are the major source of infection of infants with AIDS, and the second most common route of transmission of AIDS to women is through heterosexual intercourse. Trends in AIDS in women may help to determine future trends for pediatric cases and may be a good surrogate for monitoring heterosexual transmission of infection. (Guinan and Hardy 1987, 2039)

This was a theme repeated in countless journal papers and scientific conference presentations, where women were routinely characterized as "vessels" of infection and "vectors" of perinatal transmission.

In September 1987, the CDC revised its AIDS guidelines and diagnostic criteria, and some researchers believed its expanded case definition would prove more sensitive in identifying signs and symptoms of HIV in women. On December 31, 1987, the CDC reported 3,751 adult females with AIDS in the United States, compared to 47,014 adult males, or 7.4 percent of the total cases among adults with AIDS. The official CDC message, nonetheless, was that although every sexually active person should be cautious, women and heterosexuals still made up only a tiny percentage of cases of HIV infection. Paradoxically, even as AIDS continued to be represented and understood primarily as a "gay men's disease," various versions of the following "urban legend" were turning up all over the United States: a straight man meets an attractive young woman at a singles bar and takes her back to his apartment where they make love (without condoms); she is gone the next morning, but written across the bathroom mirror in bright red lipstick he reads, "Welcome to the World of AIDS!" (Fine 1987). This contaminated woman was a cultural icon with a life of its/her own, a story waiting to run.

And run it did, in late 1986 and early 1987. In the last months of 1986, three different biomedical reports on AIDS—from the U.S. Surgeon General, the Institute of Medicine/National Academy of Sciences, and the World Health Organization (WHO)— collated available data and reached the same conclusion: the AIDS epidemic was urgent, global, increasingly transmitted through sex between men and women, and required immediate intervention. The reports received enough media coverage to launch major stories on AIDS as a threat to "all of us" in *Newsweek*, the *Atlantic*, the *Village Voice*, and elsewhere. On the *U.S. News and World Report* cover, a young white urban professional couple stared somberly out at the reader over the caption "What *You* Need to Know about AIDS" (Jan. 12, 1987); *Time*'s cover story, called "The Big Chill," showed a giant wave about to crash (Feb. 16, 1987). The tabloids got into the act. The *Weekly World News* on May 12, 1987, produced a morality tale about a female surgeon who put HIV in her husband's tomato juice: "Wife Murders Hubby with AIDS Cocktail" (the subheading: "He should have had a V-8!"). "Farewell, Sexual revolution. Hello, New Victorianism," trumpeted *The Futurist* magazine. Condom manufacturers reported dramatically increased sales.

The *Reader's Guide* listed 231 articles on AIDS in 1987; women, with five articles, finally got their own sub-category in the listings (nine articles were on children). A cover story in the February 1987 *Atlantic Monthly*, "Heterosexuals and AIDS," showed a man and a woman huddled separately under their blankets, arms crossed protectively around their legs. Writer Katie Leishman warned against three "sub-populations" who constitute the danger for heterosexuals: Catholic priests, married gay men, and single, sexually active bisexuals (Leishman 1987). A similar theme was struck in *The Real Truth about Women and AIDS* by New York sex therapist Helen Singer Kaplan. The 1987 book spelled out the implications for women, arguing that their "moist vulnerable mucous membranes" put them at high risk for HIV. In Kaplan's view, women were the hoodwinked victims of individual men and a duplicitous federal government, who were selling them a bill of goods about "safe sex." "There are no safe behaviors, only safe partners," she wrote. In an August *Newsweek* interview on the book, Kaplan said, "I felt like Cassandra" (Seligman 1987).

1988

In January 1988, Cassandra was trumped. *Cosmopolitan* magazine published an article by Dr. Robert E. Gould designed to reassure Cosmo's women readers about AIDS: "There is almost no danger," wrote Gould, "of contracting AIDS through ordinary sexual intercourse," that is, unprotected penile-vaginal intercourse with an infected man. Gould, a psychiatrist with no special expertise in AIDS research or treatment, argued that a "healthy vagina" was protection enough against the virus. If it were not, he reasoned, the prevalence of AIDS in the U.S. heterosexual population would by now be extensive. To account for the existence of widespread HIV infection among heterosexual men and women in Central Africa, Gould offered two explanations: homosexuality among African men was common but taboo and therefore not acknowledged to investigators; and "many men in Africa take their women in a brutal way, so that some heterosexual activity regarded as normal by them would be closer to rape by our standards" (Gould 1988, 146).

Though Gould's article was not unique in making categorical claims about women and AIDS based on limited research and experience (see Treichler 1988b), none had appeared in so widely read a publication as *Cosmo*. ACT UP immediately picketed and protested, calling attention to the article and calling for a boycott of *Cosmo*. The controversy was picked up by other media; Gould appeared on local and national talk shows, given automatic credence in some cases by his M.D. degree. On *ABC's Nightline*, however, Gould appeared with *Cosmo* editor Helen Gurley Brown, who claimed that while risk of HIV for normal heterosexual women was virtually nonexistent, *Cosmo*'s message was that women should "be safe—use condoms." "I'm sorry to contradict you," responded Ted Koppel, "but I read the article very carefully and that is precisely what you *don't* say."

These texts about women, such as they were, went largely unchallenged. Neither mainstream nor medical media took the time or responsibility to analyze and account for competing claims. They simply published them in serial order, touting each as "news." Indeed, the *Cosmo* splash had barely subsided when noted sex researchers William Masters and Virginia Johnson, with Robert Kolodny, declared in their book *Crisis: Heterosexual Behavior in the Age of AIDS* (Masters, Johnson, and Kolodny 1988) that "the AIDS virus is now running rampant in the heterosexual community." Hard on the heels of *Crisis* came Michael Fumento's book *The Myth of Heterosexual AIDS* (1990), which claimed there was no scientific evidence that HIV could be acquired through normal heterosexual intercourse.

As of August 1990, the number of women (adult and adolescent) in the United States officially diagnosed with CDC-defined AIDS totaled 13,807, or about 9 percent of total cases; of these, 4,824 were reported in the prior year (and more than half of the total had been reported in the two prior years). The total included about 7,000 women who were black, 3,500 who were white, 2,500 who were Hispanic, 75 who were Asian or Pacific Islander, and 30 who were Native American. The number of additional women in the United States with HIV infection and HIV-related symptoms was estimated to be much larger; it was estimated that in 1988 about 100,000 women were HIV-infected, with the total number of reported AIDS cases expected to reach 22,000 to 30,000 by 1991. These numbers conformed to earlier CDC predictions of a gradual increase of AIDS cases in the "heterosexual population."

The Women's and Feminist Glossies

1981–1983

How did mainstream women's and feminist magazines frame the AIDS crisis during this same period? No articles appeared in these outlets during 1981 or 1982. In 1983, three articles were listed in the Reader's Guide: one in *Ms.* in May and two in the *Ladies Home Journal* in November. The *Ms.* story, by Lindsy Van Gelder, was titled "The Politics of AIDS." Though it assumed that "a good many lesbians are monogamous" (and therefore not at risk for AIDS?), it examined the politics of funding and the problems of racism and homophobia (Van Gelder, 1983). In the *Ladies Home Journal*, "AIDS: The Latest Facts," by Bibi Weinhouse, presented AIDS as an epidemic still confined to the familiar "high risk groups" but nevertheless as news, and as a potential personal health issue for women (Weinhouse 1983). The other AIDS story in that issue, "AIDS: What It Does to a Family," by K. Barret, was a sympathetic profile of the widow of a bisexual man who died of AIDS. "People need to understand that there are children involved," said the widow, "and wives and mothers. . . . I'm tired of hearing about AIDS as a gay disease. It doesn't matter how it's transmitted. What matters is how much AIDS victims suffer and how their families suffer" (Barret 1983). These two articles signaled the coverage that would predominate in the glossies: "what women need to know" was the first kind of story; the second was human interest or personal narrative. We first trace coverage in the glossies, than backtrack to outline the feminist coverage.

Women's Glossies

1984–1985

As early as 1984, such magazines as *Glamour, Mademoiselle,* and *Ladies Home Journal* indicated that women were perhaps at risk for AIDS. (*Ms.* was not to address personal risk or social politics for many years.) The six articles listed for 1985, for example, included a September story by Chris Norwood in *Mademoiselle* titled "AIDS Is Not for Men Only" (Norwood's book on women and AIDS would appear in 1987.) In November, *Good Housekeeping* based a story on the findings of the Project AWARE study (4 percent of the "high risk" women studied were found to be HIV positive), warned readers that antibody testing should not replace safer sex precautions, and gave the number of the 24-hour CDC hotline ("AIDS: What Women Must Know Now!" 1985).

1986–1987

In 1986, 12 articles appeared; as in the mainstream and medical media, condoms were a major issue, as were the cultural changes they implied. A January article in *Vogue* by Ellen Switzer (Switzer 1986) was titled "AIDS: What Women Can Do," and introduced a theme that would be picked up in biomedical and popular discourse: "The killer disease called acquired immune deficiency syndrome (AIDS) not only has begun to strike women, but its control and eventual conquest are probably in their hands, in the opinion of Michael Gottlieb, M.D." (222). The article quoted Dr. Gottlieb: "In such battles women have historically been our best allies. They want to protect their families and themselves, so they pay attention to what science can tell them about any new threat, and act accordingly" (222). In Gottlieb's scenario, women could be counted on to get the facts: "What we need desperately right now is an informed public . . . and that is where women can help us" (222).

A different spin was given to women's role by long-time feminist writer Barbara Grizzuti Harrison in February's *Mademoiselle*. "It's Okay to Be Angry about AIDS," wrote Harrison, and specifically okay to be angry that some gay men have had "as many as 50 sexual partners a week: Is that normal? I don't think promiscuous gay men have a right to demand that we think the way they live is fine and dandy; their business is now our business, and we are under no obligation to find it lovely. . . . Even, however, if we acknowledge our anger—and/or our aesthetic and moral revulsion—does it follow that we don't extend succor and compassion to AIDS

victims? Of course not. They suffer; they must be helped" (Harrison 1986).
An example of a personal narrative appeared in the November 1986 *Ladies
Home Journal*, "I'm Fighting for My Life," by a woman who contracted
AIDS through a transfusion (Sloan 1986). The ambiguity of gender in the
article—though the person with AIDS was a woman, transfusion was usually not a gendered route of transmission (transfusion during childbirth
being an exception)—was echoed in a sidebar that updated AIDS statistics
on people diagnosed with AIDS: 70 percent were homosexual and bisexual
men, 17 percent were intravenous drug users, and 2 percent were adults
who contracted the disease through blood transfusions. Accounting for 89
percent of the people diagnosed with AIDS, the article omitted the
remaining 11 percent: the heterosexuals not infected through drug use or
blood products, whether male or female.

In 1987, 14 articles appeared in the women's magazines. This was the
year of the big heterosexual "spread of AIDS" scare, and women's risk and
the problems of negotiating safe sex were taken up in women's media. If a
man won't wear a condom, wrote Barbara Seville in *Today's Chicago
Woman*, "[o]bviously he cares little for your emotional well-being, and
more for satisfying his own physical needs. Give him a piece of liver and
send him on his way" (Seville 1987). In *Mademoiselle*, three articles spoke
to women's concerns: "Is there a man in your man's life?" asked the magazine in July 1987; "Never love a stranger," it warned in September (p.
214); and in October, a fresh theme at last—"The New Foreplay."

Four books were published in 1987 on women and AIDS: Diane
Richardson's *Women and AIDS* was published in London. Chris Nor-
wood's *Advice for Life: A Woman's Guide to Aids Risks and Prevention* [this is
how Norwood spelled AIDS so the large caps wouldn't be scary] from
Pantheon was the first book on women and AIDS published in the United
States. Helen Singer Kaplan's widely publicized book, *The Real Truth about
Women and AIDS: How to Eliminate the Risks without Giving up Love and
Sex*, called upon women to be the conscience of the nation, using their
monogamy to contain the infection and preserve relationships from the
tides of men's sexual rampages:

> We women form the "bridge" that are virtually the only avenue by which
> the AIDS virus can escape from its current confinement to the small, highly
> concentrated pool of infected high-risk men and spread out to the general
> population, which is still largely uncontaminated. . . . Women do not mind
> monogamy and sexual exclusivity as much as gay men do; in fact, many pre-
> fer sex in a committed relationship. Women as a group have always been

more interested in the quality of sex rather than the quantity provided by different partners (Kaplan 1987).

Much less widely distributed was the pamphlet *Making It: A Woman's Guide to Sex in the Age of AIDS*, by Cindy Patton and Janis Kelly, a realistic and humorous pro-sex tract in which neither sex nor gay male sexuality was criticized or blamed for AIDS (Patton and Kelly 1987).

Feminist Glossies

1981–1988

How did the mainstream feminist press cover the AIDS epidemic over this same period, 1981–1988? By 1988, the mainstream women's magazines— "the big glossies"—had run a total of 58 articles on AIDS (19 articles appeared in 1988). Despite the "gee whiz, is it safe to date?" tone at times, these articles generally provided more substance than the mainstream feminist magazines (*Ms.*, *New Woman*, *Self*, etc.). Until 1988, which was a turning point of sorts for the mainstream feminist media, three premises remained fairly constant in these magazines, particularly *Ms.*: (1) women prefer monogamy; (2) men are duplicitous; (3) getting tested—"the only way to know for sure"—is the answer to your prayers (Van Gelder 1987). Such a perspective only strengthened the dominant message that AIDS, "a gay men's disease," was a direct consequence of men's hedonistic, promiscuous, appetitive, destructive behavior. It failed to articulate the social and political aspects of the epidemic. Indeed, not only did feminist journals fail to produce an effective counternarrative, they often repeated, endorsed, and even magnified the standard account.

Ms. magazine, for example, the mother of mainstream feminist publications and still the most consistently feminist of all the glossies, was listed as running a total of 10 articles on AIDS between 1983 and 1988, most less than a page. And most of these articles, instead of undermining or challenging the homophobic and racist rhetoric of mainstream reports, instead adapted it to *Ms.*'s own preoccupation—the sterile "heterophobic," or anti-heterosexual sex, discourse of the new celibacy. Indeed, in the discourse of mainstream feminism, AIDS became a "good-news, bad-news" disease. The bad news was that thousands of people worldwide were dying, with no end in sight, and this was scary. But the good news, repeated in magazines from *Ms.* to *New Woman*, was that "women don't get AIDS." This interpretation fit nicely with the revisionist take on female sexuality: the sexual revolution, something forced on women by men, had been brought to an end by AIDS. Women had always preferred heterosexual monogamy, these magazines suggested, and AIDS was the ticket back to what women always wanted: a lifetime, monogamous partner or maybe no sex at all.

In a 1986 article in *New Woman*, Erica Jong, creator of the zipless fuck, used AIDS to celebrate the new celibacy. "For some women," she wrote, "the AIDS crisis may be a way to come to terms with the fact that they never really liked multiple-partner sex in the first place." Parroting a conservative's dream of the ideal woman, she observed that "in our dreams and fantasies, promiscuity seemed to bring freedom from hypocrisy and repression. In reality, it often did not. . . . Nor was it always a pleasure to have sex demystified and deromanticized. . . . Many women were glad for an excuse to turn away from casual sex."[13] And what, in Jong's opinion, replaced casual sex? Chastity, family, gardening, and needlepoint. (She doesn't explain how chastity produces children—a basic family requisite.) A sidebar was entitled "Good News (for Women) about AIDS." Jong's point of view was echoed in other mainstream feminist publications. And AIDS brought home a lesson women have always known but may temporarily have forgotten. As *Ms.* stated it: "Brace yourself for a shocker. Men lie to get laid" (Van Gelder 1987, 71).

For some feminist journals, *Ms.* included, AIDS served to reinforce favored notions of disempowered global sisterhood. In 1986, in its fourth piece ever on AIDS, *Ms.* reported that "an anthropologist with the University of California" believed "the spread of Acquired Immune Deficiency Syndrome (AIDS) in Africa may be connected to the practice of female genital mutilation." The anthropologist, actually a doctoral candidate who had read some of the literature on AIDS, contended that in those areas of Africa where AIDS was prevalent, "intercourse between men and prepubescent girls is also common," noting, too, that because of infibulation, anal intercourse was a common alternative to penile-vaginal penetration (Hornaday 1986). With little supporting scientific evidence, the article blindly reproduced familiar themes about Africa (e.g., social and sexual oppression of women, oppressive cultural traditions), joining them to the familiar "us/them" dichotomy of "4-H Club" rhetoric.[14] Other feminist authors (e.g., Fran Hoskens in her *International Women's Health Newsletter*) continued to claim that AIDS was caused by female genital mutilation and other forms of male sexual exploitation.

It was not until April 1987, well after the publication of the books on women and AIDS noted above, that *Ms.* offered its first piece suggesting that women in the United States might be at risk for HIV. AIDS, the journal noted, had become the leading killer of women between the ages of 25 and 29 in New York City. The article did not mention race or poverty as factors, but instead assaulted "the media" for "priss[ing] on about things like 'the exchange of bodily fluids' without specifying what any sexually active person really needs to know: which ones?" (Van Gelder 1987, 71). But if you did want to know which ones, *Ms.* wasn't telling either.

In May, *Ms.* ran a short article, perhaps as a hasty corrective to April's, that mentioned racism and the isolation of women with AIDS (Bray 1987). In September, "Condoms: A Straight Girl's Best Friend" appeared, a commonsensical, straightforward discussion of current realities that included a buyer's guide and generally avoided blaming men (Hendricks 1987). In February 1988, *Ms.* ran a short article, "Women and AIDS: Who's at Risk?" (Sweet 1988), briefly summarizing the outcome of several reputable studies (by Cohen and Wofsy). In July, Chris Norwood reported in *Ms.* that deaths of women from respiratory diseases had risen dramatically and that women with HIV or AIDS might be significantly under-counted because they showed different symptoms than men (Norwood 1988a).

Meanwhile, *Self* published a test, developed by Chris Norwood, enabling readers to assess their likelihood of exposure to HIV; in contrast to the usual boilerplate recitation of "risk factors," Norwood translated these factors into everyday experience and emphasized *degree* of risk (*possibility* of exposure) rather than a clear-cut division between "risk" and "no risk" (Norwood 1988b, 150). In July, *Self* reported that 31 percent of women responding to a survey said they had not changed their behavior in response to AIDS; the article emphasized the danger to women from bisexual men.

In 1991, the "new *Ms.*" arrived—ad-free and self-proclaimed to be "more feminist"—and published its first serious cover story on the scope, politics, and gender implications of the AIDS epidemic ("Women and AIDS" 1991).

In sum, for most of the 1980s, mainstream feminist publications gave the AIDS crisis scant attention. By the time *Ms.* got serious, other groups and institutions—including the glossy women's magazines, front-line health and service agencies, predominantly male AIDS organizations like Gay Men's Health Crisis and ACT UP, and feminist writers writing outside standard feminist outlets—had done more, written more, and acted more effectively on behalf of women.

Alternative and Academic Feminist Media

Alternative Feminist Media

The Alternative Press Index, which covers about 215 alternative magazines and newspapers, listed more than 2,000 total articles on AIDS
between 1982 and 1988. Of that total, only 100 of them appeared in a
feminist or lesbian publication or mentioned "women" or "heterosexuals"
in the title; and nearly one-third of the total concerned with women
appeared in a single publication, the Boston-based *Gay Community News*,
mostly written by feminist and gay activist Cindy Patton.

Not unexpectedly, the first women concerned about AIDS and AIDS
organizing emerged from organizations of prostitutes like COYOTE,
from women's health clinics and programs, and from lesbian communities
in cities with high rates of AIDS. Activist prostitutes, organized geographically and internationally for two or more decades, took the lead in identifying AIDS as a serious public health problem—for themselves as well as
society—and calling for non-punitive efforts to assess seroprevalence and
reduce risk among prostitutes. At a 1985 international conference in Ams-
terdam they drew up a series of demands for their protection including
regular health care, required use of condoms, and legal sanctions against
non-compliant clients.[15]

1981–1983

Women's clinics began producing brochures on women and AIDS as early
as 1983, the same year that the Women's AIDS Network (WAN), a volun-
teer organization grounded in San Francisco, sponsored its first AIDS
forum on women; the network encompassed COYOTE as well as gay and
lesbian organizations. Lesbians provided an early feminist take on the epidemic from within the gay community: their gay male friends were sick or
dying; they were seeing a rise in homophobia against both men and
women; they feared that AIDS hysteria posed broad threats to civil rights;
and at first, they also feared that this "gay disease" might spread to them.[16]

Throughout 1983, sporadic commentaries on AIDS and on women
and AIDS appeared in the alternative feminist press. Sue O'Sullivan, writing in May in the British feminist journal *Spare Rib*, criticized a BBC1 program on herpes and AIDS for its naturalized conflation of the biomedical
with the moral; moreover, she began to articulate the importance of a
feminist analysis: "This notion that somehow 'nature,' the 'natural,' had
been offended against buried any idea that it was and is specifically socially

constructed sexual practices which have to be looked at and criticized. And that's something feminists have been saying for a long time" (O'Sullivan 1983). Back in the United States, the *Women's Press* of Eugene, Oregon, urged readers in its July/August issue to confront homophobia and write their congresspersons about AIDS: "What we don't know hurts us and our sisters and brothers" ("Raid Kills Bugs Dead" 1983). The Women's Caucus of the San Diego Democratic Club held a "Blood Sisters" drive, attracting almost 200 women (Patton 1985c). In September, Cindy Patton warned that the AIDS epidemic was producing both homophobia and erotophobia, not only from outside, but also internalized within the gay and lesbian community (Patton 1983)—a theme she later elaborated in her book *Sex and Germs* (1985c). The following month, *GCN* reported 147 cases of women with AIDS, attributing 51 percent to IV drug use, 49 percent to sexual contact.

1984–1988

In 1984, the Alternative Press Index listed 166 articles on AIDS, 10 of them, just under 6 percent, in women's or gay/lesbian publications. Seven of these stories involved women or women's issues. In March 1984, for example, Patton suggested in *GCN* that lessons for the AIDS crisis could be drawn from women's reactions in the crisis over Toxic Shock Syndrome (Patton 1984). *On Our Backs*, a lesbian publication whose title, a play on that of the more politically orthodox *Off Our Backs*, adapted its pro-sex politics to AIDS, asking how the epidemic was affecting women and wondering why no one had posed this question in print before. In an article "AIDS—Should We Care?" *Spare Rib* identified sources of tension between gay men and lesbians in San Francisco as they worked together to fight AIDS (Miller 1984). Some lesbians believed "men brought it on themselves" with their "fast-lane" lifestyle; at the same time they shared political beliefs, bonds of friendship, and concern over homophobia in the society at large. Another concern involved the practice by lesbians of obtaining sperm (in vitro or in vivo) from gay male friends in order to have children: with HIV transmissible through semen and the latency period between exposure and symptoms often years, artificial insemination might provide a "bridge" to the lesbian community; yet alternatives were not obviously apparent. Other tensions within the left emerged as well. In June, Patton reported in *GCN* that 340 women in the United States had AIDS; nevertheless, she wrote, "the feminist movement at large has yet to take on AIDS as a women's health issue" (Patton 1984). Efforts initiated at the 1983 Denver National Lesbian and Gay Health Conference, she noted, had foundered; more important, "most of the discussion by women to date has revolved around how women can support their gay brothers. We must move that dialogue . . ." (Patton 1984).

In July 1985, Marea Murray questioned women's lack of interest in AIDS in a letter to the editor of *Sojourner*, a Boston-based newspaper:

> Women's lack of interest strikes me as odd and reflective of the common presumption that AIDS is a gay men's disease. Women who use needles, who receive transfusions, and, probably most of all, who are partners of bisexual men are all at risk for exposure to and contagion by this dreaded illness. . . . I continue to be astounded by the lack of information and stereotypes I encounter among otherwise aware women and lesbians around AIDS. There have been intimations that women should work on "women's issues," and questions like, "Why should we help the boys? Would they do the same for us?" (Murray 1985).

In an October 1985 article, also in *Sojourner*, Cindy Patton charged that "Feminists Have Avoided the Issue of AIDS"; the efforts of the Women's AIDS Network, she argued,

> were hampered by the lack of institutional support and the unwillingness of the feminist activist community to perceive AIDS as an important health and political issue. . . . Feminists have not mounted an organized effort to cope with the AIDS epidemic or its political aftermath. There are simple and complex reasons why feminists around the country have avoided the issue of AIDS, including burnout from other work, persistent homophobia, sex-negative attitudes, and fear of confronting such an unprecedented health problem. . . . As a feminist and a gay activist, the denial I see in the women's community feels very much like the denial among gay men five years ago. (Patton 1985b, 19)

Many early women AIDS activists were brought up short when they encountered the same mantra from their feminist and lesbian colleagues that gay men had long been hearing from the right, from politicians, from mainstream media, and from spokespersons for "the straight community": it's your problem, not ours. Patton called for a change in consciousness:

> Those feminists who have been involved in AIDS organizing experience frustration and anger at our sisters' callous attitudes and refusal to believe the magnitude of the political and health problems caused by the AIDS epidemic. It can happen here and it is happening here. . . . Five years into the

AIDS epidemic, feminists should make good on the promise of "global feminism." (Patton 1985b, 20)

But other feminists and lesbians were having none of it. Jackie Winnow (1989), working with people with AIDS and their caregivers in the Bay Area, was one of the first to see the AIDS epidemic as the thief of resources for women's health problems and to make a direct comparison between AIDS and breast cancer; seeing all the human and monetary resources being poured into AIDS, and the exhaustion in the community of women caring for AIDS sufferers, Winnow feared for women who were sick, for nothing was there for them (Winnow 1989; for discussion, see also Stoller 1995, 280–281). Patton was criticized for her presentation of the lesbian/gay community as a harmonious united front—and, in her call to activism, not articulating the understandable ambivalence of many lesbians, toward, for instance, male sexuality (Cayleff 1989).

Yolanda Retter, a feminist activist and lesbian separatist, put it this way:

> I still think that lesbians are going to inherit the earth, because males, straight and gay, can't control themselves. They're very self-destructive. . . . The boys are still asking for Mommy to come help them, and when lesbians want to play Mommy, I really despair. . . . One thing that made me very angry was when someone told me that 48,000 women per year die of breast cancer—that's more per year than have died of AIDS. And who's mobilizing for them? Nobody. I wanted to cry. I thought, "That's it, don't even talk to me about AIDS." (quoted in Limmer 1988)

When biomedical researchers suggested that lesbian sex was too gentle, infrequent, or boring to transmit HIV, lesbians and AIDS activists at an international AIDS conference staged a public kiss-in and distributed safer sex brochures aimed at lesbians (Crimp with Rolston 1990). Yet the feminist activist paper *Off Our Backs* responded with a 1991 story by Beth Elliot: "Does Lesbian Sex Transmit AIDS? GET REAL!" Any move to focus on women's own behavior, especially sexual behavior, raised a highly contentious question—what was "women's sexuality"? Did the notion encompass the whole range of sexual practices that women, in their infinite diversity, might engage in? Or did it define only the sexual practices that are wholesome, ethical, and politically appropriate? Many versions of this question (e.g., can a lesbian have sexual intercourse with a man and still be "a lesbian"?) cropped up repeatedly.

For the most part, the AIDS epidemic did not open a feminist-lesbian conversation about sexuality, and the voices calling for a reexamination or

restructuring of sexuality were few. Notable exceptions were United
Kingdom feminists Susan Ardill and Sue O'Sullivan, writing in *Spare Rib*:

> AIDS touches off deeply buried fears or ignorance of sex. . . . The negative
> aspect of the AIDS crisis—don't do this, avoid that, change or you may
> die—strikes at the heart of sexual acceptance and celebration. For women,
> the acceptance of the body—for oneself, of the other—is such a break-
> through. Separating out sexual pleasure, procreation, and marriage was a
> huge step towards women seizing control of their lives. This was what
> makes our fear now so heart rending and what we, as feminists, must seize
> hold of and attempt to turn round (Ardill and O'Sullivan 1987).

Ardill and O'Sullivan called for collaboration among gay men, lesbians,
AIDS activists, and feminists in rethinking and restructuring sexuality. In
Z magazine, Cynthia Peters and Karen Struening argued, similarly, for a
view of sexuality as socially constructed and hence open to discussion and
rethinking:

> A "new morality" should not stress monogamy and celibacy, but the value
> and importance of sexual desire in our lives. The importance of sexuality as
> a political issue should not be underestimated by the Left. While main-
> stream culture (and even the Left) interprets sex narrowly as a physical plea-
> sure analogous to other leisure time activity, and as easily commodifiable,
> feminists and gay and lesbian activists have pointed to the importance of
> sexual desire and its centrality to the formation of identity. A social con-
> struction of women that makes us invisible does not leave us well-equipped
> to take on the active re-creation of sex so desperately needed in the age of
> the AIDS epidemic. Safer sex requires that, in the context of sexuality,
> which is so often (and incorrectly) mythologized as a depoliticized zone
> devoid of rules and norms, women be active subjects of desire, constructing
> sex in order to be safe. (Peters and Struening 1988, 135).

To fill in our chronological story: in 1985, the Alternative Press Index
listed 278 AIDS articles, 13 of them (4.5 percent) about women, heterosexuals, or in a lesbian or feminist publication. On September 24, 1985,
the *Village Voice*, a national "alternative" publication, ran "Women with
AIDS: Untold Stories," a long article by Peg Byron on AIDS and women,
the first of its kind in anything approaching a mainstream magazine. In
1986, 356 articles on AIDS appeared in alternative media, 14 (4 percent)
on women or in feminist-lesbian publications. For the first time, titles
were explicit: "Women and AIDS Update," "AIDS: The Risks for
Women," "Lesbians and AIDS." In 1987, of 422 articles on AIDS, 16 (3.6

percent) were on women or in women's/feminist publications. *Making It: A Woman's Guide to Sex in the Age of AIDS*, by Cindy Patton and Janis Kelly, was promoted by the Women's Caucus of ACT UP/New York as a "hopeful, humane alternative" to prevention campaigns emphasizing abstinence or monogamy; Helen Singer Kaplan's book, *The Real Truth about Women and AIDS* (1987), was boycotted for its racism and its blaming of those in "high risk groups" for the advent and spread of AIDS.

In early 1988, the ACT UP/NY Women's Caucus brought the issue of women and AIDS to national attention and, though not immediately transforming a confused discourse into a coherent one, provided a new model for feminist AIDS activism and cultural work. The provocation was psychiatrist Robert E. Gould's assertions in *Cosmopolitan* magazine (noted earlier) that women were in no danger of AIDS from "ordinary sexual intercourse." A protest action outside *Cosmo*'s offices challenged the view of AIDS as a "gay men's disease" and led to media appearances, a video, a handbook on women and AIDS, and more demonstrations including a protest in Shea Stadium, where the women (and men) of ACT UP passed out condoms and unfurled banners with messages like "Men: Don't balk at condoms" and "No glove, no love" (Treichler 1992; Crimp with Rolston 1990; Juhasz 1995; Maggenti and Carlomusto 1988; and ACT UP/NY Women and AIDS Book Group 1992). Feminist silence and ambivalence began to give way to diverse responses and organized action.

Academic Feminist Media

1981–1988

The story of women and AIDS was much the same in academic feminist publications as in mainstream feminist publications—absent. In the women's studies literature, there was virtually no story at all. *Studies on Women Abstracts*, an international index covering about 250 specialized journals, listed no articles on AIDS between 1982 and 1986. Yet, for comparison, there was no dearth of articles on other topics in women's health: in 1986, for example, the *Abstracts* listed 13 articles on abortion, 10 on anorexia and bulimia, and 20 on menstruation and menopause. It was not until 1987 that five articles on AIDS finally appeared in the women's studies academic press; five more were listed in 1988 (e.g., Scott 1987; Lindhorst 1988). There were feminist voices in the earlier academic literature, but few were accessible through standard feminist listings like *Studies on Women Abstracts*. Based on a 1985 conference on AIDS organized by San

Francisco psychologist Leon McKusick, for instance, a collection of published papers (McKusick 1986) included the groundbreaking feminist
work on women and AIDS by sociologists Nancy Shaw and Lyn Paleo.
Chapters on women in several published AIDS collections of predominantly biomedical and epidemiological papers made strong, if not radical,
arguments on behalf of women (e.g., Guinan and Hardy 1987; Schneider
1988; Campbell 1990a; Stephens 1989; Cohen and Wofsy 1989). Additional research on women was represented by abstracts and papers at
international AIDS conferences and at professional disciplinary meetings.
Some of the most interesting feminist work on AIDS was interdisciplinary
and generally reflected the influence of critical and cultural theory, postmodernism, postcolonialism, and what was to become queer theory (e.g.,
Patton 1985c; Hammonds 1987; Richardson 1987; Treichler 1988b). Such
work found a home where it could, in odd journals, special journal issues,
and conferences in fields like cultural studies, art history and criticism,
media studies, sociology and history of science, and cultural anthropology.
But it found little welcome in women's studies.

For many, AIDS became an occasion for analyzing the dominant feminism of the 1970s and 1980s, even a test case for its assumptions—which
in some cases were found wanting. "It is inherently assumed that women
are weak, powerless and dependent on men while we maintain sexual relationships with them," wrote Peters and Struening. "It stopped us from
looking at women's power and sexual pleasure within heterosexual relationships" (Peters and Struening 1988, 135). AIDS, in fact, intensified
questions many feminists had been asking since the late 1970s: when we
say we are feminists, who are the "we," and at what price?

We have cited examples that document debate, conflict, and analysis in
the alternative feminist and lesbian media; they also show—for better or
for worse—the greater fragmentation of ideas in media that lack national
distribution and institutional hierarchies. Debate and cultural critique are
often fresh, unexpected, and diverse; yet they may also be local, parochial,
and highly individualized. Thus on the one hand, some oppositional
voices challenged, analyzed and re-interpreted the dominant us-versus-
them reading of AIDS as a rigidly gendered epidemic and instead took it
up as "our" epidemic, not "theirs." But other voices, just as "oppositional,"
not only accepted, but capitalized upon the dominant reading. For some,
it exacerbated and indeed justified the sometimes troubled relations
between lesbians and gay men; for others it represented and further naturalized an even deeper divide perceived between male and female. AIDS,
in this account, was just another chapter in the long bitter battle of the

sexes: men hogging the resources, calling the shots, erasing women, and demanding nurturing, caretaking, and sacrifice. Clearly, responses to AIDS within the alternative and academic feminist media testify to the existence of feminisms, plural, and lesbianisms, plural. They showed, too, the growing strain of maintaining the fiction of an undivided lesbian-feminist, multi-ethnic, multi-racial, woman-identified "we."

Discussion

This chronological sketch of three broad types of media coverage suggests that data about women with AIDS, though somewhat ambiguous, were available from the very early years of the epidemic; the mainstream media took little leadership in exploring AIDS' potential threat to women and women's interests. Feminist publications, too, took little leadership in the epidemic: they largely failed to challenge mainstream neglect of women, to clarify the data on gender, to articulate for their constituencies "women's interests" in relation to the epidemic, or to counter the conservative forces that were aggressively constructing the social meaning of AIDS.

Several points warrant discussion. First, the process of actually constructing a chronology (or chronologies) of AIDS media coverage poses some problems. While chronologies appear to chronicle history, they also create it—through selection, emphasis, language choice, and omission. To try, in 1998, to disentangle the threads of "women" from the various patterns and fabrics into which they have been woven over the years is an extremely difficult, perhaps impossible, task. Our account here does not transcend the problems of constructing any chronology. Though individual researchers, like sociologist Carole Campbell, tried to keep separate statistics for women, they found themselves creating "shadow chronologies" that remained largely unpublished, private, and not easy to maintain as statistics, geographical sites, and surveillance categories shifted and proliferated.[17] In addition to these problems and ambiguities, HIV statistics in general are still the subject of intense political, disciplinary, and institutional debate and professional investment. Some commentators, therefore, hold fast to accounts of the epidemic that discount heterosexually acquired cases among women, attributing them (as Gould and Fumento did) to drug use, lying, pathological clinical conditions, or what are perceived as non-ordinary or stigmatized sexual practices (rape, anal intercourse, sado-masochism, etc.). At this point, too, the long accumulation of inconsistent terminology and reporting protocols problematizes any claims and findings about "women." Researchers, clinicians, and surveillance agencies may use the term "women" more or less interchangeably with "prostitutes," "heterosexuals," "women at risk," "sex partners," and/or "sexually active women." They may define any single unmarried sexually active woman as a prostitute, establish no clear definition for "sex with multiple partners," "promiscuity," or "prostitution," lump as one risk factor "sexual contact with multiple partners, including prostitutes," and in some health jurisdictions classify cases in this category as "heterosexual transmission," in others as "no identifiable risk" or "other." Such confusions make it impossible to sort out the potentially salient issues of risk and prevention that each term connotes, and render much research on "women" and AIDS meaningless.

Terminology, a second important issue, has erased women in another way. The standard chronologies of AIDS, produced in the 1980s and tracing the evolution of the epidemic, typically encompass scientific, epidemiological, clinical, and legislative and policy events. In the United States, AIDS first appeared among homosexual men (with various speculations as to where they acquired it), then spread to other individuals and groups by the familiar "modes of transmission." While no chronologies focus specifically on the epidemic's movement among women, virtually all describe the inexorable spread of HIV to families, sexual partners, and infants. Yet even in accounts of the "heterosexual scare" of 1986–1987, explicit mention of women (i.e., the actual words "woman," "women," "female," or "she") is rare, and almost always confusing. The gender-neutral term *PWA*, person with AIDS, for example, does nothing to undo the perception that the PWA is male.[18]

Could an AIDSWATCH for women have been established early on to track, analyze, explain, and disseminate the statistics of the epidemic? Could the CDC have been pressured to set up more sensitive tracking mechanisms? At the least to establish a category for multiple sources of exposure for women? Could the CDC or a comparable agency have been required to regularly produce alternative scenarios? Or depart from the "gender-neutral" and presumed politically correct language to use the word "women" when it was pertinent? To accomplish any of these outcomes would have required organized lobbying, not just by individual researchers and clinicians, but by feminist and women's health institutions and organizations. And that, in turn, would have required a radically different formulation of the AIDS epidemic.

Let us turn to a third general issue, that of perspective, or framing. The concept of "media frames," developed by Stuart Hall, Todd Gitlin, Gaye

Tuchman, Anne Karpf, and others, seeks to explain how hegemonic discourse selects, orders, or excludes certain versions of reality in its effort to organize the world according to its own purposes. Karpf, drawing on the assumptions of this body of work in her 1988 study of media approaches to medicine and health, argues that the media production process inevitably transforms material and data into a recognizable, accessible form; this form (frame, approach, peg) defines the scope of the piece, determines the approach to the subject, and invites the viewer to ask certain questions and not others. Frames are "principles of selection, emphasis, and presentation composed of little tacit theories about what exists, what happens, and what matters"—theories that also help us understand "what and how alternative frames or approaches are regularly excluded" (Karpf 1988, 3). What, then, is "dominant"? "Oppositional"? What is the "hegemonic" truth the "alternative" press is positioned to critique? Scholarly work on "the media" is typically concerned with the "mass media," which it often reifies as a monolithic institution with few nuances and internal distinctions. Simultaneously, the "alternative press" is viewed, often approvingly, as contestational to the dominant hegemonic order. The dichotomy assumes, implicitly, that the "alternative media" can be trusted to identify and adequately cover "alternative issues" of interest to "the community." A 1996 symposium on alternative press coverage of women's and feminist issues, for example, clearly articulated this expectation: "Stories that appear for the first time in so-called 'feminist' or 'women's'" outlets just don't get 'buzzed about' as much as comparable stories elsewhere" (Flanders 1996, 6). Editor John Stoltenberg charged that mainstream and progressive editors have a "responsibility to pay attention to the feminist press and to echo it. . . . It's not a female ghetto that you can afford to ignore" (quoted in Flanders 1996).

But is this familiar charge born out by AIDS media coverage? The chronological record compiled by the gay (male) media clearly supports the view that editors should "pay attention to," even echo, the voices on the ground captured by the alternative press. To take only one example, Larry Mass, a gay physician and fledgling journalist in Manhattan, was the first to publish a story or report on AIDS. Quoting directly from CDC officials who basically denied the problem, "Disease Rumors Largely Unfounded" appeared on page 7 of the alternative gay newspaper *The New York Native*, on May 18, 1981. When the *MMWR* report appeared on June 5, 1981, confirming the "unfounded" rumors, Mass, with the backing of *Native* editor Charles Ortleb, determined in the future not to trust official spokespersons to track down the real facts firsthand. Mass's second report for the *Native*, "Cancer in the Gay Community" (July 27, 1981), was on page 1 and heralded the *Native*'s central role in covering the epidemic and providing an early—if usually unacknowledged—source for mainstream media (see Kinsella 1989 for more information). But this is not the record compiled by the feminist alternative press (nor, it should be added, of the progressive alternative media in general). As we noted above, of 2,000 articles on AIDS listed in the Alternative Press Index between 1981 and 1988, fewer than 100 were either by, for, or about women. And, as we have suggested, stories in feminist (and alternative) outlets were more likely to "echo" mainstream sources than the other way around.

Anne Karpf identifies four "persistent frames (or approaches) used in the media coverage of health and illness" (Karpf 1988, 3): the medical approach, the consumer approach, the self-help/alternative approach, and the environmental/systemic approach—approaches readily applicable to media coverage of the AIDS epidemic. What we call here medical/mainstream coverage consistently embodied the medical approach. As we have seen, the glossy women's magazines took up medical/mainstream information about AIDS and repackaged it for their female readership—as health news that women, as sexually active health consumers, needed to know. These magazines embodied the consumer frame, and with it broad assumptions about society—for example, that federal agencies can generally be trusted, that most women are, have been, or will be sexually active, probably with men, and that most women are willing to take responsibility for their health. Gay publications, and especially AIDS activist groups, incorporated medical/mainstream and consumer perspectives, but filtered it through a fairly explicit alternative frame that could be termed "What do people with AIDS need now?"—a frame that in turn led to an environmental/systemic frame that called for a broad-based strategy that included political action. The glossy feminist press, however, seemed unable to carry out any comparable tasks for its readers: presumably deeming the "4-H club" categories irrelevant to its readership, it chose not to challenge the categories themselves nor to revise or update its own understanding of a "feminist frame."

What might this revision have encompassed? As Clay Stephens (1989) has long argued, AIDS showed us, early on, the state of women's health in microcosm: women are low priority; if they are valued, it is in their roles as wives, caretakers, and mothers; they are readily stereotyped; and few resources are provided for them. AIDS should have gone to the heart of feminist inquiry, for it raised fundamental questions about how sex, gender, sexual identity, and sexual worthiness are described and understood.[19]

But, in fact, not a single woman had to acquire HIV or die of AIDS to establish that the epidemic embodied stereotypes and blaming practices that feminism had sought to combat for decades. As soon as AIDS was linked to sexual transmission, female prostitutes were blamed for the epidemic; even when prostitutes failed to oblige by coming down with AIDS en masse, the media ran stories in which alarmed experts voiced the fear that they *would* acquire it at any moment, by which time it would be too late: AIDS would have spread to respectable men and to their innocent families everywhere. Reinforced by murky photographs of working girls on the job, these stories revealed the legacies of cultural memory even as they updated them. So what if the HIV/AIDS epidemic in the United States never "exploded" as predicted among female sex workers? Feminists should have heeded the warning signs of stigma and persecution: the familiar virgin-whore discourse appropriated from earlier epidemics, the focus on prostitutes rather than their clients as carriers of disease, the use of stock photographs as evidence for favored "spread-of-AIDS" hypotheses, and so on. AIDS discourse, in other words, readily came to reenact many of the semantic and political battles that had characterized relations between women and biomedical science since at least the mid-nineteenth century.

Mostly, however, feminists at last reaped a Pyrrhic victory from decades of virgin/whore discourse: while homosexual and bisexual men stood in for women and were assigned women's historical roles and images, women—including women who were longtime feminists—for the most part stood by and let the men be the whores this time. Breathing deep sighs of relief, perhaps, they accepted for women the much more sympathetic virgin roles: helpmate, caretaker, mother, deceived wife or lover, puzzled daughter, compassionate physician. To this list, we can now add unsullied feminist, complacent about images of women as moral saviors of the nation. AIDS coalesced with "the new femininity/monogamy/abstinence" to reinstate oppressive gender stereotypes and warn women that if they were careerist and sexual, like Glenn Close in the 1987 movie, *Fatal Attraction*, they would die the terrible death they deserved, while the pure survived, happy and healthy.[20] What one might normally and approvingly term "oppositional discourses" within feminist media operated in their own hegemonic fashion within the feminist communities involved. These frames worked to organize, select, or exclude information to order to sustain a particular reality, a reality that shared some features with the dominant ideological discourse and divided on others.

What does it mean when feminists act to corroborate, by default, a dominant account? In closing, we wish to address the phenomenon of silence and, with regard to the AIDS epidemic, the role of silence and omission within the feminist media. By the early 1980s, the feminist movement may have been fragmented, but it was far from powerless. The movement had the resources, the channels of discourse, and the ability to speak out and gain attention on many issues. Where AIDS was concerned, they chose not to; yet AIDS represented a crisis of morality, sexuality, and structural inequality, issues that feminism had addressed for more than 100 years. Moreover, medical discourse had played its part in that history, inventing and sustaining gender distinctions that for the most part did not further women's stature as independent human subjects. Feminist interventions into that discourse have altered medicine's linguistic and cultural constructions of women and reshaped medical practice in a number of ways—epistemological changes brought about by a social movement (noted Donna Haraway, "I don't think epistemological changes can happen without social movements," cited in Darnovsky 1991, 76). The feminist critique of science and medicine demonstrates how feminist process, feminist activism, feminist research, and feminist theory interconnect. Indeed, the strength and current sophistication of feminist work comes from this history of feminist process and activism, where science, technology, and constructions of race, class, and gender meet. So why, in the AIDS epidemic, did feminists have so little to say? Why, when they had the tools to intervene, did they choose not to? The lengthy and voluble history of medical discourse that represented women's bodies as pathological and contaminated is matched by a history of silence—silence in which women are virtually non-existent, their interests and health concerns simply ignored. To understand what it means for feminism to collude in the silence surrounding women and AIDS requires us to examine not the power *to intervene*, but the power *not to*.

Silence, when it is linked to power, has mostly been understood as the domain of the oppressed, not the putative oppressor. Such classics as Paulo Freire's *Pedagogy of the Oppressed* (1970) helped establish an understanding of this. The erased voice of the oppressed has been well theorized, especially within feminism. That work first posited a silence that was "unnatural," that came from oppression: being a woman, being black, being poor. Feminist criticism developed and refined this model substantially over the years, recovering the "lost," undervalued, misrepresented, suppressed woman's voice, in history, in literature. This recuperative work of feminism in the 1970s and early 1980s theorized numerous types of gendered silences: "silence because women are not speaking, silence because their voices are not heard, silence because their voices are not understood, silence because their voices are not preserved" (Balsamo and Treichler 1990, 6).

What tends to be elided in these accounts, which focus on language and discourse as the consolidating point of power, is the power of silence. We are familiar with the concept of the silenced victim, that is, of someone *being silenced*. We are familiar, too, with *silencing*—the power of the powerful to silence others. But a third element exists: the silence of the powerful themselves. The ability to keep an area silent and virtually unexamined is an important, if not ultimate, key to institutional power (Warren 1996). In this trilogy of silence, the first two kinds of silence could not occur without the third. Hence to the gendered silences with which feminists must be concerned, we can add another category: silence because women choose not to speak. This notion has an implicit power in it, a notion of choice (Hedges and Fishkin 1994; Lewis 1993) that transforms the "silencing of" into "the silence of" and grants some degree of power to the silent. Such a notion of silence bridges the divide between the erased voice of the oppressed and the voice of the powerful—voluntarily suppressed. Feminists who chose not to speak out in the early stages of the AIDS crisis are on that bridge.

Tracing the feminist silence about AIDS presumes links that need to be made more explicit. This is relevant to questions of race, class, sexuality, and gender, for dominant constructions of those subject positions depend implicitly on the selective silences of the powerful. It is the three formations of silencing—the silence of the weak, the silencing of the weak by the powerful, and the silence of the powerful themselves—that provide a foundation for structures of power. None of these silences exists separately; their interdependence is implied when Lewis terms the silence of the powerful themselves a "double-cross-reversal, that is, the privilege of the dominant to talk at great length about that which is not and to stay silent about what which is" (Lewis 1993, 191).

Any institution, in other words, has areas it vigilantly ignores, black holes that constitute nodal points of power. The black hole, for *Ms.* and much of the feminist media by the 1980s, involved the founding notion of "women" as a self-evident category. Through internal policing, feminist publications ultimately acted to suppress emerging narratives that threatened to dissolve such treasured identities as "woman," "lesbian," "feminist," "victim of sexual oppression," and so on. Feminist omissions and silences surrounding AIDS were produced out of a complex nexus of tangled loyalties and stereotypes involving sexuality, sexual orientation, race, and class issues. But in the face of the AIDS epidemic, this complex feminist nexus became simplified into Victorian dualisms: women represented virtue and men represented vice. AIDS was simply the latest item on a long deadly list of men's acts—including sexual harassment, incest, pornography and rape. Lying somewhere between repression and power, feminist non-intervention worked ultimately against women as well as men infected with HIV, collaborating with medical and social discourses about contamination and contributing to the lack of action by health and government agencies. And when the various feminist silences began to break, it was too little and too late. By the time they got the message that condoms were okay, for example, and that it was politically respectable to say so, the feminist media had been scooped—by *Vogue*, the *Ladies Home Journal*, and even *Consumer Reports*.

Finally, it is important for us to better understand media institutions and the work they do. One continuing effect of the media in the AIDS epidemic, including feminist media, was to obscure structural inequalities. Effective feminist activism, regardless of its specific object and subject, has long worked to bring such inequalities to light. But we have argued here that mainstream feminism's ability to enforce silence about AIDS and keep the epidemic virtually unexamined can be seen as a key index of its power. In ignoring AIDS and hence problematic aspects of the category "women," mainstream feminism preserved silence about its own foundations and protected its power to define its corporate mission. When we, as feminists, regard "the dominant media" as patently manipulative and our own "alternative media" as transparently trustworthy, we limit the value of progressive commentary and compound the consequences of silence.

Conclusion

In this essay, we have reviewed U.S. media coverage of women and the AIDS epidemic, emphasizing the critical years 1981 to 1988. In doing so, we have sought to better understand the silence and invisibility that have made the story of women and AIDS so slow to emerge and so difficult to hear. At a time when the AIDS crisis was in grave danger of being high-jacked by the right, many battles were fought by and on behalf of the many constituencies affected by the epidemic; and indeed, a number of projects and agencies during these years attempted to alert women to their potential risk of contracting HIV, to devise programs and services appropriate to women's needs, and to put out a call to arms on behalf of solidarity and progressive politics. But the media generally failed to cover or amplify these initiatives and hence participated in the wider failure to link AIDS and HIV to other significant social problems. We conclude that the silence of mainstream feminism contributed to this wider failure by uncritically adopting the widespread but problematic proposition that "AIDS is—and is likely to remain—the price paid for anal intercourse." By adopting the view of AIDS as a "gay men's disease," feminist leaders missed a major opportunity to articulate the AIDS epidemic to long-standing feminist concerns, to influence the development of AIDS-related resources, to identify and address a range of women's health concerns, and to capitalize on existing women's networks and infrastructures to disseminate AIDS/HIV information and guidance.

Women's rights are being challenged today in a discouragingly cyclical manner on a multitude of fronts, so certainly, activist feminists have other things to do than untangle AIDS narratives. Yet feminist silence has had powerful effects, in part by facilitating and legitimating a range of anti-feminist and anti-woman interests. We cannot strictly quantify what was lost in those years of relative silence about AIDS between 1982 and 1988, or what difference an active coherent challenge would have made. The fragmentary and contradictory information about women and AIDS continues to cloud efforts to address problems specific to women. AIDS, in summary, is one of the premier symbolic battlegrounds of our time. It needs articulation by all feminists—not just those on the front lines, not just those whose friends are dying, and not just those concerned about "women" as the monolithic category championed by dominant feminism.

Notes

1. This essay first appeared in *The Gendered Epidemic*, ed. Nancy L. Roth and Katie Hogan (New York: Routledge, 1998). We thank the editors and publisher for their permission to include it in this collection.

2. The Centers for Disease Control published its first "Update" on the epidemic in the United States in the *Mortality and Morbidity Weekly Reports* (*MMWR*) in September 1982. Officially adopting the term "AIDS" and listing cases among women for the first time, the Update reported a total of 693 cases to date; of these 34, or 5.1 percent, were among women (*MMWR* 24, no. 31 [Sept. 24, 1982]: 607–614). By December 1982, 67 adult women had been diagnosed with AIDS, or 6 percent of the total cases. In this essay, subsequent citations from the *MMWR* will be documented internally.

3. ABC World News Tonight with Peter Jennings, Sept. 7, 1993.

4. This early framing and potent shorthand of AIDS as a "gay disease," widespread in the 1980s and persisting to some degree even now, has seemed impervious to repeated challenges—including epidemiological counter-evidence, public attacks from left and right, the "heterosexual panic" ironically triggered by the news that Rock Hudson had AIDS, extensive media coverage of "innocent [i.e., non-homosexual] victims," news that AIDS in Haiti and elsewhere appeared to be transmitted through sex between men and women, and a public health doctrine that declared HIV to be transmitted through specific behaviors regardless of gender, age, race, or ethnicity. A critical overview of public information campaigns can be found in Flora et al. (1995).

5. See, for example, Shilts 1987; Panem 1988; Fumento 1990; Arno and Feiden 1992; Kinsella 1989; Lupton 1992; and Farmer, Connors, and Simmons 1996.

6. The ambiguity of data is not a trivial factor in trying to account for inattention to the issue of women and HIV. Had large numbers of women emerged with symptoms suddenly and in some setting in which they were likely to be identified, the history of AIDS might have unfolded very differently. A sharp contrast in terms of media coverage is provided by Toxic Shock Syndrome (TSS) in 1979; developing acute symptoms suddenly and dramatically, women began showing up in emergency rooms around the country, a health care setting where emergent conditions and illnesses are reported promptly to the Centers for Disease Control in Atlanta. With 136 cases showing up each month, and some patients dying of an as-yet unidentified disease, TSS made headlines fast and was as rapidly taken up by women's health groups and feminist journals. Even so, women's health interests were not automatically given top priority. When it was determined that toxic shock was most typically triggered by the use of super-absorbent tampons, women's lobbies had to work intensively to reduce blame-the-victim media coverage (women are too cheap—ignorant—lazy—whatever to change their tampons often enough; if God had wanted women to wear tampons . . . ; and so on) and to convince the FDA to require manufacturers to package tampons with warning inserts and with information about absorbency capacity. The unexpected difficulties of bringing about these sensible changes led one feminist journal to suggest that TSS stood for Tough Shit, Sweetie.

7. For women, this has already brought about court-ordered cesarean-sections, penalties for health care providers who provide contraceptive information, incarceration for drug-using pregnant women, and calls for an end to legal abortion. For a fuller analysis, see Hunter 1992; ACT UP/NY Women and AIDS Book Group 1992; Campbell 1990b; Stoller 1995; and Gorna 1996. For women in many third world countries, surveillance and repressive legislation are even more widespread with fewer protections available. See Berer with Ray 1993; Mann and Tarantola 1996.

8. See Mann and Tarantola 1996. The CDC's 1992 revised definition of AIDS and HIV infection attempted to provide criteria that will better identify and track potential manifestations of HIV infection specific to women; these diseases, which appear to occur at a higher rate in HIV-infected women, include cancer of the

cervix, vulvovaginal candidiasis, cervical dysplasia, and pelvic inflammatory disease (Douglas and Pinsky 1996, 60; see also Kloser and Craig 1994, 18–31). Meanwhile, experts continue to debate the accuracy of statistical estimates and the value of models for arriving at those estimates. We refer interested readers to the Appendices in Mann and Tarantola (1996).

9. Many good collections of papers on the AIDS/HIV epidemic reflect such coalitions, cutting across biomedicine, caregiving, community service, policy and politics, activism, and academics in relevant fields. See, for example, Crimp (1988); Aggleton and Homans (1988); Fee and Fox (1988); and Fee and Fox (1992).

10. This research is based primarily on the following sources. The *Reader's Guide to Periodical Literature*, which indexes about 176 periodicals in the United States and Canada, was the main source for identifying mainstream AIDS coverage. Mainstream (glossy) women's and feminist magazines are listed in the *Reader's Guide to Periodical Literature*. Though we are categorizing magazines like *Self* and *New Woman* as "feminist" on the grounds that they emphasize women's professional lives over fashion and personal issues, only *Ms.* offers an explicit feminist politics. The main source for coverage in the alternative feminist/gay/lesbian press was the Alternative Press Index, which covers about 216 alternative magazines and newspapers. Two subcategories were broken out: feminist journals and gay/lesbian journals. For the academic feminist press, the indexes searched were the *Studies on Women Abstracts*, an international index that covers about 260 specialized journals. Searched by computer using the key words AIDS, WOMEN, POLITICS, FEMINIST, LESBIAN, HIV, PROSTITUTE, and IMMUNO- were the *Social Science Citation Index* from 1973 to present, *Dissertation Abstracts* from its inception through October 1990; and *Sociological Abstracts* from 1963 through 1990. Secondary sources that were particularly helpful include Kinsella 1989; Colby and Cook 1992; Lupton 1994; Watney 1996; Dearing and Rogers 1988; and McAllister 1990.

11. These figures are based on the quantitative investigation of AIDS coverage by James Dearing and Everett Rogers at the University of Southern California in leading U.S. media from 1981 through 1987. By "leading national media" they meant the *New York Times*, the *Los Angeles Times*, and the *Washington Post*, and the three major television networks (CBS, NBC, and ABC). By "every story" they meant those that could be identified via standard computer databases. The research papers based on this study (e.g., Dearing and Rogers 1988) are informative, and show that media coverage of AIDS was not consistently triggered by such "real world indicators" as number of cases or scientific discoveries. Still, the Dearing and Rogers chronology misses some crucial points through its decisions about what to count. Gay outlets including *The New York Native*, *The Advocate*, *Christopher Street*, and *Gay Community News* covered the epidemic earlier and more consistently than the national media; these stories, together with Randy Shilts's reporting in the *San Francisco Chronicle*, provided historical and cultural background, informed sources, and professional goad for subsequent national stories.

12. See Treichler (1988b) and Treichler (1992) for more discussion of representation of people with AIDS. For example, women through most of the 1980s were largely represented as loving companions or caring moms who humanize the gay men in their lives, a role they shared with stuffed animals and pets; women with AIDS/HIV were invisible by default.

13. Erica Jong (1986). See Treichler (1988b) for more extensive discussion of Jong's article and its use of Langone (1985) as a source.

14. Research by Jenny Kitzinger and David Miller at the Glasgow Media Project (1991) shows that both journalists and their audiences drew on stock white cultural images of black Africa in structuring their understanding of AIDS in Africa, but that the media are neither "all powerful" nor their output "one dimensional." Audience understandings were shifted and negotiated given new information, and alternative media accounts played a role. Yet the process of "scapegoating" is clearly evident in a "mock" news report prepared by a young, white lesbian, who notes that "AIDS is said to have spread though the homosexuals in America and a lot of the practices they participate in whereas in fact it could have originated from Green Monkeys in Africa, spreading from the heterosexual population over to America."

15. The conference was reported in *World Wide Whores News*, a mimeographed newsletter, not available at the corner newsstand. Though some of the presentations from the conference trickled up to more accessible outlets here and there, the example points out that established indexes will miss instances of "alternative media" that are published irregularly, presented locally, or circulated privately. See Delacoste and Alexander (1987) for more on prostitutes' organizations.

16. Cindy Patton indicated, in a personal conversation with Catherine Warren, in April 1991, that before the HIV virus was identified, "it seemed possible that we'd be next." Not until the frame of the disease shifted from immunology to virology and legitimated the STD model did tendencies to blame gay men emerge (paralleling the pattern that Allan Brandt documents in his historical analysis of venereal disease).

17. In a December 1990 conversation with Catherine Warren, Carole Campbell said her article tracing the epidemiology of women and AIDS was motivated by her mounting frustration with contradictory, partial information. A similar frustration was expressed by physician Janet Mitchell at the Los Angeles 2nd Annual Conference on Women and HIV (Nov. 14, 1993). Based at Harlem Hospital in New York City, Mitchell saw a growing number of women patients with AIDS-like symptoms throughout the 1980s, and become convinced that they were infected primarily through heterosexual transmission. The voices of individual clinicians, however, were no match for the machinery of epidemiological surveillance, which already attributed such cases to "IV drug use" or "no identified risk." Gena Corea (1992) recounts similar experiences of women researchers, clinicians, and social service workers.

18. For example, James Kinsella's timeline of medical, political, and media events (1989, 269–270) runs from the beginning of the epidemic through early fall 1989; in its 116 entries, persons with AIDS or at risk for AIDS are referred to 90 times. Out of the total 90 references to those who have acquired or might acquire HIV infection, 88 are gender-neutral or are gendered male. While gender-neutral language is often admirable in challenging sexist stereotypes, it is no help when information about gender should be communicated and emphasized.

19. Beth Schneider has argued similarly that (1) AIDS among women necessarily raises a host of issues that do not emerge clearly when the focus is on men, including gay men: reproductive, sexual, economic, historical, family, kinship issues. It is a microcosm of women's social relationships and arrangements; (2) Women are not a class worldwide; and (3) wherever there is AIDS, the fault lines and deficiencies of systems are revealed. Responses to AIDS reveal a great deal about gender systems of specific cultural locations and their potential for change (1988).

20. Laurie Stone (1987, 79), among others, observed that the 1987 film told women that they should stay at home, that single, working women were damaged, barely human. "This is a fairly tale for the age of AIDS if there ever was one."

References

ACT UP/NY Women and AIDS Book Group (1992). *Women, AIDS, and Activism*. Boston: South End.

"AIDS: What Women Must Know Now!" (1985). *Good Housekeeping* (Nov.): 245–246.

Aggleton, Peter, and Hilary Homans, eds. (1988). *Social Aspects of AIDS*. New York: Falmer Press.

Ardill, Susan, and Sue O'Sullivan (1987). "AIDS and Women: Building a Feminist Framework." *Spare Rib* 178 (May): 40–43.

Arno, Peter S., and Karyn L. Feiden (1992). *Against the Odds: The Story of AIDS Drug Development, Politics and Profits*. New York: HarperCollins.

Balsamo, Anne, and Paula A. Treichler (1990). Feminist Cultural Studies: Questions for the 1990s. *Women & Language* 13 (1): 3–6.

Barnes, E., and A. Hollister (1985). "The New Victims." *Life* (July): 12–19.

Barret, K. (1983). "AIDS: What It Does to a Family." *Ladies Home Journal* (November): 98+.

Berer, Marge, with Sunanda Ray (1993). *Women and HIV/AIDS: An International Resource Book*. London: HarperCollins.

Brandt, Allan M. (1987). *No Magic Bullet: A Social History of Venereal Disease in the United States Since 1880*. New York: Oxford University Press.

Bray, Fiona (1987). "Facing the Fear: Help for Women with AIDS." *Ms.* (May) 31.

Byron, Peg (1985). "Women with AIDS: Untold Stories." *Village Voice* Sept. 24: 16–19.

Campbell, Carole A. (1990a). "Prostitution and AIDS." In *Behavioral Aspects of AIDS*, ed. David Ostrow. New York: Plenum.

Campbell, Carole A. (1990b). "Women and AIDS." *Social Science and Medicine* 30 (4): 407–415.

Campbell, Carole A. (1991). "Prostitution, AIDS, and Preventive Health Behavior." *Social Science and Medicine* 32 (12): 1367–1378.

Campbell, Carole A. (1995). "Male Gender Roles and Sexuality: Implications for Women's AIDS Risk and Prevention." *Social Science and Medicine* 41(2) (July): 197–210.

Cantarow, E. (1984). "AIDS Has Both Sexes Running Scared." *Mademoiselle* (February): 158–159+.

Cayleff, Susan E. (1989). "The Politics of a Disease: Contemporary Analysis of the AIDS Epidemic." *Radical History Review* 45: 172–180.

Chin, James (1990). "Challenge of the Nineties." *World Health* (Nov./Dec.): 4–6.

Cohen, Judith and Constance Wofsy (1989). "Heterosexual Transmission of HIV." In *AIDS Pathogenesis and Treatment*, ed. Jay A. Levy. New York: Marcel Dekker, 135–157.

Colby, David C., and Timothy E. Cook (1992). "The Mass-Mediated Epidemic: The Politics of AIDS on the Nightly Network News." *In AIDS: The Making of a Chronic Disease*, ed. Elizabeth Fee and Daniel M. Fox. Berkeley and Los Angeles: University of California Press, 84–122.

Corea, Gena (1992). *The Invisible Epidemic: The Story of Women and AIDS*. New York: Harper Collins.

Crimp, Douglas, ed. (1988). *AIDS: Cultural Analysis, Cultural Activism*. Cambridge: MIT Press.

Crimp, Douglas, with Adam Rolston (1990). *AIDS Demo Graphics*. Seattle: Bay Press.

Darnovksy, Marcy (1991). "Overhauling the Meaning Machines: An Interview with Donna Haraway." *Socialist Review* 21(2): 65–84.

Dearing, James W., and Everett M. Rogers (1988). "The Agenda-Setting Process for the Issue of AIDS." Conference paper, International Communication Association, May 28–June 2.

Delacoste, Frederique, and Priscilla Alexander, eds. (1987). *Sex Work: Writings by Women in the Sex Industry*. Pittsburgh: Cleis Press.

Douglas, Paul Harding, and Laura Pinsky (1996). *The Essential AIDS Fact Book*. New York: Pocket Books.

Echols, Alice (1984). "The Taming of the Id: Feminist Sexual Politics, 1968–83." *In Pleasure and Danger*, ed. Carol Vance. Boston: Routledge & Kegan Paul, 50–72.

Elliot, Beth (1991). "Does Lesbian Sex Transmit AIDS? GET REAL!" *Off Our Backs* 21 (10) (November): 6.

Farmer, Paul, Margaret Connors, and Jamie Simmons, eds. (1996). *Women, Poverty, and AIDS: Sex, Drugs, and Structural Violence*. Monroe, ME: Common Courage Press.

Fee, Elizabeth, and Daniel M. Fox, eds. (1988). *AIDS: The Burdens of History*. Berkeley and Los Angeles: University of California Press.

Fee, Elizabeth, and Daniel M. Fox, eds. (1992). *AIDS: The Making of a Chronic Disease*. Berkeley and Los Angeles: University of California Press.

Fine, Gary Allen (1987). "Welcome to the World of AIDS: Fantasies of Female Revenge." *Western Folklore* (July): 192–197.

Fischoff, B., S. Lichtenstein, P. Slovic, S. I. Derby, and R. L. Keeny (1981). *Acceptable Risk*. New York: Cambridge University Press.

Flanders, Laura (1996). "How Alternative Is It? Feminist Media Activists Take Aim at the Progressive Press." *Extra!* (May/June).

Flora, June A., et al. (1995). "Communication Campaigns for HIV Prevention: Using Mass Media in the Next Decade." In *Assessing the Social and Behavioral Science Base for HIV/AIDS Prevention and Intervention, Workshop Background Papers*. Washington: Institute of Medicine, 129–154.

Foucault, Michel (1976). *The History of Sexuality*. New York: Vintage Books.

Freire, Paulo (1970). *The Pedagogy of the Oppressed*. Trans. Myra Bergman Raymos. New York: Continuum.

Fumento, Michael (1990). *The Myth of Heterosexual AIDS*. New York: Basic Books. (2nd edition Washington DC: Regnery Gateway, 1993.)

Gitlin, Todd (1980). *The Whole World Is Watching: Mass Media in the Making and Unmaking of the New Left*. Berkeley: University of California Press.

Gorna, Robin (1996). *Vamps, Virgins, and Victims: How Can Women Fight AIDS?* London and New York: Cassell.

Gould, Robert E. (1988). "Reassuring News about AIDS: A Doctor Tells Why You May Not Be at Risk." *Cosmopolitan* (January): 146–147.

Guinan, Mary E., and Ann Hardy (1987). "Epidemiology of AIDS in Women in the United States: 1981–1986." *Journal of the American Medical Association* 257(15): 2039–2042.

Gupta, Geeta Rao, and Ellen Weiss (1993). "Women's Lives and Sex: Implications for AIDS Prevention." *Culture, Medicine, and Psychiatry* 17 (4): 399–412.

Hammonds, Evelynn (1987). "Race, Sex, AIDS: The Construction of 'Other.' " *Radical America* 20(6): 28–37.

Harrison, Barbara Grizzuti (1986). "It's Okay to Be Angry about AIDS." *Mademoiselle* (February): 96.

Hedges, Elaine, and Shelley Fisher Fishkin (1994). *Listening to Silences: New Essays in Feminist Criticism*. New York: Oxford University Press.

Hendricks, Paula (1987). "Condoms: A Straight Girl's Best Friend." *Ms.* (September): 98, 100, 102.

Hornaday, Ann (1986). "New Theory: AIDS and Women." *Ms.* (November): 28.

Hunter, Nan D. (1992). "Complications of Gender: Women and HIV Disease." In *AIDS Agenda: Emerging Issues in Civil Rights*, ed. Nan D. Hunter and William B. Rubenstein. New York: New Press, 5–39.

Jong, Erica (1986). "Women and AIDS." *New Woman* (April): 42–48.

Juhasz, Alexandra (1995). *AIDS TV*. Durham: Duke University Press.

Kane, Stephanie, and Theresa Mason (1992). "AIDS Research, Anti-Drug Policies, and Ethnography." In *The Time of AIDS*, ed. Gilbert Herdt and Shirley Lindenbaum. Beverly Hills: Sage.

Kaplan, Helen Singer (1987). *The Real Truth about Women and AIDS: How to Eliminate the Risks without Giving up Love and Sex*. New York: Simon & Shuster, Inc.

Karpf, Anne (1988). *Doctoring the Media: The Reporting of Health and Medicine*. London: Routledge.

King, Edward (1993). *Safety in Numbers*. London: Cassell.

Kinsella, James (1989). *Covering the Plague: AIDS and the American Media*. New Brunswick, NJ: Rutgers University Press.

Kitzinger, Jenny, and David Miller (1991). "In Black and White: A Preliminary Report on the Role of the Media in Audience Understandings of 'African AIDS,' " a paper presented at the 5th Conference on Social Aspects of AIDS, South Bank Polytechnic, March.

Kloser, Patricia, and Jane Maclean Craig (1994). *The Woman's HIV Sourcebook: A Guide to Better Health and Well-being*. Dallas: Taylor Publishing.

Langone, John (1985). "AIDS: The Latest Scientific Facts." *Discover* (December): 27–52.

Leishman, Katie (1987). "Heterosexuals and AIDS: The Second Stage of the Epidemic." *Atlantic* (February): 39–58.

Lewin, Tamar (1995). "Fears, Suits and Regulations Stall Contraceptive Advances," *New York Times* Dec. 27: A1–A9.

Lewis, Magda Gere (1993). *Without a Word: Teaching beyond Women's Silence*. New York: Routledge.

Limmer, Melissa (1988). "A World Apart." *Advocate* Oct. 10: 26–27.

Lindhorst, Taryn (1988). "Women and AIDS: Scapegoats or a Social Problem?" *Affilia* (Winter): 51–59.

Lupton, Deborah (1994). *Moral Threats and Dangerous Desires: AIDS in the News Media*. London: Taylor & Francis.

Maggenti, Maria, and Jean Carlomusto (1988). *Doctors, Liars, and Women: AIDS Activists Say No to Cosmo*. Video. Gay Men's Health Crisis. Color, 28 min.

Mann, Jonathan M. and Daniel J. M. Tarantola, eds. (1996). *AIDS in the World II: Global Dimensions, Social Roots, and Responses*. New York: Oxford University Press.

Marmor, M., et al. (1986). "Possible Female-to-Female Transmission of Human Immunodeficiency Virus" (letter). *Annals of Internal Medicine* 105: 969.

Masters, William, Virginia Johnson, and Robert Kolodny (1988). *Crisis: Heterosexual Behavior in the Age of AIDS*. New York: Grove Press.

McAllister, Matthew (1990). Medicalization in the News Media: A Comparison of AIDS Coverage in Three Newspapers. Doctoral dissertation. University of Illinois at Urbana-Champaign.

McKusick, Leon, ed. (1986) *What To Do about AIDS: Physicians and Health Professionals Discuss the Issues*. Berkeley: University of California Press.

Miller, Barbara (1984). "AIDS—Should We Care?" *Spare Rib* (April): 28.

Murray, Marea (1985). "Too Little AIDS Coverage" (letter). *Sojourner* (July): 4.

Norwood, Chris (1985). "AIDS Is Not for Men Only." *Mademoiselle* (September): 198–99, 293–296.

Norwood, Chris (1987a). *Advice for Life: A Woman's Guide to AIDS Risks and Prevention*. Pantheon Books: New York.

Norwood, Chris (1988a). "Alarming Rise in Deaths." *Ms.* (July): 65+.

Norwood, Chris (1988b). "How Real Is *Your* Risk?" *Self* (June): 148–151.

Oleske, James, et al. (1983). *Journal of the American Medical Association* 249: 2345–2349.

O'Sullivan, Sue (1983). Reviews: "Panorama." *Spare Rib* (May): 38.

Panem, Sandra (1988). *The AIDS Bureaucracy: Why Society Failed to Meet the AIDS Crisis and How We Might Improve*. Cambridge, MA: Harvard University Press.

Patton, Cindy (1983). "Taking Control: Women, Sex, and AIDS." *Gay Community News*, Sept. 17: 5.

Patton, Cindy (1984). "Illness as a Weapon." *Gay Community News* June 30: 5.

Patton, Cindy (1985a). "Heterosexual AIDS Panic: A Queer Paradigm." *Gay Community News* Feb. 9: 1.

Patton, Cindy (1985b). "Feminists Have Avoided the Issue of AIDS." *Sojourner* (October): 19–20.

Patton, Cindy (1985c). *Sex and Germs: The Politics of AIDS*. Boston, South End Press.

Patton, Cindy, and Janis Kelly. (1987). *Making It: A Woman's Guide to Sex in the Age of AIDS*. Ithaca, NY: Firebrand Books.

People with AIDS Coalition of New York (1995). *Newsline*. Special issue on HIV/AIDS and pregnancy (July/August): 6–32.

Peters, Cynthia, and Karen Struening (1988). "Talking with Women about AIDS." *Z* (July/August): 133–137.

Public Media Center (1995). *AIDS Stigma and Discrimination: The Attitudes of National Experts and Influentials*. Public Media Center in Association with the Ford Foundation and Joyce Mertz-Gilmore Foundation.

"Raid Kills Bugs Dead/AIDS Kills Gays Dead" (1983). *Women's Press* [Eugene, OR] (July/August): 3.

Randolph, Laura B. (1988). "The Hidden Fear: Black Women, Bisexuals and the AIDS Risk." *Ebony* (January): 120–126.

Randolph, Laura B. (1997) "Cookie Johnson on the Magic 'Miracle': 'The Lord Has Healed Earvin.'" *Ebony* (April): 72–76.

Redfield, Robert R., et al. (1985). "Heterosexually Acquired HTLV-III/LAV Disease (AIDS-Related Complex and AIDS)." *Journal of the American Medical Association* 10 (18): 2094–2096.

Richardson, Diane (1987). *Women and AIDS*. London and New York: Methuen.

Rudd, Andrea, and Darien Taylor, eds. (1992). *Positive Women: Voices of Women Living with AIDS*. Toronto: Second Story Press.

Schiller, Nina Glick (1993). "The Invisible Women: Caregiving and the Construction of AIDS Health Services." *Culture, Medicine, and Psychiatry* 17 (4): 487–512.

Schneider, Beth E. (1988). "Gender and AIDS." In *AIDS 1988: AAAS Symposia Papers*, ed. Ruth Kulstad. Washington, DC: AAAS, 97–106.

Scott, Sara (1987). "Sex and Danger: Feminism and AIDS." *Trouble and Strife* (Nov.): 13–18.

Seligman, Jean (1987). "A Warning to Women on AIDS: Counting on Condoms Is Flirting with Death" (interview with Helen Singer Kaplan). *Newsweek* Aug. 31: 72.

Seville, Barbara (1987). "Aids [*sic*] and Women." *Today's Chicago Woman* (September): 33.

Shaw, Nancy S., and Lyn Paleo (1986). "Women and AIDS." In *What to Do about AIDS: Physicians and Health Professionals Discuss the Issues*, ed. Leon McKusick. Berkeley: University of California Press, 142–154.

Shilts, Randy (1987). *And the Band Played On: Politics, People, and the AIDS Epidemic*. New York: St. Martin's Press.

Sloan, Amy (1986). "I'm Fighting for My Life." *Ladies Home Journal* (November): 22–23.

Sobo, E. J. (1993). "Inner-City Women and AIDS: The Psycho-social Benefits of Unsafe Sex." *Culture, Medicine, and Psychiatry* 17(4): 455–485.

Stephens, Clay (1989). "U.S. Women and HIV Infection." In *The AIDS Epidemic: Private Rights and the Public Interest*, ed. Padraig O'Malley. Boston: Beacon Press. 381–401.

Stoller, Nancy E. (1995) "Lesbian Involvement in the AIDS Epidemic: Changing Roles and Generational Differences." In *Women Resisting AIDS: Feminist Strategies of Empowerment*, ed. Beth E. Schneider and Nancy E. Stoller. Philadelphia: Temple University Press, 270–285.

Stone, Laurie (1987). "The New Femme Fatale," *Ms.* (December): 78–79.

Sweet, Ellen (1988). "Women and AIDS: Who's at Risk?" *Ms.* (February): 26.

Switzer, Ellen (1986). "AIDS: What Women Can Do." *Vogue* (January): 222–223+.

Switzer, Ellen (1988). "AIDS: Fear and Loathing." *Vogue* (March): 326+.

Treichler, Paula A. (1988a). "AIDS, Homophobia, and Biomedical Discourse: An Epidemic of Signification." In *AIDS: Cultural Analysis, Cultural Activism*, ed. Douglas Crimp. Cambridge: MIT Press, 31–70.

Treichler, Paula A. (1988b). "AIDS, Gender, and Biomedical Discourse: Current Contests for Meaning." In *AIDS: The Burdens of History*, ed. Elizabeth Fee and Daniel M. Fox. Berkeley: University of California Press, 190–266.

Treichler, Paula A. (1992). "Beyond Cosmo: AIDS, Identity and Feminist Activism." *Camera Obscura* (28): 21–76.

Tuchman, Gaye (1978). *Making News*. New York: Free Press.

Van Gelder, Lindsy (1983). "The Politics of AIDS." *Ms.* (May): 103.

Van Gelder, Lindsy (1987). "AIDS." *Ms.* (April): 64, 71.

Vance, Carole S. (1984). *Pleasure and Danger: Exploring Female Sexuality*. Boston: Routledge & Kegan Paul.

Warren, Catherine A. (1996). First, Do Not Speak: Errant Doctors, Sexual Abuse, and Institutional Silence. Doctoral dissertation, University of Illinois at Urbana-Champaign.

Watney, Simon (1996). *Practices of Freedom: Selected Writings on HIV/AIDS*. Durham, NC: Duke University Press.

Weinhouse, Bibi (1983). "AIDS: The Latest Facts." *Ladies Home Journal* (November): 100, 202.

Winnow, Jackie (1989). "Lesbians Working on AIDS: Assessing the Impact of Health Care on Women." *Out/Look* (Summer): 10–18.

Wofsy, Constance (1987). "Human Immunodeficiency Virus Infection in Women" (editorial). *Journal of the American Medical Association* 257(15): 2074.

"Women and AIDS" (1991). Special section. *Ms.* (January/February): 16–33.

Worth, Dooley, and Ruth Rodriguez (1987). "Latina Women and AIDS." *Radical America* 20(6): 63–67.

Anne K. Eckman

4

Beyond "The Yentl Syndrome"

Making Women Visible in Post-1990 Women's Health Discourse

Sometime in the 18th century, sex as we know it was invented. The reproductive organs . . . [became] the foundation for incommensurable difference: "women owe their manner of being to their organs of generation, and especially to the uterus," as one eighteenth century physician put it.

—Laqueur, 1990, p. 149

[Studies carried out exclusively on men] have suffered from the underlying assumption that men are the normative standard, and such studies have served to reinforce the myth that heart disease is unique to men. I refer to this practice as the Yentl syndrome.

—Healy, 1992b, p. x

First constructed as an article on the pages of the *New England Journal of Medicine* (NEJM) in 1991 by then National Institutes of Health (NIH) Director Bernadine Healy, "The Yentl Syndrome" indexes a concerted attempt to shift medicine's fundamental construction of sexual difference from its long association, since "sometime in the 18th century," with reproductive organs to the whole of men's and women's bodies. "The Yentl Syndrome" argues that medicine has failed to adequately diagnose heart attacks because of a flawed assumption that significant medical differences between men and women are related to reproductive organs alone. And it asserts that for women to receive equal medical treatment, medicine must instead see women's entire bodies as different from men's.

The date marking this attempted shift is widely agreed upon: not sometime in the twentieth century or even sometime in the late twentieth century, but June 18, 1990. "That's what June 18, 1990, did for us," says Florence Haseltine, M.D., the director of NIH's Center for Population Studies and founder of the Society for the Advancement of Women's Health Research (SAWHR). "It changed the way we think. And that's far more powerful for us than any law" (Nechas & Foley, 1994, p. 230). Or, as Nechas and Foley write in their 1994 popular press book *Unequal Treatment: What You Don't Know About How Women Are Mistreated by the Medical Community*, "June 18, 1990 marks the day that women became visible."

June 18, 1990—" 'D-day' for women's health," as the American Medical Association's vice president described it in his March 1993 *Good Housekeeping* column (J. S. Todd, p. 102)—specifically refers to a Government Accounting Office (GAO) report to the United States Congress. In it, the GAO detailed the National Institutes of Health's failure to implement its 1986 research protocols policy, designed to meet the recommendation of the 1985 *Report on the Public Health Service Task Force on Women's Health Issues* that "biomedical and behavioral research should be expanded to ensure emphasis on conditions and diseases unique to, or more prevalent in, women in all age groups" (p. 76). To document the NIH's failure, the June 18, 1990, report included, among other examples, the clinical trial that had demonstrated aspirin's protective effect against cardiovascular disease without including one woman among its 22,000 subjects (Nadel, 1990).

Though previous reports had addressed the potential problems of all-male research populations (e.g., Ramey, 1982; Hamilton, 1985), and though previous critiques of medicine had advocated for "a new view of women's bodies" (Federation of Feminist Women's Health Centers, 1981; see also, e.g., Davis, 1983; Dreifus, 1977; Ehrenreich & English, 1973), the definitive and pervasive identification of June 18, 1990, has marked it as a "watershed" for women's health (e.g., T. Johnson & Fee, 1994; Nechas & Foley, 1994; Pinn, 1992c; Rock, 1993; Ulene, 1991a, 1991b). "Within two weeks of that date," write Nechas and Foley (1994), "nearly every newspaper and news magazine in the country had written about the all-male aspirin study, the all-male aging study, the all-male uterine study and the all-male laboratory rats" (p. 219). Within three months of that date, the Office for Research on Women's Health (ORWH) at the National Institutes of Health was created at the direction of Congress, with the explicit mandate of ensuring that the NIH conduct and coordinate research relevant to the "diseases, disorders and conditions that are unique to, more prevalent among, or far more serious in women" (Kirschstein, 1992, p. 1). And within little more than a year, not only had "The Yentl Syndrome" appeared in the *New England Journal of Medicine*, but the groundwork for institutionalizing this changed understanding of women's health within medical education, clinical practice, and the production of new knowledge about women's health had been laid as well.

Some of the most notable of these developments include the following: the NIH has designed a study, known as the "Women's Health Initiative," designed to be "the most definitive, far-reaching study of women's health ever undertaken" (Healy, 1991b, p. 567). Policy makers have revised long-standing clinical trial guidelines that functioned to exclude women, and especially pregnant women, from participating in clinical research (Mastroiaionni, Faden, & Faderman, 1994a, 1994b; Merkatz et al., 1993). Advocates have proposed the creation of a new medical specialty in "women's health" that would treat the whole of women's health, as opposed to women's reproductive and obstetrical needs alone (e.g., Cain, 1993; K. Johnson, 1992). The need to establish minimum clinical competencies in women's health for all practicing physicians has also been proposed (Henrich, 1994), and established medical specialties have begun to develop their own training and competencies in "women's health" (American College of Obstetricians and Gynecologists, 1993; Joint Ad Hoc Committee, n.d.; Krasnoff, 1992a). The American Medical Women's Association (AMWA) has designed and implemented a continuing medical education curriculum in women's health (AMWA, *History*, n.d.). Individual medical schools have begun to develop women's health courses (Bickel & Quinnie, 1993; Henrich, 1994; Levison, 1994) and the Medical College of Pennsylvania (MCP)—with the aid of federal funding—has created a women's health curricula designed to serve as a national model for integrating women's health throughout medical school curricula (MCP & Hahnemann University School of Medicine, 1994–1995, p. 5). And the United States Congress has requested a survey that assesses the adequacy of women's health curricula at all U.S. medical schools (S. Rep. No. 102-397 to accompany H.R. 5677, 1993; H.R. Rep. No. 103–56 to accompany H.R. 5677, 1993).

These developments have been extensively covered both by mainstream medical journals and by popular and mass media. Medical journals such as the *New England Journal of Medicine* and the *Journal of the American Medical Association (JAMA)* have regularly reported on the initiatives surrounding women and biomedical research, women's health conferences, and debates over the establishment of, for instance, a medical specialty in women's health (e.g., Angell, 1993; Cotton, 1990a, 1990b; Healy, 1992b; Skolnick, 1992). These journals have also published recommended changes and new research relevant to post-1990 women's health concerns, including reports such as "Gender Disparities in Clinical Decision Making" (American Medical Association [AMA], 1991), research about differential clinical diagnoses and interventions for women and coronary heart disease (Ayanian & Epstein, 1991; Steingart et al., 1991), a theme issue devoted to "women's health" (*JAMA* [268], 1992), and findings such as "Sex and Gender Bias in Anatomy and Physical Diagnosis Text Illustrations" (Mendelsohn et al. 1994).

Finally, as part of the effort to consolidate and disseminate a new understanding of women's health, women's health advocacy groups have founded two new academic medical journals, *Women's Health Issues* and the *Journal of Women's Health*.

Similarly, major news magazines and newspapers not only covered the 1990 GAO report and the immediate outrage that it generated, but have also published regular features on the ongoing attempts to define and refine "women's health." In the three years following the report, coverage of "women's health" in the popular and mass media more than doubled.[1] For instance, *New York Times* articles concerning medicine's need to reorganize its care for women—"Doctors Consider a Specialty Focusing on Women's Health" and "Does Fragmented Medicine Harm the Health of Women"—made front-page news in both 1992 and 1993 (Lewin, 1992; Rosenthal, 1993). Furthermore, popular portrayals of these efforts have marked these changes as historic. In the popular press, Laurence and Weinhouse have written in their 1994 book, *Outrageous Practices: The Alarming Truth About How Medicine Mistreats Women*, that "health care is promising to become *the* women's issue of the nineties, the 'next wave' of feminism" (p. 10). Popular magazines articles have labeled the current initiatives part of a "decade of women's health" (see, e.g., J. S. Todd, 1993). And a full-page drop quote in *Ladies Home Journal* went even further, stating that "women's health is our modern-day suffrage movement" (Rock, 1993, p. 138).

Such discussions have served not only to document the new initiatives but also to help institutionalize a new understanding, both for the medical community and for a broader public, of the stuff that women's health is made of. The *Index Medicus*, the National Library of Medicine's annual bibliographic index that designates and categorizes medical knowledge, reflects this change. Prior to 1991, medical knowledge about women was categorized and organized through the prism of women's reproduction. By contrast, the 1991 *Index Medicus* listed a new term: women's health. Medical knowledge specific to women was indexed under the broad categories of "obstetrics" and "gynecology" or specific categories such as "menstruation" and "pregnancy," with the occasional study of a disease's different etiology or manifestation in women listed with other entries about those diseases. An article in the *American Journal of Preventive Medicine* by Vivian Pinn, the director of the ORWH, speaks to the pervasiveness of this new understanding of women's bodies as wholly different from men's: "Most biomedical research has assumed that women are just like men. Now, we witness a dramatic shift in perspective. Not just professional and scientific journals, but newspapers, television and radio productions, community and religious organizations, and even social conversations convey the urgency of women's health concerns" (1992a, p. 324).

Understanding this dramatic shift in both medical and public understandings of women's health and bodies is the subject of this chapter. The effort to shift medicine's perspective is not new. In fact, using the term "women's health" to challenge traditional medical perspectives can be dated to the women's health movement of the late 1960s and 1970s. But it is the June 19, 1990, GAO report that has effected a widespread realignment in the understanding of women's health. It is thus important to ask the following: Why has "women's health" been taken up at this time and in this form? What constellation of forces has encouraged this realignment? How have these forces affected whose health concerns are legitimated and whose are not?

While many aspects of this watershed moment warrant analysis, I want here to focus my questions around the newly visible image of women's bodies that emerged in the wake of the June 18, 1990, GAO report. In particular, I want to consider how this image has been constructed and to assess the progress that such constructions promise women. Thomas Laqueur (1990) has written in reference to the shift from a one-sex to a two-sex model of humans "sometime in the eighteenth century" (p. 149) that "sex, in both the one-sex and the two-sex worlds, is situational; it is explicable only within the context of battles over gender and power" (p. 11). Laqueur's claim relies on two related arguments of importance here. One is that "no set of facts ever entails any particular account of difference" (p. 19)—and thus that "no historically given set of facts about 'sex' entailed how sexual difference was understood and represented at the time" (p. 19). The other is that facts become understood as foundational to certain constructions of difference as the result of cultural processes. A long line of feminist critiques has elaborated the processes by which certain facts become foundational to the construction of differences that mark women's health and women's bodies (e.g., Bleier, 1986; Davis, 1983; Ehrenreich & English, 1973; Gilman, 1985; Harding, 1993). These critiques have further shown that battles over gender as well as race, class, ethnicity, sexuality, and nationality shape the processes by which differences are constructed. For us to understand what this new body of women's health promises, we thus must understand current battles over gender and how they are inextricably imbricated with race, class, nationality, ethnicity, sexuality—and power. How does the particular representation of women's bodies that has appeared in conjunction with many post-1990 developments draw upon, and reshape, these battles?

To answer this question, I first examine the commonsense understanding of the need for medicine to change its view of women's bodies, and the key images and facts that have anchored this commonsense as it has emerged in popular, policy, and medical accounts subsequent to the June 18, 1990, report. Joan Scott (1988) understands gender as "a useful category of historical analysis." Following her lead, I analyze the reconstruction of women's bodies in terms of "the cultural symbols in use at a particular time, the normative concepts that try to establish and contain symbols' meaning, the political organization of social institutions by which and for which meanings are mobilized, and the socio-economic conditions that govern these processes" (Scott, 1988, pp. 42–22). After examining the common sense and its key images, I then use the concepts of hegemony and articulation to analyze how these images, when linked in this new vision, have rearticulated the battles over gender and power that have marked both women's bodies and health care critiques during the early 1990s. As Stuart Hall (1986) has written, "it is not the individual elements of a discourse that have political or ideological connotations, it is the ways those elements are organized in a new discursive formation" (p. 55).

Using articulation theory provides one window on the contradictory nature of social change. As I will show, a good part of the popularity of the new discourse of woman's health as "more than a woman's reproductive organs" derives from a distancing of body parts and critiques that have been understood as "politically difficult"—body parts and critiques vital to a vision that includes the social contingencies and inequalities that shape so many women's struggles for better health. My question thus is not whether reform within mainstream institutions necessitates cooptation. Nor is it how more radical versions of feminism have been "perverted" into yet one more add-women-and-stir recipe for change. Rather, I am interested in how the particular forces structuring this new image of women's bodies have forged—or broken—connections between women's health and feminist critiques. It is my hope that understanding how these images are working at present will significantly aid feminist efforts to articulate a fuller vision of women's health.

The Making of "The Yentl Syndrome"

When the GAO report on NIH's failure became public on June 18, 1990, so too did the aspirin study in which, as almost all reports concerning women's health initiatives noted subsequently, no women were included among the 22,000 subjects of biomedical research for whom aspirin was shown to be beneficial. There was no necessary guarantee, to use Stuart Hall's (1983) phrase, that heart attacks should become so strongly linked to the identification of women's health inequalities or to a new image of what women's health should be. For instance, the high incidence of cardiovascular disease in women as well as men had, in fact, been raised in the 1985 *Report of the Public Health Services* (Hamilton, 1985)—and had garnered no particular public attention then. Moreover, there were no lack of other conditions for which clinical trials had excluded women. The 1990 GAO report itself listed other studies from which women had been excluded, such as the Baltimore Longitudinal Aging Study ("Women Left Out at NIH," 1990). When referred to in the press, often the background information concerning the lack of clinical data would note that "a number of treatments now recommended for men and women—from cholesterol-lowering drugs and diets to AIDS therapies and antidepressants—have been studied almost exclusively in men" (Purvis, 1990a, p. 66). However, it is the lack of knowledge concerning heart disease that has anchored much of the dramatic change in perspective that followed the GAO report.

To outline briefly, the following commonsense logic has linked heart attacks to this new view of women's bodies:

- Problem: The lack of biomedical research specific to women's health conditions, especially evidenced by the fact that little to no data exists for analyzing women's leading cause of death—heart disease—in women.
- Cause of problem: The extrapolation of clinical data from male subjects to female subjects, due to biased views of medical bodies.

- Solution to problem: Medical understandings of women's bodies need to be redifferentiated so as to ensure equality in women's health research and, hence, women's health. Most importantly, all of a woman's body needs to be seen as different from and equally important to that of a man.

The lead for *Time* magazine's "Women Face the 90s" feature on medicine provides the outlines of this common sense as it has appeared in much media coverage. It highlights the dilemma of a woman who, having just reached menopause, wanted to know whether she should start taking aspirin. It reads:

> One morning two years ago, a 60-year-old woman in Madison, Wis. asked her doctor what seemed like a simple question. The patient had just reached menopause and wanted to know whether she should start taking aspirin daily. She had seen the newspaper and TV reports claiming that the pills lower the risk of heart attack, and she knew such risks increase dramatically for women after they stop menstruating. "My answer was dead silence," says the woman's physician, Dr. Elizabeth Karlin, who teaches at the University of Wisconsin medical school. A week later, after scouring the literature, Karlin came to what she called an "appalling" conclusion: the finding, trumpeted in some newspapers as a lifesaver for everyone, was based entirely upon research on men. "There were simply no data to say this was safe for women." (Purvis, 1990a, p. 66)

Here, the health inequalities faced by women are focused around the lack of available biomedical data—data unavailable to well-informed physicians as well as laypeople—about preventing heart disease in women.

Subsequent popular articles on women's health have also often featured cardiovascular disease as the prime example of women's health inequities (Gordon, 1992; Silberner, 1990). Medical reports concerning "disparities in clinical decision making," and the media's coverage of these, have highlighted the relevance of heart attacks and the lack of biomedical research to the question of "equal rights for women's health," to quote a 1991 *New York Times* headline. Two studies published in the July 25, 1991, *NEJM* (Ayanian & Epstein, 1991; Steingart et al., 1991)—and widely covered by the mass media—reported that women with coronary artery disease receive less aggressive treatment than men do, providing "evidence that there is sex bias in the management of coronary heart disease" (Healy, 1991c, p. 274). The 1991 AMA report, "Disparities in Clinical Decision Making," similarly starts with the example of cardiovascular disease in women to which other types of gender bias—both in other types of medical procedures and illnesses (e.g., hysterectomies and cesarian sections) and in the treatment and evaluation of women (e.g., patient-physician communication)—are linked.

In popular and medical discussions of women's health following the GAO report, lack of attention to heart attacks in women has thus functioned as a primary index of medical bias against women. More than this, though, the lack of biomedical research about women has also crucially functioned to produce a new narrative about the source of women's inequality—a narrative that foregrounds the need for medicine to embrace a new view of women's bodies. As Healy's "Yentl Syndrome" editorial especially illustrates, the common sense generated around the GAO report has also positioned the lack of attention to heart attacks as the prototype for women's unequal treatment by medicine. That is, the need to see heart attacks as a disease of women has also become the key site in reference to which a new construction of women's bodies has been produced.

"The Yentl Syndrome" opens by setting the stage for the entrance of women's bodies:

> Yentl, the 19th-century heroine of Isaac Bashevis Singer's short story, had to disguise herself as a man to attend school and study the Talmud. Being "just like a man" has historically been a price women have had to pay for equality. (p. 274)

Of the two *NEJM* studies on heart disease in women for which "The Yentl Syndrome" served as the editorial, Healy explains that their findings "demonstrate the Yentl syndrome at work. That is, once a woman showed she was just like a man, by having severe coronary artery disease or a myocardial infarction, then she was treated as a man would be" (p. 274). Thus, writes Healy,

> the problem is to convince both the lay and the medical sectors that coronary heart disease is also a woman's disease, not a man's disease in disguise. We must be challenged by the example of coronary artery disease to examine critically the extent to which the Yentl syndrome pervades medicine and medical research and to respond promptly whenever its influence is evident. (p. 275)

The rhetoric proffered by Nechas and Foley (1994)—that June 18, 1990, "marks the day women became visible" (p. 219)—resonates with the concrete image of women's visibility that the Yentl syndrome calls forth. What have previously been hidden from view are diseases that have been regarded as unsexed and consequently attached to men, of which heart

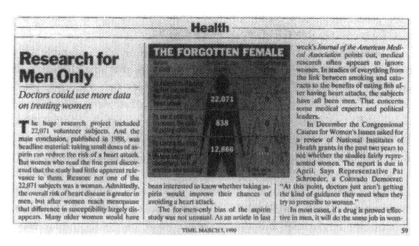

Figure 4.1   *Time*, March 5, 1990: 59. Used with permission of *Time* magazine.

disease serves as a prime exemplar. Women's lack of visibility, and hence women's source of inequality, has resulted from medicine's failure to accord women a complete set of organs and, correspondingly, to pay as full attention to these organs in women as they have in men. As the metaphor of the Yentl Syndrome suggests, women's equality is tied to Yentl's coming forth on the stage of medicine with a fully visible and complete set of organs.

In drawing upon the images of women and heart attacks, and the commonsense logic connecting them, "The Yentl Syndrome" can be understood to have crystallized a specific vision of a new body of women's health, reconstructed so that women receive equal medical care. Indeed, the logic animating Healy's editorial can be seen in a host of complementary images at work in media, policy, and medical accounts about women's health initiatives where, matched against the outlines of a male body, a woman's body is considered in every respect equal to, yet different from, a man's.

To take one example, *Time* magazine's "Research for Men Only" (Purvis, 1990b) article [Figure 4.1] is illustrated as follows: The body of the male is outlined by a solid line—made possible, the graphic suggests, by the research available for all regions of a male body. The body of the female is depicted similarly, with her outline comparable in size and shape. However, her body is outlined by a dashed line—as a result, the graphic suggests, of "missing" research for these regions of a woman's body. Here, what had been the previously universal and standard body of medical research has been reconstructed as a specifically male body, simultaneously creating the need for a comparable female body and norm.

In other post-1990s discussions, the reconstruction of comparable male and female norms has been similarly explicit. In showing that clinical trials have been conducted on men only, critics pointed out that in clinical practice the standard referent for calculating appropriate drug dosages and making clinical decisions has been the "70-kilogram male." Since then, the "standard" 70-kilogram male has become a shorthand reference for the practice of defining male physiology as the norm upon which all medical knowledge is based. *Outrageous Practices'* concluding paragraph quite literally evokes the new image of women in terms that mirror that of the "male norm": "And so we celebrate the new female norm: the 60-kilogram woman. She has breasts and a uterus and a heart and lungs and kidneys" (Laurence & Weinhouse, 1994, p. 354).

Discussions in popular and medical journals thus have envisioned constructing women's bodies in reference to, and against, a male norm identified and criticized as such by post-1990s women's health discourse. A *Harper's Bazaar* 1992 article, tellingly titled "Their Bodies, Our Selves," states that "[b]iology can be destiny: Men and women sometimes show different symptoms for the same disease, and a drug that cures men may have side effects that hurt women" (Gordon, 1992, p. 384). And the editor's column in *JAMWA* asks, "Women's Health: Is Anatomy Still Destiny?" before arguing that the answer is unclear and awaits further biomedical research (Goldrick, 1990).

The self-conscious reworking of the Freudian adage that "anatomy is destiny" suggests the extent to which biomedical research about women has been linked to constructing a new body of women's health. Biology and anatomy in the above examples refer to the whole of women's bodies, as opposed to Freud's reference to women's reproductive anatomy. Just as significantly, biological and anatomical destiny understood this way—as the biophysiological differences between men and women—has been positioned as a crucial fact for rectifying the medical discrimination that women have faced. The promise is that inequality in health will be conquered as the result of the human body's division into two different, physiologically distinct entities.

The post-1990 common sense concerning women's health, condensed into the image of "The Yentl Syndrome," has thus profoundly rearticulated two long-standing medical assumptions about women's health and bodies. As the image of Yentl both reflects and helps to construct, the common sense formed around the June 18, 1990, report disarticulates the location of biological sex from its traditional links to sexuality and the reproductive organs and reextends its influence to include the whole of a woman's body. Sex, in other words, has been reunderstood as residing biologically throughout the body, not merely at the anatomical sites of primary and secondary sex differences. According to this common sense, the problem with medical understandings of women's bodies is anything but a Freudian one: it is not a penis women lack, but a heart.

The second rearticulation effected by the Yentl syndrome is related and equally profound: biological sex, understood as residing throughout a woman's body, has been constructed as the difference that most determines women's health. Pinn (1992c), writing as director of the NIH's Office for Research on Women's Health, reflects this new construction of differences between women and men—and, by implication, between men's and women's health—as, at root, due to the differences between two different biological systems. Pinn (1992c) writes that "there will always be differences between men and women because of their normal physiology and hormonal milieu. Therefore there will always be a continuing need for women's health research, but with fewer blatant knowledge gaps left to address" (p. 63).

It is this image of women's bodies as completely physiologically distinct from, but comparable to, men's that has served as the key image around which advocates have argued for changes not only in biomedical research protocols but in medical education, clinical practice, and the organization of health care services as well. Indeed, the major women's health proposals and initiatives that have followed in the wake of the GAO report—from changes in clinical trials policies, to changes in medical curricula and clinical training, to proposed normative standards for medical textbooks—define and legitimate a female norm by making comparisons to "the male norm":

- The federal government has directly mandated that medical schools assess their women's health training: "They [the House and Senate] recognize that almost all medical schools use the 70 kg male as their model and that medical practitioners have gaps in their knowledge about the special health needs of women" (MCP & Hahnemann University School of Medicine, 1994–1995).
- Congresswoman Nita M. Lowey (D–N.Y.), calling for a congressionally sponsored survey of women's health medical school curricula, states that "because of a lag in research on women's health, and because almost all medical schools use the 70-kilogram man

as their model, women's health is not integrated into general training" (1994).

- The report of the American Medical Association Council on Ethical and Judicial Affairs (1991), "Gender Disparities in Clinical Decision Making," published in *JAMA*, expresses concern "that medical treatments for women are based on a male model, regardless of the fact that women may react differently to treatments than men or that some diseases manifest themselves differently in women than in men. The results of medical research are generalized to women without sufficient evidence of applicability to women" (p. 559).

- The Institute of Medicine report on the ethical and legal issues of including women in clinical studies concludes that "male bias (observer bias caused by adopting a male perspective and habit of thought) and the male norm (the tendency to use men as the standard and the tendency to see females as deviant and problematic, even in studying diseases that effect both sexes) . . . have been thought to contribute to a predominant focus on men's health and on men as research participants" (Mastroianni, Faden, & Federman, 1994a).

- "Sex and Gender Bias in Anatomy and Physical Diagnosis Text Illustrations" (Mendelsohn et al., 1994), appearing in *JAMA* and authored by women medical students and faculty associated with women's health education program at the Medical College of Pennsylvania, argue that "the finding that males are depicted in a majority of nonreproductive anatomy illustrations may perpetuate the image of the male body as the normal or standard model for medical education (p. 1267). . . . Publishers and illustrators should be urged to correct this imbalance in medical texts by representing females and males equally and by normalizing women through the inclusion of equal numbers of females and males in nonreproductive chapters. . . . [And] although neutral illustrations avoid bias by portraying neither sex, they do not address the known physical and functional differences between the sexes" (p. 1270).

The Remaking of the Body of Women's Health

This new body of women's health discourse has undeniably changed our understanding of women's bodies and health care needs. Resexing women's bodies radically challenges a previous order of medical understandings that had equated women, per se, with their reproductive organs, subsuming everything else under the male-defined rubric of "human." Accordingly, this reconstruction potentially acknowledges significant problems within existing women's health policy and interventions. In addition to a greatly increased public recognition of the incidence of heart disease in women, this redefinition of women's health to include more than strictly reproductive health concerns extends support to advocated changes in policies and research related to other diseases, such as AIDS, that have been traditionally thought of and defined as "male." Although not popularly framed in these terms, this redefinition also seems consistent with the need—especially identified by women who are not white and middle-class—for attention to serious medical conditions, such as heart disease, diabetes, lupus, and other chronic health conditions that have much higher rates among African American women than white women (e.g., Avery, 1990; Davis, 1990; Leigh, 1994; White, 1998). And this redefinition potentially responds to activist arguments that the earlier women's health movement, so visibly focused around gynecology and obstetrics, could usefully be extended to other health concerns and medical specialties (e.g., Marieskind, 1980; Ruzek, 1978), and that many of the most visible women's health movement constructions of health and reproduction largely reflected the concerns of white middle-class women (e.g., Davis, 1983; Pollner, 1973; Smith, 1982).

But there is another way to consider the changes advocated for, and promised by, the new image of women's bodies and the host of initiatives it has licensed. As Hall and colleagues (1978) have written,

> "Public images," at one and the same time, are graphically compelling but also stop short of serious, searching analysis. They tend to appear *in place of analysis*— or analysis seems to collapse into the image. Thus, at the point where further analysis threatens to go beyond the boundaries of the dominant ideological field, the "image" is evoked to foreclose the problem. (p. 118)

If we consider "The Yentl Syndrome" as Hall suggests, we can ask what may this redefinition of women's health have foreclosed? Analyzing this new public image of women's health shows that, at the same time that it successfully changes our view of women's bodies and garners support for these changes under the language of a "movement," it also works to distance body parts and analyses of women's health that are visibly associated with "difficult" politics.

Body Politics

We can better understand these deferred body parts and politics by examining the 1985 Public Health Service (PHS) report on women's health,
which recommended more biomedical research into "conditions and diseases unique to, or more prevalent in, women of all age groups" (p. 76)
and hence provided the acknowledged foundation for the June 18, 1990,
GAO report. First, the 1985 PHS report's recommendations for biomedical research were directly linked to contraception, as well as "cancer of
the breast and reproductive system; sexually transmitted diseases; arthritic
conditions, including lupus; osteoporosis; and certain mental disorders"
(p. 76). Second, of the fifteen recommendations made by the 1985 PHS
report to improve women's health, only five were explicitly related to
research. And third, of the five recommendations for research, only one—
the one taken up by the June 18, 1990, GAO report—focused on the need
for biomedical research. The others instead focused on the interaction of
behavioral and social factors with biological factors and called for better
data on health distinctions among different women's health, workplace
health hazards, and cultural conditions and socialization factors as they
affect women's health (p. 76). This agenda matched the report's introduction, which emphasized the influence of environmental factors on health
and questioned the explanatory power of biological models alone.

Considered in the context of the 1985 PHS report, the 1990 GAO
report and its subsequent reception raise obvious questions: Where is the
Public Health Service's concern with women's reproductive processes
and related concern with sexuality, contraception, and STDs? And where
is the consideration for social structures that shape women's lives and
research to address these concerns? The answer is: virtually nowhere.
This is certainly true of the immediate reception of the GAO report. The
following sentence, buried in the middle of *Time*'s article, is one of the
only references to biomedical research on contraceptives in media
reports about the GAO report: "Meanwhile, no new contraceptive
method has been approved in the U.S. since the 1960s" (Purvis, 1990a, p.
67). References to the effects of race and income on women's health
research are also absent. For instance, even though reports published
shortly before the GAO report had demonstrated that black men receive
less intensive treatments for heart disease than white men (AMA Council
on Ethical & Judicial Affairs, 1990), these reports of racial inequalities
were not linked to evidence of women's unequal treatment. Nothing
inherent in these discussions of medicine's sex bias, in other words, would

preclude its links to other systemic discrimination; yet these links were largely avoided.

In this regard, the metaphor of the Yentl syndrome is worth a second look for the cultural work that it does, especially in reference to the image of women's bodies that it has helped to reconstruct. The Yentl syndrome argues that for women to achieve equality, medicine needs to pay attention to the sex differences in parts of women's bodies that it had *not* previously seen as gendered—parts other than those traditionally associated with women's reproduction. In calling for women to be accorded a complete set of organs, the metaphor is calling especially for women to be seen as having organs other than those related to reproduction. While a woman's reproductive organs are ostensibly included in this public image, the need to identify sex differences in women's body parts not previously sexed has ironically positioned women's reproduction—a site already fully differentiated according to sex differences, albeit interpretations of these differences continue to be a site of considerable struggle—as peripheral to current efforts to secure equal health and health care for women. Picturing women as having had to wear male garb in order to be seen by medicine thus effectively cloaks another history of women's overly visible, deviantly interpreted, status as a "vagina surrounded by a woman" (Vance, 1990)—and the continuing contests over this prior history.

Indeed, as a second look at popular press and policy and medical texts suggests, much of the widespread support for women's health as it became visible on June 18, 1990, derives from its depoliticization of gendered health issues. Current news reports and feature stories indicate that there is little for any politician not to support. As *U.S. News and World Report* concluded its article on "Health: Another Gender Gap": "At least part of the reason for the speed of the response is the absence of opponents. No politician or scientist has gone on record saying that it is a wise thing to ignore women's health problems" (Silberner, 1990, p. 55). Or, as Irma Meban—an epidemiologist at NIH's Heart, Lung and Blood Institute and board member of SAWHR—said when interviewed in a *Chicago Tribune* article ("Bad Medicine: Health-care Groups Urge Remedies for Inequities"): " 'Women's health' sounds like 'motherhood and apple pie' " (Baurac, 1991).

Information made available after President Clinton's 1992 election indicate that certain specific issues were excluded from discussions of women's health and how it would be institutionalized because they were politically difficult to support—in particular, the issues of women's reproductive issues, sexuality, and poverty. The 1993 position paper by SAWHR states that the society planned "to capitalize on the opportunity that a new administration and Congress [would] provide," concretely list-ing "heretofore taboo topics such as adult and adolescent sexual behavior, contraception, fetal tissue research, and abortion," which it hoped to slate for research (T. L. Johnson, 1993, p. 97). Similarly, the NIH strategic plan, released in May of 1993, calls for both reproductive health and behavioral science research that, as the *New York Times* reported, "some scientists say had been neglected during the Bush administration" (Burd, 1993, p. A22).

Similarly, although advocates for women's health initiatives recognized that poverty crucially determines the health status of many women, directly identifying and advocating for poor women's health issues was deferred as a "politically difficult" issue. A *JAMA* news column, for instance, reports Pinn's statement that health for all women means recog-nizing that "most of those who have not been part of studies or who do not have access to care or who have the greatest health problems are those who are either economically disadvantaged or from the nation's minority groups" (Cotton, 1992, p. 470). But it qualifies that statement with the following observation by Florence Haseltine: "So many factors that affect health are related to poverty. We have to admit that, and it becomes polit-ically difficult" (p. 470).

In this political context, two things have especially served to disarticu-late contraception, sexual politics, and structural inequalities from the body of women's health: the focus on women's heart attacks and the pre-occupation with the problematic 70-kilogram male. Heart attacks, given their previous understanding as a condition almost exclusively affecting men, evoke few images of sexuality and reproduction. The norm of "the 70-kilogram male," constructed as the template against which a woman's body should be filled in, further elides social determinants of health. Instead, it focuses women's health initiatives on the task of filling physio-logical knowledge gaps, and constructs biological sex as the key determi-nant of health. With regard to the question "how many ways must we slice and dice in the interest of fairness?" asked in 1993 by Marcia Angell in *NEJM*, Laurence and Weinhouse (1994) argue that "the answer, for now, is at least *two*: male and female. Before the pie can be served, it must first be cut in half" (p. 76). The implication is that the health of the 60-kilo-gram female, like the 70-kilogram male, is not significantly affected by inequalities such as race, class, ethnicity, or sexuality.

The newly visible body of women's health has further displaced consid-eration of these inequalities by its articulation to a specific demographic address. The new women's health discourse—through the declaration that medicine has omitted half of the population by not including women in clinical trials for heart attacks—links women's health to menopause. Women's risk for heart attacks rises dramatically after a woman reaches menopause. Furthermore, estrogen replacement therapy, and its long-debated value for women in menopause, has enjoyed a new life as research explores whether it protects against heart disease in postmenopausal women. Indeed, the NIH's Women's Health Initiative focuses on determinants of women's health during and after menopause, including the effects of estrogen (Cotton, 1992; Healy, 1991b). Similarly, the Continuing Medical Education Program in Women's Health—designed to cover a different stage of a woman's lifespan each year—concentrated its first year's course, held in November 1993, on the health of women in menopause (American Medical Women's Association Foundation, n.d.).

The strong articulation of post-1990s women's health with menopausal women has provided a body for women's health that is not linked with questions about pregnancy and childbearing, nor with concerns about women's access to economic resources. Pinn's assurance that "another priority area for research will be reproductive functions and diseases" acknowledges that, as of 1992, the Office for Research on Women's Health had not focused on reproductive concerns (in Cotton, 1992, p. 469). Moreover, not only has the new body of women's health been strongly associated with women who are entering menopause, but these women have been constructed as quintessential baby boomers—replete, so the common sense assumes, with an unprecedented amount of political and economic clout. Far from raising concerns about the economic inequalities that many women face, the media, marketers, and even medicine have identified menopausal baby boomers as a "gold mine" (e.g., Braus, 1993; Foreman, 1992; Skelly, 1992). In their "Menopause Megatrend" chapter in *Megatrends for Women*, Aburdene and Naisbitt (1992) thus explain the post-1990 origins of a "new" women's health movement as follows: "A generation of activists is now approaching an age when medical sexism can threaten their lives" (p. 143). In so portraying this new movement, Aburdene and Naisbitt imply that women have, and do, experience equality in health care prior to the age of menopause. They also imply that the menopausal women who will tackle this sexism will do so from a position of economic security and political power.

Accordingly, in post-1990s discussions, women's health often appears as a final frontier on which equality needs to be achieved, as opposed to one place among many others where women experience profound inequity. Laurence and Weinhouse (1994) imply in *Outrageous Practices* that women already have achieved equality in arenas other than medicine, writing that "women may have won the right to be seen as more than wives and mothers in society, but in medicine the old beliefs still persist" (p. 7). In an interview that appeared in *Ladies Home Journal*, Bernadine Healy's framing of current women's health initiatives pictures women's health still more explicitly as building upon a position of equality achieved elsewhere:

> Advancing women's health is sort of our modern-day suffrage movement. In the first third of the century, the focus was on getting the vote. Then in the middle part of the century women moved into gaining education and economic opportunities. Now we are worried about quality-of-life issues, which include women's health. (Rock, 1993, p. 187)

The emphasis on making women "equal scientific citizens" (Gordon, 1992, p. 385) thus often occurs in conjunction with the assumption that women have achieved equality in other realms. From this perspective, the most egregious inequality visible is seen as follows: "In all of the NIH's and FDA's new guidelines, one glaring omission remains. Currently, neither NIH nor the FDA has guidelines for including *female* animals in scientific research" (Laurence & Weinhouse, 1994, p. 76). While it *is* outrageous that female lab rats have been banned from clinical trials because of their more troublesome "female" physiology, that it is pictured as the most "glaring omission" suggests how limited the grounds of women's inequality are taken to be.

The equality promised by this newly visible body of women's health must therefore be read in light of the particular conditions within which this image of women's health has taken shape—namely, the constraints of a conservative federal government and a popular understanding of women's social status that elides systematic social inequalities. Instead, the new view of a woman's body as equal and opposite to a man's construes a woman—especially in the niche of menopausal baby boomer—as possessing social, political, and economic power equal to that of the independent, income-earning man who suffers a heart attack. Considered in terms of other current public images, this new image of women's bodies and health is in many ways the polar opposite of the popularly scapegoated, and thoroughly demonized, image of women—as young, poor, pregnant, of color, and "dependent" on welfare. As such, this new image is fundamentally separated from battles over women's basic rights to reproductive freedom, support for childbearing, and economic security.[2]

Knowledge Politics

The popularly articulated body of women's health has both named systemic medical sexism and contained its account within the bounds of bodies that are imagined independent of social forces. Similarly, the newly institutionalized body of women's health knowledge both identified the need to systematically reconstruct women's health knowledge and primarily restricted this reconstruction to the creation of new biomedical research that imagines itself independent of social processes.

This popularly constituted body of women's health has thus provided a commonsense logic about women's health research in which gender has been equated with biological sex differences; research about women's health in general, and biological sex differences in particular, have been seen as independent of other social processes; and the knowledge most important to understanding women's health—knowledge about the physiological differences between men and women—has been divorced from prior and ongoing critical accounts of health and the production of health knowledge. Accordingly, this new body of women's health knowledge has worked to obscure questions and critiques concerning the design, production, and interpretation of women's health knowledge in general and biomedical research in particular. Even more significantly, it has created a framework that not only distances the project of creating new women's health knowledge from prior and ongoing efforts that foreground these concerns, but also profoundly misreads their critiques.

Although the critique of women's exclusion from clinical trials and biomedical research has relied upon feminist scholarship that has shown the constructed nature of women's bodies, the power of gendered analysis has been reduced to a question of biological sex differences. As the newly visible body of women's health has constructed a well-bounded set of female organs, "gendered" health has once more been defined in terms of sex differences, albeit sex differences that are no longer linked to women's reproductive organs alone. Biological sex, extended throughout the whole of a woman's body, has been repositioned as the foundational truth from which women's health research should start.

As a result, important questions about the construction of sexual differences as a category of analysis within research—questions at the heart of a well-elaborated feminist and radical critique of science (e.g., Bleier, 1986; Hubbard, 1990; Harding, 1986, 1993; King, 1992)—have not been linked to the production of new biomedical knowledge. A critical history of the interpretation of biological differences in ways that legitimate economic and political inequalities has been divorced from post-1990 women's health discourses. Given that questions of gender's construction initiated the spate of current initiatives, that history should be easily articulated to women's health biomedical research. Rather, general biomedical research and a newly naturalized account of sexual difference have emerged in the place of such critique.

At the same time, the image of a new body of women's health distances questions concerning who controls the process of research, biomedical or otherwise. As popular images and revised research protocols have suggested, the post-1990 initiatives focus on including women's bodies—with a full set of organs—in biomedical research and clinical trials. But, again, the highly visible image of a woman's body replete with a full, bounded set of physiological organs has stood in for—and largely displaced—long-standing feminist concerns with transforming research to reflect and produce knowledge relevant to women's lives and women's needs and with restructuring the research process so that women have control over the production and distribution of research knowledge. While women's inclusion in clinical trials is vital for transforming women's health, much of the post-1990 women's health discourse has limited women's "participation" to a subject position that feminist critics of science have roundly critiqued: women as research object, albeit an object with more than reproductive organs.

This containment of feminist critique has been achieved through a related commonsense understanding. The Yentl syndrome's emphasis on making visible what had not been visible before has effectively implied that knowledge created prior to June 18, 1990 is not relevant to post-1990s women's health discourse. Florence Haseltine's opening statement to the 1994 Symposium on Women's Health in Medical Education is typical of post-1990s accounts of the origins of women's health. As the symposium's proceedings reported it: "Dr. Haseltine stated that there is a great deal of confusion surrounding the origins of interest in women's health, which began with three fortuitous events. The first was the Government Accounting Office (GAO) audit" (Nieman, 1994, p. 366). Rather than envisioning its work as an extension of attempts initiated by the women's health movement and other radical critiques of health to transform the production and control of health knowledge, current women's health initiatives envision women's health research and the reconstructed image of women's bodies that guides it as new ground separate from and independent of prior women's health critiques.

Most initiatives have accordingly implied that the knowledge most pertinent to women's health is "to be created" by current initiatives. In the opening paragraph of the first issue of the *Journal of Women's Health* (1.1), Bernadine Healy suggests that research important "to getting what we want—improved health for all women—is only now beginning to appear" (1992a). The AMA Council on Ethical and Judicial Affairs' report, "Gender Disparities in Clinical Decision Making" (1991), follows up on this logic. The report argues that forthcoming biomedical research on women's health will provide a baseline of "appropriate biomedical or medical indications" for differences in clinical treatments and, as such, will provide a reliable measure for gauging discrimination, even though an extensively developed body of feminist literature already exists that documents the role of biomedical culture in constituting and reproducing inequities on the basis of class, race, and gender.[3] By implication, not only does biomedical knowledge maintain its position as the authoritative source of knowledge regarding health but it is also positioned as the yardstick by which discrimination within medicine can, and should, be judged in the future.

The result is that prior analyses of women's health research—including efforts that were directly related to changing official research agendas and professional programs of training—are themselves being treated as nonexistent at best, and inadequate at worst. Notably, when detailing available work relevant to women's health, official reports on the women's health research agenda (e.g., National Institutes of Health, Office of Research on Women's Health, 1992; Henrich, 1994) omit references to the 1975 *Women and Their Health: Research Implications for a New Era* (Olesen, 1975). This report, cosponsored by the National Center for Health Services Research and the Health Resources Administration in conjunction with the University of California at San Francisco's School of Nursing, was in many ways an encoding of the "old" women's health movement agenda in an official document. The report explicitly laid out key women's health research questions posed by feminist, community health, and other grassroots movements as well as by the then emerging critical health scholarship.[4] Similarly, fully developed clinical programs in women's health by professions other than medicine—principally by the field of nursing, especially in conjunction with the women's health movements of the late 1960s and 1970s—are neither referenced nor considered.[5]

In its most problematic formulation, this new vision of women's health has created a new body of women's health knowledge that not only fails to acknowledge feminist work, but also profoundly misrecognizes crucial

women's health movement critiques and concerns. Such dismissal of critically important concepts about the construction of gender and the nature
of women's participation in research has both shaped, and been shaped by,
an explicit portrayal of the women's health movement as "narrow." More
specifically, several popular accounts of post-1990 initiatives criticize the
old women's health movement for reducing women to their reproductive
organs, when one of the movement's central projects was precisely to contest such reductions. Both *Outrageous Practices* and *Unequal Treatment* provide similar descriptions of the "old" women's health movement.
Laurence and Weinhouse (1994) write:

> While many of the criticisms the feminists heaped on the medical establish-
> ment were valid, in at least one way the feminist movement itself was guilty
> of what it accused physicians of doing—genitalizing women's health. . . .
> They, too, ignored women's bodies from the waist up. It took women *within*
> the system—people like National Institutes of Health Director Bernadine
> Healy and ob-gyn Florence Haseltine—to blow the whistle and agitate for
> change. (p. 9)

Nechas and Foley (1994) offer a related assessment:

> Even in the early days of modern feminism, women's health was a political
> issue of narrow parameters. During that time, the Boston Women's Health
> Book Collective published its groundbreaking book, *Our Bodies Ourselves*,
> the feminist health collective movement was born, and the National
> Women's Health Network was founded by a group of women concerned
> with the mounting death toll from the pill. But those groups were more
> concerned with reproductive matters and with how women were treated in
> the examining room than in how they were treated in the laboratory and the
> corridors of political power. (pp. 23–24)

This rhetoric, by severing the previously visible link between feminist
challenges to traditional reproductive care, not only avoids "difficult politics" but fundamentally misrecognizes the goal of redistributing the access
to, control over, and distribution of medical knowledge and health care.
Lost from this new body of women's health is the understanding, hard
fought for by the women's health movement, that women's bodies are also
sites of societal struggles. Rather, assessing the relative power of the two
health movements relies upon an arithmetic in which the "old" women's
health movement appears "less than" the new movement because of its
focus on fewer body parts—where number of visible body parts provides
the measure of how fully a woman's health interests are represented.

Beyond *"The Yentl Syndrome"*

As this chapter has argued, the body of women's health made visible in the wake of the June 18, 1990, GAO report has largely legitimated a vision of women's health that obscures the social conditions that structure women's health and women's experiences. Having argued this, though, I must emphasize that other efforts to transform structures and institutions have certainly extended beyond—yet are now affected by—the vision of women's health sanctioned by the Yentl syndrome. With this in mind, I want to conclude my analysis by considering post-1990 efforts to radically reshape medical education, a site key to medical culture's reproduction.

Current Attempts and Contests

Many post-1990 efforts to transform medical education and practice have explicitly challenged the existing institutional structure of medicine and how it defines, produces, and disseminates knowledge about women's health. The report to the Council on Graduate Medical Education, for instance, reflects the consensus that successful women's health "depends on fundamental changes in medical education that . . . run counter to the structure of traditional medical institutions" (Henrich, 1994, pp. 38–39). As these attempts have unfolded, they have drawn upon radical conceptions of women's health that have, with varying degrees of contradiction and success, helped to shape the emergent post-1990 commonsense understanding of women's health.

Proposals for a medical specialty put forward since the June 18, 1990, GAO report show the force with which popular articulations of the new body of women's health have foreclosed explicitly feminist approaches. For example, since the early 1980s, psychiatrist Karen Johnson (1992) has been developing and attempting to institutionalize a proposal for a women's health specialty. Her proposal calls for knowledge from a range of disciplines—including nursing, the history of medicine, the sociology of knowledge, and women's studies—to be integrated into women's health in the medical curricula. In terms of institutional change, Johnson's proposal for a woman's health specialty follows the path established twenty years earlier by the creation of women's studies departments within universities. After June 18, 1990, her proposal gained national attention, in conjunction with other post-1990 women's health initiatives. Not only the *Journal of Women's Health*, the *Journal of the American Medical Association*

(Clancy & Massion, 1992; Skolnick, 1992), and the *Journal of the American Women's Association* (Harrison, 1990; K. Johnson & Dawson, 1990; Wallis & Klass, 1990), but also the front pages of the *New York Times* and other newspaper and news magazines covered debates surrounding a proposed medical specialty.

However, in the words of feminist psychiatrist and researcher Jean Hamilton (1993), discussions of a women's health specialty have since "taken on a life of their own." Johnson proposed a specialty that would have institutional links with feminist scholarship, past and present, and, as such, would be "a logical extension of the women's health movement that began in the 1960s" (K. Johnson, 1992, p. 97). But as these proposals were debated, questions about how to integrate the diverse sets of knowledge proposed by Johnson were displaced by a debate over the cultural construction of women's bodies, how they should be reconstructed, and how a specialty could be set up to match the body parts included in the new woman's body. That is, the proposal to radically integrate knowledge long silenced by medicine—the social context of women's lives and women's experiences—has again become largely invisible as questions about the appropriate rereading of women's body parts have moved to center stage.

Accordingly, both supporters and opponents of a woman's health specialty have sounded surprisingly similar as the debate over how to best reconstruct women's bodies has displaced questions central to Johnson's proposal over how to address the context of women's lives and social situations. For instance, a *New York Newsday* article (Ochs, 1993) quotes Eileen Hoffman's support of a woman's health specialty: "Women's health goes beyond gynecology. There needs to be a way to reintegrate [a woman's] reproductive parts back into her whole body and to see her as a total person. . . . We don't have a discipline that looks at the whole constellation" (p. 22). Michelle Harrison (1990), writing in opposition to a specialty, counters "The linking of breast with pelvis, as in obstetrics-gynecology, is an example of a cultural definition of the body, rather than a physical one . . . other than the breast and pelvis, male and female bodies tend to work or not work the same" (p. 225). The question of how to see a woman's body, and whether it includes nonreproductive as well as reproductive organs, has emerged as the central topic of discussion—a topic where connections to feminist knowledge and institutional transformation are by no means essential. In popular and medical discussions, how best to repackage all of these parts into a whole body has become the grounds for different specialties to argue that, with a little tweaking, their specialty could incorporate all of a woman's body parts.[6]

The 1994 article "Sex and Gender Bias in Anatomy and Physical Diagnosis Text Illustrations" (Mendelsohn et al., 1994), appearing in *JAMA* and authored by women medical students and faculty associated with the women's health education program at the Medical College of Pennsylvania, also illustrates the conceptual limits that this new body of women's health has placed on institutionalized feminist critiques. The article cites Scully and Bart's (1973) send-up of gynecology textbooks as its inspiration and takes their work as a model of feminist analysis appropriate for challenging sexism as it is institutionalized within official medical knowledge. Yet it also relies upon the commonsense notion of gendered difference articulated in the Yentl syndrome: it equates gender differences with physiological sex differences extended throughout the body and accordingly takes representations of women's whole bodies as the gold standard for ensuring women's equal treatment in medicine. It thus concludes that women's bodies suffer underrepresentation in medical texts and urges publishers to "correct this imbalance in medical texts by representing females and males equally and by normalizing women through the inclusion of equal numbers of females and males in nonreproductive chapters" (p. 1270).

Such claims follow logically from the Yentl syndrome parameters of their study and the focus on institutionalizing a new image of women's bodies. But when taken as a standard in and of itself, this new body obscures the processes by which knowledge about women's health is produced and distances past and present struggles over the ways in which different women's bodies have and have not been made visible, and understood, within medicine. The myopia of this approach becomes clear in two subsequent *JAMA* letters to the editor, letters that question the article's assumption that greater visibility of body parts means greater equality (Denman, 1995; Passaretti, 1995). Both writers refer to their memory of Becker et al.'s *The Anatomical Basis of Medical Practice* (1971) where women—overrepresented and overexposed—were posed with beach balls and other pin-up props as they showed off their anatomy. The reason, explained in the textbook's preface, lay in the fact that "only on rare occasions will the attractive well-turned specimen appear before him [the physician] for consultation. He should be prepared for this pleasant shock."

But the reconstruction of women's health based on the new vision of women's bodies, while powerful, has not been monolithic in its effects. Indeed, the complexity and unpredictability of the processes of articulation are suggested in some instances in which post-1990 women's health initiatives, starting from notions centered on the new body of women's health, have sought available women's health resources and models and found themselves making links to community women's health groups and "difficult" politics generally excluded from the new body of women's health. For instance, some individual medical schools, in seeking what's available for women's health training in their communities, have established links with existing grassroots women's health programs—programs with feminist and antiracist roots (see, e.g., Bickel & Quinnie, 1993; Center for Research on Women and Gender, 1995; and Krasnoff, 1992b). Similarly, although the model Medical College of Pennsylvania's Women's Health Education Program did not originally include a "women's studies specialist" in its proposed organizational structure, it created one at the suggestion of a Fund for the Improvement of Secondary Education (FIPSE) coordinator who, as a former women's studies professor in a liberal arts college, recognized the value of institutionalizing such a position (L. B. Weiss, personal communication, October 1995). And some medical students and physicians, in considering the lack of women's health knowledge within medicine, have reintroduced questions about the adequacy of physicians' knowledge about reproductive health issues, including abortion, as well as their knowledge of historical and ongoing social struggles over these issues (Levison, 1994). However, these more radical links have occurred at individual institutions, and without a more public framework—in the form of a women's health agenda—to evaluate why and how these more radical links might be important *for* women's health, they will remain individual and largely unseen. As the head of the AMWA reproductive initiative notes, her program "hasn't gained the same widespread attention that other efforts have" (S. Eisendrath, personal communication, October 1995).

Still, there have been signs within more official realms of a shift toward making visible not just the body parts that "women's health" should attend to, but the broader processes that structure how women's health knowledge is produced. With the advocacy efforts of groups such as the National Women's Health Network (NWHN), participation in the agenda setting process has begun to include community and advocacy groups (C. Pearson, NWHN, personal communication, November 1995).[7] And in 1993, the *Journal of Women's Health* notably reported that

> initially the Society [SAWHR] envisioned its agenda as a laundry list of diseases and conditions in dire need of research attention. However, throughout our consumer roundtables and professional conferences, the Society was continually struck by the number of questions and concerns related to the

research *process* and *institutions*. . . . Hence, our Women's Health Research Agenda is intended to respond to these procedural concerns. (T. L. Johnson, 1993, p. 96)

Along these lines, the *Journal of Women's Health* devoted half of its Winter 1993 issue to the proceedings from the Center for Research in Women and Gender's (CRWG) Reframing Women's Health conference. These proceedings directly tie women's health to the women's health movement and the politics of women's lived experiences. The introduction explicitly cites definitions of health that emphasize the importance of women's subjective experiences and structural inequalities to understanding women's health (see also Ruzek, 1993). And it argues that the essential components of women's health are those that illuminate complex understandings of social context: links with grassroots women's groups, women's studies and feminist theory.

As these examples suggest, it is far from settled how these initiatives will integrate concerns that extend beyond the currently privileged body of women's health discourse, and how critical perspectives and connections will be formed or foreclosed. The examples do, however, show that the popular understanding associated with the new body of women's health—that of making women's nonreproductive body parts foundational to women's health—in and of itself has not facilitated links to other knowledges and perspectives crucial to meeting women's needs. In fact, it is evident that this popular understanding has at times worked against concerted attempts to make these links. These examples also indicate that links to understandings, programs, and practices that transform the relations through which medical knowledge is produced have occurred alongside of—rather than as an integral part of—the new image of women's health and its emphasis on nonreproductive organs. The struggle thus remains that of winning more space for a definition of women's health that links "more than" women's reproductive parts with these "difficult politics" and critical knowledges.

Future Visions

It is no small matter for women's health to be redefined so that it is no longer assumed to be coterminous with women's reproduction. If we take Laqueur's (1990) account as our historical reference point, it is in fact a watershed moment in a two-hundred-year history of constructing medical

sexual difference. However, as I have argued here, how such a reconstructed vision of women's bodies reconfigures the resources available to
women is intertwined with the specific links and alliances—both symbolic
and material—that are made at this historically specific conjuncture. That
is to say, the effects of a new construction are "never guaranteed," to use
Stuart Hall's (1983) phrase. Rather, these effects depend on what, within a
given social formation, is reconfigured as integral to such a vision—and
what, within this configuration, is immediately legitimated.

The conclusion of *Outrageous Practices* offers what is in many ways a
representative condensation of the current moment and its orderings. The
book celebrates "the new female norm. She has breasts and a uterus and a
heart and lungs and kidneys." Yet the book concludes with these sentences: "But she's much more than that. No longer a metaphor for disease,
she's the model for health: The time is right for a new woman-centered
health care movement" (Laurence & Weinhouse, 1994, p. 354). This ending affirms a vision of "woman-centered health" that extends beyond a
woman's physiology. But as the "new" indicates, this affirmation remains
explicitly divorced from the politics and struggles, either past or present,
that have fought for better women's health.

We might summarize the new logic and ordering licensed by this new
discursive body as follows: Women's health first and foremost needs to
attend to the biological workings of body organs and systems heretofore
ignored. Having done this, women's health should consider how to reintegrate all body parts—including women's reproductive organs—into some
sort of whole knowledge. Whatever else remains beyond these parts—
whatever concerns of politics or economics or race relations—can be
added on if and as needed. Though an admittedly crude rendition, this
logic is the inverse of what a well-developed and diverse body of feminist
critique has argued: for women's health to serve women, it needs first and
foremost to be viewed in terms of the complex and often contradictory
social forces of race, class, ethnicity, and a host of other determinants that
structure women's lives and health. Thus, although the new body licensed
by the June 18, 1990, watershed has made visible more diseases that affect
women, it has also done so in a political environment that has limited
understanding of the social inequalities structuring the production and
distribution of women's health and knowledge about women's health.

However, just as there are no guarantees that connections to prior and
ongoing radical critiques will be integral to the emerging body of women's
health, there are also no guarantees that the new body of women's health
cannot itself be rearticulated. Understanding how the popularly licensed

image of women's health has reordered what is most immediately understood to constitute women's health allows us to better understand the particular context in which attempts to rearticulate women's health in more radical ways have occurred since 1990. It suggests how the focus on "more than" reproductive organs has often displaced concerns with "other than" biomedically defined concerns. It thus also suggests that linking "more than" reproductive concerns to the contexts structuring women's lives—especially the intensifying effects of structural inequalities and the field of ongoing inequalities that women face with regard to reproduction as well as other health conditions—is crucial for a feminist rearticulation of the current body of women's health discourse.

Not that this will be easy. The popularity of the new body of women's health has been facilitated by politics that have done little to make visible, much less address, the structural inequalities of women's lives. But there does exist a rich body of feminist, antiracist, and pro-economic-justice work that well describes these inequalities and the complex ways in which they affect women's health. And there also do exist many community women's groups that, in diverse and powerful ways, have continued to voice women's needs from the ground up. The task here, in working to reshape the current body of women's health, is to preserve and support such critiques and resources so that the links that they make—among bodies, knowledges, politics—themselves become visible as women's health.

Notes

1. This estimate of increased coverage is based on the following search strategy. Using the Lexis/Nexis database for *Time, Newsweek, U.S. News and World Report*, the *New York Times*, and the *Washington Post*, I searched for the number of articles in which the phrase "women's health" appeared three or more times between January 1, 1987, and January 1, 1990, and between January 1, 1990, and January 1, 1993. Between 1987 and 1990, 25 articles appeared, whereas between 1990 and 1993, 62 articles appeared; that is, the number of "women's health" articles increased two-and-a-half fold.

2. For an extremely illuminating, and detailed, analysis of the connotations of "dependence" that have emerged especially since the late 1980s, see Fraser, 1993; and Fraser & Gordon, 1994.

3. This body of literature is extensive. For feminist critiques from the women's health movement, see, e.g., Corea, 1977; Dreifus, 1977; Ehrenreich & English, 1973, 1978; and Smith, 1982. For a theoretical overview of woman's health movement critiques, see Fee, 1983; for a more comprehensive historical overview of the

women's health movement, see Ruzek, 1978, 1980. Historical studies of women and health have been crucial to understanding the role of class, race, sexuality, and ethnicity in constructing women's health care; see, e.g., Leavitt, 1984; and Apple, 1992. Sociolinguistic analyses have also detailed the role of race, class, and gender in the current construction of provider-patient interactions; see, e.g., Fisher, 1986; Todd, 1989; and West, 1984. For a current overview of women's health in medicine—written in the wake of the post-1990 women's health initiatives—see Rosser, 1994.

4. Ruth Zambrana (1987) has critiqued this conference for its lack of attention to and inclusion of women of color's health issues.

5. *Outrageous Practices'* gloss of the University of California at San Francisco (UCSF) School of Nursing program in women's health reflects the marginalization of nursing in popular accounts of women's health: "to meet women's increased demands for nursing services, the University of California, San Francisco, School of Nursing now offers a woman's primary care program, one- and two-year courses of study for nurse-practitioners interested in graduate training in women's primary health care" (Laurence and Weinhouse, 1994, p. 250). The fact that nursing as a field—and UCSF's Department of Social and Behavioral Science as a particular institution—had developed "women's health" programs in association with the women's health movement, and thus as the result of events prior to the 1990 GAO report, is obscured. Also obscured is the particular history of the UCSF women's health program—a program that cosponsored with the Department of Health and Human Services the 1975 conference "Women and their Health: Research Implications for a New Era" and has developed one of the most extensive feminist lists available regarding women's health as part of their Women, Health and Healing project.

6. The National Women's Health Network's (NWHN) working paper, "Research to Improve Women's Health Research: An Agenda for Equity" (1991), while supportive of national initiatives to advance women's health research, had concluded that laywomen and community groups were excluded from the initial national agenda-setting process (p. 17).

7. For a detailed discussion of the emergence of women's health as a profitable medical marketing strategy, see "Negotiating a Model of Women's Health: Feminist Contests and Market Constraints in the 1980s and 1990s" in *From JANE to the Journal of Women's Health: Women's Health as an Emergent Body of Medical Knowledge* (Eckman, 1996, pp. 162–248).

References

Aburdene, P., & Naisbitt, J. (1992). *Megatrends for women*. New York: Villard Books.

American College of Obstetricians and Gynecologists. (1993). *The obstetrician-gynecologist and primary-preventive health care*. Washington, DC: Author.

American Medical Association Council on Ethical and Judicial Affairs. (1990). Black-white disparities in health care. *Journal of the American Medical Association, 263*, 2344–2346.

American Medical Association Council on Ethical and Judicial Affairs. (1991). Gender disparities in clinical decision making. *Journal of the American Medical Association, 266*, 559–562.

American Medical Association Council on Long Range Planning.(1989). *The environment of medicine.* Chicago: American Medical Association.

American Medical Women's Association. (N.d.). *The reproductive health initiative: Improving reproductive health care by improving medical student training* [brochure]. Arlington, VA: Author.

American Medical Women's Association. (N.d.). *History: Advanced curriculum on women's health* [brochure]. Arlington, VA: Author.

American Medical Women's Association Foundation. (N.d.). *The women's health curriculum: Training specialists on women's health needs* [brochure]. Arlington, VA: American Medical Women's Association.

Ames, K. (1990, December 17). Our bodies, their selves: A bias against women in health research. *Newsweek, 116*, 60.

Angell, M. (1993). Caring for women's health—What is the problem. *New England Journal of Medicine, 329*, 271–272.

Apple, R. D. (1992) *Women, health and medicine in America: A historical handbook.* New Brunswick, NJ: Rutgers University Press.

Association of American Medical Colleges. (1995, January). *Medical curriculum questionnaire.* Washington, DC: Author.

Avery, B. Y. (1990). Breathing life into ourselves: The evolution of the national black women's health project. In E. C. White (Ed.), *The black women's health book: Speaking for ourselves* (pp. 4–10). Seattle: Seal Press.

Ayanian, J. Z. & Epstein, A. M. (1991). Differences in the use of procedures between women and men hospitalized for coronary heart disease. *New England Journal of Medicine, 325*, 221–225.

Baurac, D. R. (1991, December 8). Bad medicine: Health-care groups urge remedy for inequities. *Chicago Tribune*, Womanews, p. 12.

Bickel, J., & Quinnie, R. (1992). *Women in medicine: Statistics.* Washington, DC: Association of American Medical Colleges.

Bickel, J., & Quinnie, R. (1993, January). Women's health curricula. *Building a stronger women's program: Enhancing the educational and professional environment.* Washington, DC: Association of American Medical Colleges.

Bleier, R. (Ed.). (1986). *Feminist approaches to science.* New York: Pergamon Press.

Braus, P. (1993, March). Facing menopause. *American Demographics, 15*, 44–48.

Braverman, P., Oliva, G., Miller, M. G., Schaaf, V. M., & Reiter, R. (1988). Women without health insurance: Links between access, poverty, ethnicity, and health. *Western Journal of Medicine, 149*, 708–711.

Burd, S. (1993, May 19). Director's strategic plan for NIH faces an uncertain future. *Chronicle of Higher Education*, pp. A19, A22.

Cain, J. M. (1993). Undergraduate and graduate medical education in women's health care: Reconsidering faculty, setting, and content. *Women's Health Issues*, 3, 104–109.

Center for Research on Women and Gender. (1995). Women's health elective set for fall 1995. *Connections* (Fall) 2. [Newsletter of the Center for Research on Women and Gender. University of Illinois at Chicago. 1640 West Roosevelt Road, Fifth Floor. Chicago, IL 60608–6902].

Clancy, C. M., & Massion, C. T. (1992). American women's health care: A patchwork quilt with gaps. *Journal of the American Medical Association*, 268, 1918–1920.

Cohen, J. (1993). Bernadine Healy bows out. *Science*, 259, 1388.

Corea, G. (1977). *The hidden malpractice: How American medicine mistreats women.* New York: Jove/Harcourt Brace Jovanovich.

Cotton, P. (1990a). Examples abound of gaps in medical knowledge because of groups excluded from scientific study. *Journal of the American Medical Association*, 263, 1051, 1055.

Cotton, P. (1990b). Is there still too much extrapolation from data on middle-aged white men? *Journal of the American Medical Association*, 263, 1049–1050.

Cotton, P. (1992). Women's health initiative leads way as research begins to fill gender gaps. *Journal of the American Medical Association*, 267, 469–473.

Davis, A. Y. (1983). Racism, birth control and reproductive rights. In A. Y. Davis (Ed.), *Women, race and class* (pp. 202–221). New York: Random House.

Davis, A. Y. (1990). Sick and tired of being sick and tired: The politics of black women's health. In E. C. White (Ed.), *The black women's health book: Speaking for ourselves* (pp. 18–26). Seattle: Seal Press.

Denman, S. J. (1995). Letter to the editor. *Journal of the American Medical Association*, 273, 1256.

Dreifus, C., Ed. (1977). *Seizing our bodies: The politics of women's health.* New York: Vintage Books.

Eckman, A. K. (1996). *From JANE to the Journal of Women's Health: Women's health as an emergent body of medical knowledge.* Unpublished doctoral dissertation, University of Illinois, Urbana-Champaign.

Ehreinreich, B., & English, D. (1978). *For her own good: 150 years of the experts' advice to women.* New York: Doubleday.

Ehrenreich, B., & English, D. (1973). *Complaints and disorders: The sexual politics of sickness.* Old Westbury, NY: Feminist Press.

Federation of Feminist Women's Health Centers. (1981). *A new view of a woman's body.* New York: Simon and Schuster.

Fee, E. (1983). Women and health care: A comparison of theories. In E. Fee (Ed.), *Women and health: The politics of sex in medicine.* (pp. 17–34). Farmingdale, NY: Baywood.

Fisher, S. (1986). *In the patient's best interest: Women and the politics of medical decisions*. New Brunswick, NJ: Rutgers University Press.

Foreman, J. (1992, June 21). Health industry sees gold mine in women's care. *Boston Globe*, pp. 1, 8.

Fraser, N. (1993). Clintonism, welfare, and the antisocial wage: The emergence of a neoliberal political imaginary. *Rethinking Marxism, 6* (2), 9–23.

Fraser, N., & Gordon, L. (1994). A genealogy of "dependency": Tracing a keyword of the U.S. welfare state. *Signs: Journal of Women in Culture and Society, 19*, 309–336.

Gilman, S. L. (1985). *Difference and pathology: Stereotypes of sexuality, race and madness*. Ithaca, NY: Cornell University Press.

Goldrick, K. E. (1990). Women's health: Is anatomy still destiny. *Journal of the American Medical Women's Association, 45*, 211–212.

Gordon, M. (1992, September). Their bodies our selves: Women ignored in medical research. *Harper's Bazaar, 58*, 382–385.

Hall, S. (1983). The problem of ideology—Marxism without guarantees. In B. Matthews (Ed.), *Marx 100 years on* (pp. 57–86). London: Lawrence and Wishart.

Hall, S., Critcher, C., Jefferson, T., Clarke, J., & Roberts, B. (1978). *Policing the crisis: Mugging, the state, and law and order*. New York: Holmes and Meier.

Hall, S. (1986). On postmodernism and articulation: An interview. *Journal of Communication Inquiry, 10* (2), 45–77.

Hamilton, J. A. (1993). Feminist theory and health psychology: Tools for an egalitarian, woman-centered approach to women's health. *Journal of Women's Health, 2*, 49–54.

Hamilton, J. A. (1985). Guidelines for avoiding methodological and policy-making biases in Gender-Related Health Research. In Public Health Service, *Women's health: Report of the Public Health Service Task Force on Women's Health Issues*, vol. II (pp. IV54–64). (DHHS Publication No. [PHS] 85–50206.) Washington, DC: U.S. Government Printing Office.

Harding, S. (1986). *The science question in feminism*. Ithaca: Cornell University Press.

Harding, S. (Ed.). (1993). *The "racial" economy of science: Toward a democratic future*. Bloomington: Indiana University Press.

Harrison, M. (1990). Woman as other: The premise of medicine. *Journal of the American Women's Medical Association, 45*, 225–226.

Harrison, M. (1992). Women's health: A deceptive solution. *Journal of Women's Health Issues, 1*, 101–106.

Healy, B. (1991a, July 29). *Women's health issues*. Speech given at a briefing on women's health issues held by the Congressional Biomedical Research Caucus, Washington, DC.

Healy, B. (1991b). Women's health, public welfare. *Journal of the American Medical Association, 266*, 566–68.

Healy, B. (1991c). The Yentl syndrome. *New England Journal of Medicine, 325*, 274–276.

Healy, B. (1992a). A celebration and a new resolve. *Journal of Women's Health*, *1*, xvii.

Healy, B. (1992b, September). Forward. In National Institutes of Health, Office of Research on Women's Health, *Report of the National Institutes of Health: Opportunities for Research on Women's Health* (Summary Report) (pp. ix–xii). (NIH Publication No. 92-345-7A). Washington, DC: Author.

Hemphill, S., & Dan, A. J. (1993). Introduction. *Journal of Women's Health*, *2*, 41–42.

Henrich, J. B. (1994). *Academic and clinical programs in women's health* [report]. Washington, DC: Council on Graduate Medical Education.

Hubbard, R. (1990). *The politics of women's biology*. New Brunswick, NJ: Rutgers University Press.

Johnson, K. (1992). Women's health: Developing a new specialty. *Journal of Women's Health Issues*, *1*, 95–100.

Johnson, K., & Dawson, L. (1990). Women's health as a multidisciplinary specialty: An exploratory proposal. *Journal of the American Women's Medical Association*, *45*, 222–224.

Johnson, K., & Hoffman, E. (1993). Women's health: Designing and implementing an interdisciplinary specialty. *Women's Health Issues*, *3*, 115–120.

Johnson, T. L. (1993). Position paper: A women's health research agenda. *Journal of Women's Health*, *2*, 95–98.

Johnson, T., & Fee, E. (1994). Women's participation in clinical research: From protectionism to access. In A. C. Mastroianni, R. Faden, & D. Federman (Eds.), *Women and health research: Ethical and legal issues of including women in clinical trials*, vol. 2 (pp. 1–10). Washington, DC: National Academy Press.

Joint Ad Hoc Committee of the American Academy of Family Physicians, the American College of Obstetricians and Gynecologists, the Council on Resident Education in Obstetrics and Gynecology, and the Association of Professors of Gynecology and Obstetrics. (N.d.) *ACOG-AAFP recommended core curriculum and hospital practice privileges in obstetrics-gynecology for family physicians* (AAFP Reprint No. 261). Washington, DC: American Academy of Family Physicians.

King, P. A. (1992). The dangers of difference. *Hastings Center Report*, *22*, 35–38.

Kirschstein, R. L. (1991). Research on women's health. *American Journal of Public Health*, *81*, 291–293.

Kirschstein, R. L. (1992, September). Introduction. In National Institutes of Health, Office of Research on Women's Health, *Report of the National Institutes of Health: Opportunities for Research on Women's Health* (Summary Report) (pp. 1–6). (NIH Publication No. 92-3457A.) Washington, DC: Author.

Krasnoff, M. J. (1992a). Internal medicine training and women's health. *Journal of General Internal Medicine*, *7*, 665–666.

Krasnoff, M. K. (1992b). Perspective: Participation in a multidisciplinary women's health study group. *Journal of Women's Health*, *1*, 185–187.

Laqueur, T. (1990). *Making sex: Body and gender from the Greeks to Freud*. Cambridge: Harvard University Press.

Laurence, L., & Weinhouse, B. (1994). *Outrageous practices: The alarming truth about how medicine mistreats women*. New York: Fawcett Columbine.

Leavitt, J. W. (Ed.). (1984). *Women and health in America*. Madison: University of Wisconsin Press.

Leigh, W. A. (1994). The health status of women of color. In C. Costello & A. J. Stone (for the Women's Research and Education Institute) (Eds.), *The American woman, 1994–95: Where we stand* (pp. 154–196). New York: W.W. Norton.

Levison, S. P. (1994). Teaching women's health: Where do we stand? Where do we go from here? *Journal of Women's Health, 3*, 387–396.

Lewin, T. (1992, November 7). Doctors consider a specialty focusing on women's health. *New York Times*, p. A1.

Liebert, M. A. (1992). From the publisher. *Journal of Women's Health, 1*, xix.

Lowey, N. M. (1994, June/July). Women's health and medical school curricula. *Academic Medicine, 69*, 12.

Marieskind, H. I. (1980). *Women and the health system: Patients, providers, programs*. St. Louis: C.V. Mosby.

Marketing to women: Lipsticks and ledger books. (1986, January). *Profiles in hospital marketing, 21*, 4–25.

Mastroianni, A. C., Faden, R., & Federman, D. (Eds.). (1994a). *Women and health research: Ethical and legal issues of including women in clinical studies*, vol. 1. Washington, DC: National Academy Press.

Mastroianni, A. C., Faden, R., & Federman, D. (Eds.). (1994b). *Women and health research: Ethical and legal issues of including women in clinical studies*, vol. 2. Washington, DC: National Academy Press.

Medical College of Pennsylvania (MCP) and Hahnemann University School of Medicine. (1994–1995). *Women's Health Education Program: Information for medical students, 1994–1995 academic year* [brochure]. Philadelphia: Medical College of Pennsylvania.

Mendelsohn, K. D., Nieman, L. Z., Isaacs, K., Lee, S., & Levinson, S. P. (1994). Sex and gender bias in anatomy and physical diagnosis text illustrations. *Journal of the American Medical Association, 272*, 1267–1270.

Merkatz, R. B., Temple, R., Sobel, S., Feiden, K., & Kessler, D. A. (1993). Women in clinical trials of new drugs: A change in food and drug administration policy. *New England Journal of Medicine, 329*, 292–296.

Nadel, Mark V. (1990, June 18). Statement. In U.S. Congress, Subcommittee on Health and the Environment. *Hearings: NIH reauthorization and proliferation of health facilities* (Serial No. 101–191, pp. 214–226.) Washington, DC: U.S. Government Printing Office.

National academy launched. (1994). *Journal of the American Medical Women's Association, 49*, 38.

National Institutes of Health, Office of Research on Women's Health. (1992, September). *Report of the National Institutes of Health: Opportunities for Research on Women's Health* (Summary Report). (NIH Publication No. 92–345–7A.) Washington, DC: Author.

National Women's Health Network. (1991, December). "Research to improve women's health: An agenda for equity." Washington, DC: Author.

Nechas, E., & Foley, D. (1994). *Unequal treatment: What you don't know about how women are mistreated by the medical community*. New York: Simon and Schuster.

Nieman, L. Z. (1994). Women's health research: Barriers and opportunity: Synopsis of plenary talk given by Florence P. Haseltine. *Journal of Women's Health, 3,* 365–366.

Ochs, R. (1993, October 4). Health care for the whole woman. *New York Newsday,* p. 57.

Olesen, V. (Ed.). (1975). Women and their health: Research implications for a new era. *NCHSR Research Proceedings Series*. Proceedings of a conference held at the University of California, San Francisco. (DHEW Publication No. [HRA] 77–3138.) Springfield, VA: National Technical Information Service.

Passaretti, A. V. (1995). Letter to the editor. *Journal of the American Medical Association, 273,* 1256.

Pinn, V. W. (1992a). Commentary: Women, research, and the National Institutes of Health. *American Journal of Preventative Medicine, 8,* 324–327.

Pinn, V. W. (1992b). Women's health research: Prescribing change and addressing the issues. *Journal of the American Medical Association, 268,* 1921–1922.

Pinn, V. W. (1992c, Spring). Women's health: Priority to reality. *Wellbeing* [publication of Beth Israel Hospital, Boston], 59–63.

Pollner, F. (1973, July/August). NWRO convention: Health care. *Off our backs, 3,* 8.

Public Health Service. (1985, January/February). Women's health: Report of the Public Health Service Task Force on Women's Health Issues, vol. I. In *Public Health Reports,* 100 (pp. 73–106). Washington, DC: U.S. Government Printing Office.

Purvis, A. (1990a, Fall). A perilous gap. *Time* (Special issue: Women face the '90s), *136,* 66–67.

Purvis, A. (1990b, March 5). Research for men only: Doctors could use more data on treating women. *Time, 135,* 59–60.

Ramey, E. R. (1982, April). The National Capacity for Health in Women. In P. W. Berman & E. R. Ramey (Eds.), *Women: A Developmental Perspective* (pp. 3–12). U.S. Department of Health and Human Services. NIH Publication No. 82–2298.

Rock, A. (1993, October). Women's health is our modern day suffrage movement. *Ladies Home Journal, 110,* 138–39, 184, 187.

Rosenthal, E. (1993, October 13). Does fragmented medicine harm the health of women. *New York Times,* p. A1.

Rosser, S. V. (1994). *Women's health—Missing from U.S. medicine.* Bloomington: Indiana University Press.

Ruzek, S. B. (1978). *The women's health movement: Feminist alternatives to medical control.* New York: Praeger.

Ruzek, S. B. (1980). Medical response to women's health activists: Conflict, accommodation, and cooptation. *Research in sociology of health care, 1,* 335–354.

Ruzek, S. B. (1993). Toward a more inclusive model of women's health. *American Journal of Public Health, 83,* 6–7.

Scott, J. (1988). Gender: A useful category of historical analysis. *Gender and the politics of history.* New York: Columbia University Press.

Scully, D., & Bart, P. (1973). A funny thing happened on the way to the orifice: Women in gynecology textbooks. *American Journal of Sociology, 78,* 1045–1049.

Silberner, J. (1990, September 24). Health: Another gender gap. *U.S. News and World Report, 109,* 54–55.

Skelly, F. J. (1992, July 27). Millions in menopause. *American Medical News, 35,* 45, 47, 49–50.

Skolnick, A. A. (1992). Women's health specialty, other issues on agenda of 'reframing' conference. *Journal of the American Medical Association, 268,* 1813–1814.

Smith, B. (1982). Black women's health: Notes for a course. In G. T. Hull, P. B. Scott, & B. Smith (Eds.), *But some of us are brave: Black women's studies* (pp. 54–68). Old Westbury, NY: Feminist Press.

Stabiner, K. (1994, April 4). In the menopause market, a goldmine of ads. *New York Times,* p. C6.

Steingart, R. M., Packer, M., Hamm, P., Coglianese, M. E., Gersh, B., Geltman, E. M., et al. (1991). Sex differences in the management of coronary artery disease. *New England Journal of Medicine, 325,* 226–30.

Todd, A. D. (1989). *Intimate adversaries: Cultural conflict between doctors and women patients.* Philadelphia: University of Pennsylvania Press.

Todd, J. S. (1993, March). Better late than never. *Good Housekeeping, 216,* 102.

Ulene, A. (1991a, February). Living smart, living health: Women's health campaign. *Good Housekeeping, 212,* 94.

Ulene, A. (1991b, February). Women and heart disease: What you need to know. *Good Housekeeping, 212,* 120, 127, 133, 140.

Vance, C. S. (1990). Negotiating sex and gender in the Attorney General's Commission on Pornography. In F. Ginsburg & A. L. Tsing (Eds.), *Uncertain terms: Negotiating gender in American culture* (pp. 118–134). Boston: Beacon Press.

Wallis, L. A., & Klass, P. (1990). Toward Improving Women's Health Care. *Journal of the American Women's Association, 45,* 219–221.

Wentz, A. C., & Haseltine, F. P. (1992). Editorial. *Journal of Women's Health Issues, 1,* xv.

West, C. (1984). *Routine complications.* Bloomington: Indiana University Press.

White, E. C. (Ed.). (1990). *The black women's health book: Speaking for ourselves.* Seattle: Seal Press.

Women left out at NIH. (1990). *Science, 248,* 1601.

Zambrana, R. E. (1987). A research agenda on issues affecting poor and minority women: A model for understanding their health needs. *Women and Health, 12,* 5–24.

Carol Stabile

5

Shooting the Mother

Fetal Photography and the Politics of Disappearance

what name shall we call our selves now
our mother is gone?
                    —Audre Lorde, "Harriet"[1]

Mommy Dearest

By late 1991, what Rosalind Petchesky had once described as "the Rightward Drift in the Courts" had become a right-wing tsunami.[2] Neoconservative Clarence Thomas was appointed to the Supreme Court, a decision was handed down in *Rust v. Sullivan* (the "gag rule") forbidding doctors in family planning clinics accepting federal funds to even mention abortion to pregnant women (even if that pregnancy threatened a woman's life). In January 1992, the Supreme Court announced that it would rule on Pennsylvania's restrictive abortion law by Election Day, thus casting further doubt on the future of *Roe v. Wade*. Of course, as Petchesky also observes, the Supreme Court does not produce ideology, but has merely reinforced the dominant political and ideological currents characteristic of the conservative restoration.

The central task of this essay is to examine the crucial ideological work performed by visual representations of fetal autonomy in the service of

New Right politics—to analyze the conditions that have made possible the ideological transformation of the female body from a benevolent, maternal environment into an inhospitable wasteland, at war with the "innocent person" within. For feminism in the nineties, this transformation offers an ideological double bind, for just as the articulation of "woman" with nature, feminized environments, and motherhood produces reactionary and regressive configurations of "femininity," so the disarticulation of "woman" and "mother" constructs an equally reactionary problematic.[3] In terms of visual and reproductive technologies, and the political interests these technologies often serve, what we are witnessing is the result not of a regression, but a progression. In short, the division between woman and fetus is historically unprecedented. Although this distinction is often based on traditional configurations of motherhood, its very novelty often makes the resulting articulations strained and fractured. This project of disarticulation, which has been underway for at least two decades, can be alternately read as anti-essentialist (insofar as it denies the material specificity of women's bodies) or as a process of humanizing technology, which then figures as the sign of paternalistic intervention. I do not want to collapse a complex set of conjunctural circumstances into the results of a single technological advance, for example, fetal visualization and technology, but I do want to analyze how visual technologies, in a society so dependent upon images, have played a crucial role in this erasure of women's bodies.

In terms of the traditional maternal environment, female interests have been historically subsumed beneath the interests of the family, but this more recent erasure has little to do with martyrdom or self-sacrifice. Instead, representations of "fetal personhood" depend upon the erasure of female bodies and the reduction of women to passive, reproductive machines, as in the highly publicized cases analyzed by Valerie Hartouni of "braindead" or comatose women who are kept alive long enough to give birth.[4] Where earlier appeals to "motherhood" worked to erase female subjectivity and sexuality, this recent disarticulation functions not through ideology, but through the repression of material female bodies. The maternal space has, in effect, disappeared and what has emerged in its place is an environment that the fetus alone occupies. In order for the embryo/fetus to emerge as autonomous—as a person, patient, or individual in its own right—all traces of a female body (as well as the embryo's presence as parasite within that body) must disappear.[5]

The enforced disappearance of female bodies is becoming more and more evident in legal cases having to do either centrally or peripherally with the notion of "fetal rights." Even when a "mother" is invoked, the proliferation of definitions activated by reproductive technologies (from "birth mother" to "genetic mother" to "surrogate mother") causes a fragmentation of this once unitary entity. Where the ideology of maternal altruism and self-sacrifice once functioned, in hegemonic terms, to gain the consent of female subjects to dominant ideologies, the contradictions produced during our particular historical conjuncture (which include limited, but symbolically weighted, gains in terms of female sexuality and reproductive rights, as well as an increasingly feminized labor force) make such traditional ideologies increasingly difficult to sustain.[6]

The once "docile body" of the mother has given way to representations of women who must fight on both domestic and economic fronts for their survival, as well as that of their children. The ideological anxieties activated by this shift can be seen in contemporary popular culture. In *The Seventh Sign* (1986), a pregnant Demi Moore repeatedly hears a voice asking: "Will you die for him?" In the conclusion, she saves the world from Armageddon by giving birth and then expiring. The main character in *Switch* (1991) redeems her/his recalcitrant soul by bearing a child (conceived through date rape, no less).[7] The child, "the only woman who loves him," is delivered, whereupon the protagonist immediately departs, presumably to Heaven. Such traditional appeals to discourses of maternal altruism are only part of the larger picture. The alternative is clearly and antithetically proposed: either the traditional, passive, self-sacrificing mother or a world in which, as Valerie Hartouni observes, "women have lost heart or touch with the deepest source of their identity and thus have become not only dysfunctional but potentially dangerous."[8] Morality plays about the dangerous and unnatural anti-mother, like *Fatal Attraction* (1988), *The Hand That Rocks the Cradle* (1992), and *Basic Instinct* (1992), vividly illustrate this dilemma.

If the docile female body can no longer be sufficiently disciplined through ideology, it must nonetheless be disciplined. And it is in the spheres of legal and medical discourses that the repressive state apparatus has begun to operate with much more evident violence. Whatever rights "women" may have had within the legal system (and historically certain groups of women, by virtue of race and class privilege, have always enjoyed a fuller subject status vis-à-vis the law than others) are dramatically being reversed in the so-called interests of an amorphous subject: the fetus, or as advocates of IVF (*in vitro* fertilization) technologies as well as anti-abortion factions put it, "the early human being." The visual technologies used to isolate the embryo as astronaut, extraterrestrial, or aquatic entity have had enormously repressive reverberations in the legal and medical management of women's bodies. A few examples of these legal repercussions will suffice to illustrate this point. In June of 1986, Angela Carder, a twenty-eight-year-old white woman, twenty-six weeks pregnant, who had twice before received a terminal prognosis for bone cancer, was ordered by the Washington court system to undergo a cesarean section. Against Carder's explicit wishes, against the opinions of her attending oncologist, against the protests of her husband and parents, the doctors refused to prescribe chemotherapy because of its possible harm to the fetus. According to Susan Faludi:

> So instead of treating her cancer, they jammed a tube down her throat and pumped her with sedatives, a strategy to delay the hour of death. Carder tried to fight this "treatment," her mother says, remembering how her daughter thrashed and twisted on the bed, fending off the doctors. "She said, 'No, no, no. Don't do that to me.'" But Carder lost the battle and was, quite literally, silenced. With the tube in place, she couldn't speak.[9]

The operation was performed shortly thereafter. Angela Carder barely lived long enough to hear that the fetus extracted from her uterus had died, if indeed it could be said to have lived at all.[10]

The postpartum version of policing has come to be known as "fetal neglect." In 1987, Pamela Rae Stewart, according to Katha Pollitt, was "advised by her obstetrician to stay off her feet, to eschew sex and 'street drugs,' and to go to the hospital immediately if she start[ed] to bleed."[11] When she gave birth to a brain-damaged child who died, she was charged "with failing to deliver support to a child." Her lover, who had apparently both had sexual intercourse with Stewart and had beaten her, was never charged.

In 1990, after the *Webster* decision ensured that gubernatorial elections would determine the outcome of abortion rights at the state level, ABC's *Nightline* broadcast a special program, entitled "Abortion: The New Civil War"; the program aired on the Thursday evening before Election Day. The designation of the abortion debates as "the New Civil War" is particularly revealing of the ideological amputation of embryos and fetuses from female bodies. In terms of a popular American context, the term "Civil War" has the added resonance of the conflict between the North (or Union) and the South (or Confederacy) over the issue of slavery. When applied to abortion rights, the analogy has a further symbolic valence. As represented on *Nightline*, it is a conflict between "pro-choice" and "pro-life" advocates (hereafter referred to as "pro-abortion" and "anti-abortion"): a conflict that, like the Civil War, can even divide the unity of families along ideological lines.[12] In a racist analogy, anti-abortion factions liken the situation of "the fetus" to that of African Americans: a group in Maryland, for example, calls themselves the "National Association for the Advancement of Preborn Children" (NAAPC).

The key to this rhetoric lies in another civil war, the groundwork for which has been steadily developing over the past thirty years: a civil war occurring not within the nation-state or body politic, but within the female body itself. While historically, the embryo/fetus has had no autonomy of its own (indeed, the "quickening" that signified "life" in the womb was a perceptual observation determined by the woman herself), since the late seventies a dichotomy between the pregnant woman as maternal environment and the fetus as a person in its own right has emerged in both popular culture and medical-legal discourses. This then is the "New Civil War," in which an erstwhile benevolent, nurturing, and ideal environment has been transformed into a hostile, infanticidal toxic waste dump, from which the autonomous (and, one might infer, autochthonous) "person" must be protected by the paternalistic arm of the government. The articulation of the embryo with victims of racism and of the Holocaust thus logically—if obscenely—proceeds from this logic.

How has the shift from a utopic to a profoundly dystopic "maternal environment" taken place? What ancillary repressions or erasures have been made to facilitate this shift? What part has the development and deployment of visual technologies played in the construction of this embryonic environment? As Hartouni observes, "It is difficult to see in the regressive and reactionary character of this decade's discourse on reproduction anything remotely resembling alternative, liberatory political possibilities."[13] However, these visual technologies and their narrativization also produce proleptic contradictions and anomalies that may yet be harnessed to the political struggles ahead.

The Penetrating Tale of the Sperm [14]

This is the first portrait ever made of a living embryo inside its mother's womb. It is one of an unprecedented set of color photographs—strikingly complete in their clinical detail but at the same time strangely beautiful—of human embryos in their natural state.

—*Life* magazine, 30 April 1965

> On these pages is our first sight of an event as common and as ancient as
> humankind—the way each of us came to be.
>
> —*Life* magazine, August 1990

In 1965, Lyndon B. Johnson had recently been inaugurated as President
for his first full term, the "military action" in Vietnam was escalating, as
were racial tensions within the United States, and the Civil Rights Act had
been passed by Congress before the summer recess. On 30 April, the
cover of *Life* Magazine displayed the photograph of a "Living 18-Week-
Old Fetus," under the dramatic caption of an "UNPRECEDENTED
PHOTOGRAPHIC FEAT IN COLOR." Cut to August 1990, twenty-
five years later. In response to an anticipated Iraqi invasion of Kuwait,
President George Bush mobilized the largest number of armed forces
since the Vietnam War to stage a military blockade in the Middle East.
The Louisiana Supreme Court was debating the terms of the most restrictive abortion bill in the United States, while other states were gearing up
for gubernatorial elections that in a number of instances hinged on the
candidates' stands on abortion rights. Many of a younger generation of
feminists could not recall a time when an abortion was legally (if not economically) denied to them, but they were gradually coming to anticipate
the worst. At this particular historical moment, *Life*—which ended in
1972 and was reincarnated in 1978—again presented "The First Pictures
Ever of How Life Begins"(figure 5.1).

Separated by a quarter of a century, these two texts provide a unique
illustration of the ideological shifts around the categories of "woman" and
"embryo"/"fetus." The narrative construction of this so-called empirical
evidence suggests that the ideological stakes are very differently motivated
in each case: that the skirmishes over, around, and through female bodies
involve varying productions of meaning. These distinctions, moreover,
cannot be reduced to or explained by technological advances, since as we
shall see, many of the photographs ostensibly represent the same, if not
identical, gestational sequence of events. Instead, these narratives invoke
visual technologies in the interests of shifting political formations. In
1965, abortion was illegal and although feminists had been protesting and
organizing since at least the late fifties, the second wave of feminism had
yet to converge politically upon the issue. What we see in 1990, on the
other hand, is the result of the conservative restoration: more than a
decade of increasing attacks on abortion rights and a strongly aligned
political movement in opposition to *Roe v. Wade*. In 1965, technology
offered readers of *Life* their first "realistic" glimpse into the hitherto

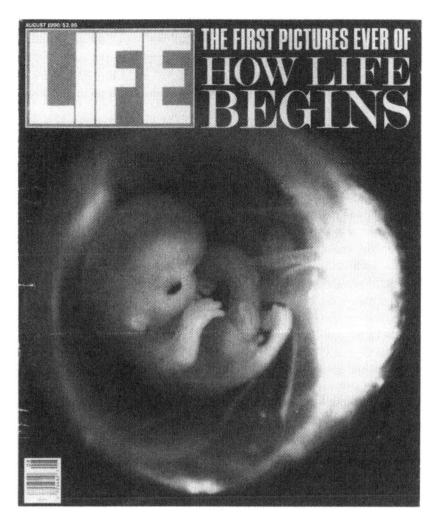

Figure 5.1 August 1990 cover of *Life* magazine.

impenetrable womb. Although for a time, X-rays had offered shadowy glimpses of a skeletal embryo, reports about the harmful effects of these had curtailed the use of X-rays by the late 1950s. And in 1965, the now familiar sonographic images had not yet appeared on the cultural scene. The cover of the magazine informs us that the dim image encased in a bubble represents a "[L]iving 18-week-old fetus shown inside its amniotic sac—placenta is seen at right." Concealed within the middle of the first page of text is the curious statement that "[T]he embryos shown on the following pages *had been surgically removed* for a variety of reasons" (emphasis added). Immediately following this disclaimer the author adds, "But, using a specially built super wide-angle lens and a tiny flash beam at the end of a surgical scope, Nilsson was able to shoot this picture of a living 15-week-old embryo."[15]

While the consistent use of the present tense works to sustain the illusion of "life," at one point the text accompanying one photograph admits that "this embryo is an imperfect one (the tissue at the right is torn and ragged)." To confuse matters even further, although the article designates eight weeks as the point at which the "embryo" becomes a "fetus," the fifteen-week-old entity, biologically a "fetus," is described as an "embryo." In attempting to construct a chronological narrative, a first, ambient portrait of life, the text foregrounds the animate status of the cover shot, thereby insinuating that all the photographs represent "human embryos in their *natural state*" (emphasis added). A careful reading of the text, however, reveals that all the photographs within the article are of autopsied embryos ("embryo had been removed from sacs," "the spongy placenta . . . has been partially peeled back here for better visibility," "the fetus has been backlighted"). What has been patched together, consequently, to simulate "life" is—ironically—death.

If attempts to represent the contents of the uterus as autonomous or separable from the female body itself ultimately break down under scrutiny, the technological and textual confusion of 1965's "Drama of Life Before Birth" is not reducible to its comparative technological simplicity, but to its different ideological purpose and positioning. In other words, questions about the status of the embryo/fetus are not ideologically urgent in the way they are after *Roe v. Wade*. "Life" exists "before birth": common sense guarantees the embryo/fetus' status as living "human being." While the article certainly works to buttress this common sense, defensive maneuvers around the ontological status of the embryo/fetus are not necessary because the woman, or mother, is not yet a threat. In other words, the fetus does not need to be separated from the woman's body in order to be protected from her.

So in 1965, the mother can be shot through, but she does not need to be erased: traces of her presence remain, both discursively and through the inclusion of the placenta in the photographs. In keeping with still dominant ideologies of motherhood, the absent body is consistently referred to as "the mother." The photographs are "the first portrait ever made of a living embryo inside its mother's womb" and although they irrevocably alter the concept of the family photo album, they remain firmly situated within traditional familial ideologies. Reminders that the mother is more than mere surface or screen—that, in fact, she is absolutely central to the processes being described—sprinkle the text: "at 3 1/2 weeks, the embryo is so tiny—about a tenth of an inch long—that the mother may not even know she is pregnant"; at eleven weeks, "as the fetus' living quarters get more cramped and as it gains steadily in strength, the mother will begin to feel the sharp kick and thrust of foot, knee and elbow," while at eighteen weeks, "It can make an impressively hard fist, and the punches and kicks are plainly felt by the mother." "Mother," in these passages, signifies a sentient, sympathetic, and self-sacrificing presence, and whatever violence taking place is enacted by the fetus itself.

The traditional warmth and benevolence of the maternal landscape is emphasized in an essay following the 1965 montage, suggestively entitled: "Pushed Out into a Hostile World." This article extols the traditional virtues of the maternal space over that of a cold, cruel world, waxing poetic about the "Marvels of the Placenta." The "tranquility of his [sic] mother's womb" and the "mother's cozy 98° F" environment are juxtaposed against "the hostile world, full of startlingly unfamiliar conditions." Against this tranquil and cozy environment, the "baby" figures as a parasitic organism. "The baby," as the text baldly puts it "is a parasite. From the day of fertilization, the embryo becomes foreign material. The woman's body does not reject the embryo because of the mediations of the placenta. She tolerates it only because of the placenta's unique ability to subvert her immunological defenses." The fact that the fetus is an organism that feeds off the mother's body, that the symbiosis is indeed one-sided, is a concept never voiced in contemporary debates in which the woman's body figures as far from tolerant, but absolutely hostile and murderous.[16]

A quarter of a century after "Drama of Life Before Birth," Swedish photographer Lennart Nilsson once again penetrated the womb to allow spectators "our first sight of an event as common and as ancient as humankind—the way each of us came to be."[17] In 1990, however, "He has embraced complex high-tech tools such as scanning electron microscopes . . . and tiny endoscopes that can peer inside a woman's womb."[18] The result of this technological intercourse? In contrast to the 1965 cover photograph of an eighteen-week-old fetus, the August 1990 cover presents a seven-week-old fetus. And within the pages of *Life*, the gestational clock has been turned back even further: from three and one-half weeks to two hours.

The earlier atmosphere of liberal tolerance, moreover, has given way to a dark, amorphous background, from which all traces of a female body, as well as any connection to a maternal environment, have disappeared. The photographs contain no traces of either the amniotic sac or placenta, while textually, the distinction between embryo/fetus and female body is elaborately reinforced. Initially referred to as "the woman" in the text, after eight days "she" is transformed into the "mother" (although women who have had "repeated miscarriages" remain "some women"). In 1965, the placenta figures as the life-sustaining link between woman and embryo/fetus: "Through the placenta the vein brings in food, oxygen and various chemical substances from the mother, while the arteries take back waste material for the mother to get rid of." In place of this circular movement of food and waste, in 1990: "The embryo has its own blood supply separate from the mother's, but the placenta brings the two systems next to each other." Instead of being a symbiotic link between woman and embryo, the placenta becomes a modem that permits communication between two distinct, and separate environments. Thus both visually and textually, the embryo/fetus enjoys a thoroughly autonomous status.

In contrast to the modest "drama" staged in 1965, 1990's "The First Days of Creation" offers a biblical epic of alienation, peril, and conflict. Mobilizing a discourse of militarism, it emphasizes the perils of an infinitely inhospitable environment, where the two-hour old, Rambo-esque blastocyte must defy and overcome a hostile system: "the 100 or so sperm cells that survived the journey up the reproductive tract are busily stripping the nutrient cells from the ovum. Over the next several hours the sperm will begin beating their tails vigorously as they rotate like drill bits into the outer wall of the egg." The sperm cells, miniaturized members of a SWAT or Special Forces team, set to their task of penetration with aggression and purpose. The woman's contribution to fertilization is reduced to the "ovum" or "egg." Reference to the word "vagina," which would imply the presence of a female body, is scrupulously avoided— instead, the sperm travel through the "reproductive tract."

Both the 1965 and 1990 articles claim an originary, authoritative status for themselves. In 1990, in particular, the article touts itself as "the culmination" of photographer Lennart Nilsson's oeuvre, by offering its readers "our first sight of an event as common and as ancient as humankind." Yet in 1983, Nilsson produced and photographed "The Miracle of Life" for PBS's science series *Nova*, a program that contains identical footage of the same events, as well as some that purport to occur even earlier (the viewer, for example, travels through the penis, accompanied by the athletic sperm, and then into the vagina and fallopian tubes in search of the passive ovum). The discourse of militarism is also evident in "The Miracle of Life." The sperm, who are the protagonists of this narrative, wait patiently in "transport canals" in the male body for "fuel" and their call to arms. Upon arousal, they begin to move into place, only to be visually propelled by means of a "propulsion system" like little cosmonauts into the battlefield: the woman's reproductive system.[19] The phalanx of sperm march through the "dangerously inhospitable" and "hostile acid environment" of the vagina (which perceives them as "alien" and "intruders"). At every turn, the woman's body provides obstacles to their success: her various "canals" all seem to contain "downward currents" and twists and turns that confuse the determined soldiers. The "women's own defense system attacks the sperm," the viewer is told. Indeed, to listen to "The Miracle of Life" it seems a wonder that fertilization occurs at all.[20]

So why the repeated claims to originality? A motivating force behind such claims seems to be to secure authority in the debates about the ontological status of the fetus. Central to the abortion debates is the concept of "viability," or when the fetus can reasonably be expected to survive outside the uterus. Fetal viability has been rapidly shifting along with associated technologies. At the time of this writing, fetal viability is said to be possible at about twenty-six weeks.[21] But the representational sleights of hand in all three visual productions are carefully constructed to deconstruct the entire notion of "viability." Like "The First Days of Creation," "The Miracle of Life" contains significant chronological gaps in fetal development, the purpose of which is to anthropomorphize and autonomize the embryo. The photographic layout in the *Life* of 1990, for example, contains insets with dates clearly labeled beneath them, but in each case the larger photograph is of an embryo/fetus gestationally much further advanced, with the date embedded in the small, accompanying print (figure 5.2). In "The Miracle of Life," the program contains a remarkable leap from eighteen weeks to birth, obscuring essential developmental processes and hinting at an early "viability" of the fetus. The purpose of this seems clear. Foregrounding the more developed organism not only erases the woman's participation, but implies that "life" occurs very early in the pregnancy. Further, it signifies that "viability" itself is a shifting concept, subject to technological advances that may soon render the term itself obsolete. Today, the photographs imply, we can now photograph "early human life," but tomorrow we may well be able to sustain it through technology.

Clearly, these and related images have worked to impose the image of the free-floating fetus and erase the reality of the pregnant bodies that

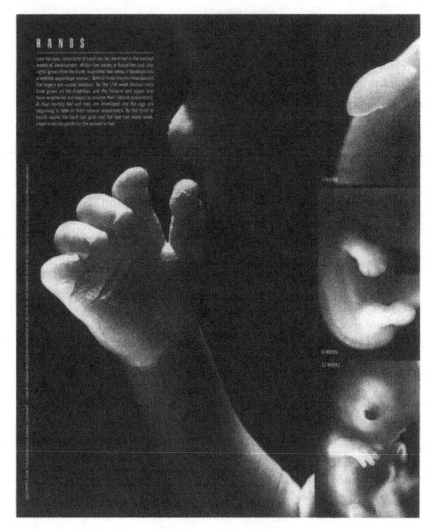

Figure 5.2   Page from "The Miracle of Life," *Life*, August 1990.

produce them. In these, the connection between representational practices and political interests is clearly revealed, for the circulation of these
images is not limited to coffee tables and readers. In the late summer and
early autumn of 1990, anti-abortion protesters were shoving the 1990 *Life*
magazine in the faces of women entering abortion clinics in Cranston,
Rhode Island.[22]

Postmodern Pregnancies

Your August cover [of pregnant Demi Moore] has provoked an intense response in our obstetrical-gynecological practice. To me, the photograph conveyed a sense of beauty and pride and I expected an overwhelmingly positive reaction from nurses and patients and their husbands. Unexpectedly, the opinions expressed were predominantly negative.

Pardon the thought of a dirty old lady — I'm seventy-two — but after showing Demi Moore's huge belly, why not on your next cover have Bruce Willis with a huge erection? After all, he made the right connection.
—Letters to the Editor, *Vanity Fair*[23]

The August 1991 cover of *Vanity Fair* contained a photograph of an extremely pregnant Demi Moore, clad only in diamonds, with her hand covering her breast (figure 5.3). The cover provoked the most intense controversy in *Vanity Fair*'s history: ninety-five television spots, sixty-four radio shows, 1,500 newspaper articles, and a dozen cartoons. Some stores and newsstands refused to carry the August issue, while others modestly concealed it in the brown wrapper evocative of porn magazines. Nevertheless, the cover displayed no more skin than magazines like *Allure*, *Cosmopolitan*, and *Vogue* do on a regular basis. What repelled and shocked viewers obviously was the vast expanse of white, pregnant belly.

Why, in an era of infinitely representable female nudity, did such a comparatively modest photograph elicit such a response? Traditionally, the pregnant female body has been the object of medical scrutiny and surveillance, as well as a mystical (if unrepresentable) reverence and awe in Western culture. The pregnant body—even clothed—is a source of abjection and disgust in popular culture: the woman is represented as awkward, uncomfortable, and grotesquely excessive. In a culture that places such a premium on thinness, the pregnant body is anathema. Not only is it perhaps the most visible and physical mark of sexual difference, it is also the sign for deeply embedded fears and anxieties about femininity and the female reproductive system. With the advent of visual technologies, the contents of the uterus have become demystified and entirely representable, but the pregnant body itself remains concealed.

It is the pregnant body's ability to shock and horrify the spectator that is conversely both its potential and its problem: an ability that interestingly transcends political and ideological lines. For a number of important reasons, the pregnant body also remains invisible and undertheorized in

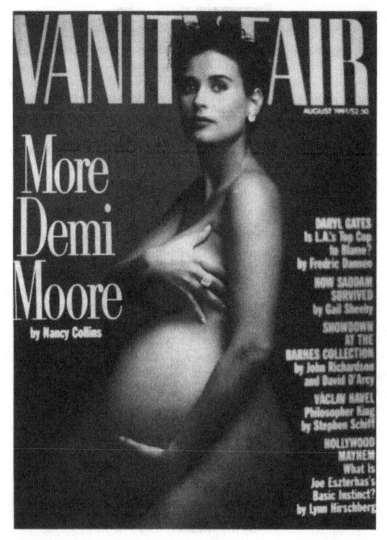

Figure 5.3 August 1991 cover of *Vanity Fair*. Courtesy of Annie Leibovitz/ Contact Press Images.

feminist theory. The resistance to theorizing pregnancy, as such, can be understood in terms of the historical trajectory of feminist activism and thought, since an overarching goal was to extricate "woman" from a purely reproductive status. Pregnancy has been traditionally predicated on an essentialism that reduces women to passive vessels, the receptacles of sperm. Pregnancy, moreover, is seemingly inextricably linked to biologism, to a particularized understanding of the female body as reproductive machine: in Hartouni's terms, it is represented as "a physiological function, a biologically rooted, passive . . . literally mindless—state of being."[24] Furthermore, when conflated with mothering, pregnancy takes on the added significance of entirely defining women's ontological state of being, her desires, her goals. As Michelle Stanworth remarks: "motherhood means different things to different women, and to identify motherhood so exclusively with pregnancy and childbirth runs the risk of blunting the cutting edge of feminist critique."[25] Mothering is thus reduced to a biological imperative and not a socially constructed labor that both women and men may choose to undertake. For feminists and non-feminists alike, pregnancy literally signifies the consequences of unprotected, heterosexual sex. For feminists, it concomitantly evokes the unavailability of both birth control and abortion and the absence of choices. To invoke the pregnant body during the struggles over abortion is also to invoke a culturally, historically, and epistemologically overdetermined concept of pregnancy as the ultimate biological goal of the female body—a Hegelian telos that dictates the proper role of the female subject. It further constitutes an apparently incommensurable and gendered division of labor. Unlike mothering, pregnancy can only be undertaken by women.

The few texts that deal, however peripherally, with pregnancy take radically divergent approaches to their subject. On one hand, there is Shulamith Firestone's claim that "pregnancy is barbaric. . . . [it] is the temporary deformation of the body of the individual for the sake of the species."[26] In this camp exist those feminists who view pregnancy as the ultimate act of female complicity, as the exemplar of feminine false consciousness. In a diametrically opposed position, Julia Kristeva deals with her own experience of pregnancy—"the immeasurable, unconfinable maternal body"—as a source of conservative power and mysticism in "Stabat Mater."[27] This polarization boils down to, in Stanworth's terms, the opposition between a positive and a negative feminist understanding of motherhood. In the former, "maternal practices are increasingly acknowledged as a source of alternative values . . . which stand in hopeful opposition to oppressive forms of thought"; while in the latter, it is suggested "that motherhood locks women into institutional and psychological structures of dependency and powerlessness."[28]

Bridging these two extremes are works that purport to deal with reproduction, but focus almost exclusively on labor and childbirth. Thus, despite critiques of the product-oriented, capitalist management of labor and childbirth, critics like Emily Martin wind up reproducing those aspects of capitalist thought that they seek to undo. In other words, by focusing on the climax of reproduction—that aspect of the process that literally introduces the product into the marketplace—the concept of labor exists only in relation to activity expended during childbirth and labor. Pregnancy, so framed, again remains only a passive ontological state.

Feminist attempts to disarticulate "women" from "pregnancy," either in the positive sense of emphasizing maternal values grounded not in biology, but in practice, or in the negative sense (pregnancy as passivity), have unfortunately participated in the larger cultural logic of removing the laborer from the site of (re)production. They have also almost entirely ceded the terrain of pregnancy to the medical profession. Pregnancy, more than either childbirth or labor, is the site for any number of mappings and various technological surveillance systems. Pregnant bodies are subjected to ultrasound to determine the gestational age of the embryo (however unreliably), amniocentesis to screen for genetic disorders like Downs Syndrome, as well as sexual selection, and Alpha Feta Protein (AFP) tests to check for neural system problems such as spina bifida.

As Emily Martin and other feminists have observed, obstetrics has functioned, since it replaced midwifery in the latter half of the nineteenth century, to control pregnancy using science and technology, as well as to dismiss women's experience and knowledge of their bodies. With the advent of reproductive technologies, however, doctors no longer have to rely on any information from the woman about her pregnancy: "As the 'iron curtain' of the mother has been swept aside revealing the womb and its contents in their full glory, it has become no longer necessary to consult mothers about their attitudes."[29] Thus "pregnant women who can pinpoint the exact date of intercourse as the time they became pregnant are met with disbelief by medical doctors, even when pregnancy testing technology (ultrasound scanning) is giving them [the doctors] obviously incorrect information."[30] The visual and symbolic exclusion of women from reproduction seems a further extension of this logic, yet another strategy for investing power in legal, medical, and other institutional bodies, while ignoring material female bodies.

In the case of unwanted pregnancies, for example, women with access to prenatal care routinely undergo ultrasounds in order to verify the gestational age of the embryo. She is admonished about the deleterious effects of repeated abortions on her body in general, and her reproductive system more specifically. Here, pregnancy is represented as the "natural" state of the female body: to disrupt this in any way is to risk irrevocable

damage to the "natural" order of things. In the case of a wanted pregnancy, the woman who can afford prenatal care sees her physician once a
month until the eighth month and with increasing frequency after that. If
she is above the age of thirty-five (or in certain areas in the United States,
over thirty), her condition is even more intensely scrutinized and pathologized. In the larger cultural sphere, she is bombarded with injunctions as
to what substances might potentially "damage" the fetus. Aside from the
labeling of cigarette packages and alcohol, she is warned about objects
ranging from VDTs (Video Display Terminals) to operating a vehicle.
Ironically, in place of pregnancy being the "natural" state of the female
body, it becomes a highly dangerous, pathological condition, subject to
intense surveillance. In the instances of both unwanted and wanted pregnancies, in short, a moral panic has been produced around the pregnant
body, but the terms of this panic are structured by different situations.

In "The Promises of Monsters," Donna Haraway claims that recent
research in the area of the human immune system has resulted in replacing
the previous system of encoding the body, a hierarchical ordering, with "a
network-body of amazing complexity and specificity." In place of a
self/other, internal/external, ordering, "a radical conception of connection
emerges unexpectedly at the core of the defended self."[31] In relation to the
struggles of people with AIDS, she observes that the positive aspects of
this restructuring are a "fundamental consequence of learning to visualize
the heterogeneous, artifactual body that is our 'social nature,' instead of
narrowing our vision that 'saving nature' and repelling alien invaders from
an unspoiled organic eden called the autonomous self."[32]

Despite such work, the pregnant body remains a potently and patently
hierarchical system that must be governed with an iron hand, from outside, but through the mediating construct of the fetus. To take a visual
example of this, in an advertisement for Volvo automobiles, an ultrasound
image takes up the larger part of the page (figure 5.4). The photograph
has calibrated lines on either side, with technical abbreviations at the top
of the page. On the left side of the page, these notations refer to the sex
and age of the embryo, while on the right, they refer to the calibration
and depth of the instrument (and remain somewhat mystifying to the
layperson). In a wavy, conical shaft of light, the fetus floats beatifically,
while the text below reads: "Is something inside telling you to buy a
Volvo?" The hail in this advertisement is seemingly pitched to the pregnant woman, but it is structured through advice given from both internal
and external hierarchies mediated through technology. The technologically generated image of the fetus "tells" her to buy a Volvo, while the

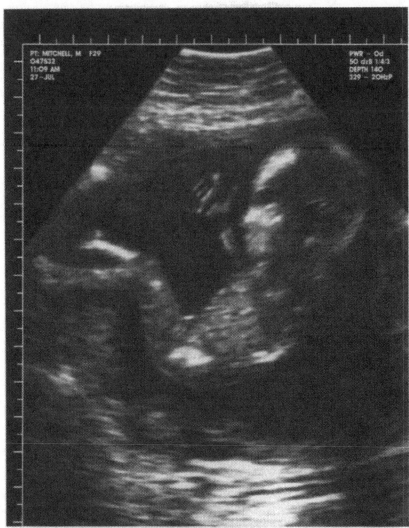

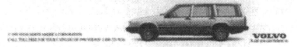

Figure 5.4   Volvo advertisement. Used by permission of Volvo Cars of North America.

safety record of the technologically advanced automobile also demands her attention.

The reinforcement of hierarchy and the consequent erasure of the pregnant female body has proved a formidable weapon in the hands of the New Right. The disappearance of the pregnant body renders female and male contributions to reproduction equivalent. For example, "The Miracle of Life" and both *Life* magazine articles begin with the apocryphal meeting of the egg and the sperm—a narrative that is structured in terms of the numerous, active sperm versus the singular, "mysterious celestial body" of the egg. The foregrounding of the sperm's quantity and activity serves to also homologize the contributions of female and male to the process of reproduction. Biological reproduction is reduced to the contribution of genetic material, the contribution of labor by the male is emphasized through the centrality of erection and ejaculation, and the female body is reduced to a single, passive ovum that waits patiently for her rendezvous. Erasing the female body, in other words, also functions to erase her contribution in terms of labor to human reproduction: nine months of labor. If reproduction is also reduced to the contribution of genetic material, further credibility is given to the "rights" of men not only in the decision to terminate a pregnancy, but in areas of child support and custody as well.

The process of naturalization, in which the fetus exists in an ideological and historical vacuum, diverts attention from material bodies, from questions about the economic situation of pregnant women, and their access to basic needs like food, shelter, and health care. The embryo/fetus exists in a nowhere land—it miraculously receives shelter and food. It exists in an environment somehow immune to racism, sexism, and economic violence—an environment without borders or boundaries. In protecting this "endangered species," the New Right can override and dismiss the material needs of the female bodies that house these cosmonauts, as well as the needs of children and their families. While the fetus needs "protection" (a thinly disguised alibi for controlling women), it doesn't ask for capital.

The "protection" proffered by the New Right also dovetails with their representational practices and strategies around issues of structural and systemic oppression. In terms of pro-life platforms, reverse discrimination arguments, welfare benefits, and so forth, the displacement of responsibility for oppression onto the oppressed has been achieved through metonymic shifts in which the New Right claims to represent the truly oppressed. Consequently, in this paternalistic maneuver, they speak for the fetus in the abortion debates, for the disenfranchised white man, for the taxpayers exploited by the alleged hordes of welfare frauds, for the citizens of

Kuwait, and for those supporters of "traditional, democratic" values silenced by the "politically correct."[33]

Haraway describes this as "a political semiotics of representation," in which "permanently speechless, forever requiring the services of a ventriloquist, never forcing a recall vote, in each case the object or ground of representation is the realization of the representative's fondest dream." Within this "political semiology of representation, nature and the unborn are even better, epistemologically, than subjugated human adults," because they can be thoroughly disarticulated from their surroundings or environment: "Everything that used to surround and sustain the represented object, such as pregnant women and local people, simply disappears or re-enters the drama as agonist."[34] The fetus hangs suspended in never-never land, for instance, while the World Wildlife Federation markets a line of silk ties (manufactured in Taiwan, no less) with prints of endangered species on them. In such scenarios, "one set of entities becomes the environment, often threatening, of the represented object. The only actor left is the spokesperson, the one who represents."[35] In terms of New Right politics, what scenario could possibly be more desirable than a world in which the only actor is the father?

What are the implications of this reinscription of paternal authority for feminist activism and theory? What potential interventions might be made, either in terms of representation or political engagements? At a recent lecture entitled "Feminism and Postmodernism: Another View," Mary Poovey described the tenuous status of women's reproductive rights as being produced by a relatively new phenomenon.[36] The problem, according to Poovey, resulted from the traditional exclusion of women from a humanist subject position that now uneasily co-exists with the partial inclusion of women in the humanist subject position forced by the feminization of the labor force. Consequently, women are held accountable to the rationality underlying humanism, while at the same time, their ability to reproduce and the traditional links between nature, femininity, and irrationality make this impossible. Although I agree with Poovey that the problem is imbrication within a humanist paradigm, her claim that gender is the primary node of oppression, which thereby "masks other hierarchies," occludes two central points. First, only certain women and men are accorded humanist subject positions under the law: others continue to be Others, that is, excluded from "humanity" by virtue of class or race. And second, what we are witnessing is a unique development: women are excluded altogether from enjoying legal rights because of the looming, newly emergent humanist subject *par excellence*—the fetus.

And here, as Poovey also pointed out, the rhetoric of "choice" becomes intensely problematic. At this point in time, feminist theorists are aware of the racial, class-based, and gender-related constraints on the discourse of choice. In regard to pregnancy and the cultural imperative for biological mothering, the notion of choice is even further complicated. As Stanworth puts it, "none of us is free in our choices until it is possible to say aloud without fear of censure, 'I don't wish to have children.' "[37] Until that time, the project is, as in the case of ecofeminism, situating the embryo/fetus *in vivo* rather than *in vitro*, as well as locating pregnant women themselves *in vivo*, understanding the ideological and material constraints on agency within specific sets of circumstances, all the time working toward an expansion of options.

Feminists have invested a great deal in theorizing mothering as work women do (but not necessarily reducible to biology) within the context of a particular social order, but they have been loath to discuss pregnancy as work women may, or may not, choose to undertake. Put bluntly, at this particular historical moment, only "women" can carry out the work that is pregnancy. Furthermore, as long as this specific laborer remains invisible, the discourse of fetal autonomy is going to be difficult to overcome. Like Poovey's, my argument hinges upon a "political resuscitation of feminism" that can only be enabled by an engagement with technoscience and questions of postmodernity, rather than withdrawal into an imaginary, nostalgic environment that depends upon appeals to traditional gender arrangements. Like Stanworth, I believe that

> it is not at all clear what a "natural" relationship to our fertility, our reproductive capacity, would look like—and it is even less clear that it would be desirable. The defense of motherhood that we ultimately construct [as well as that of pregnancy] will be stronger if we resist the temptation to use nature as a territory on which to stake our claims.[38]

The options are neither a pro- nor anti-natalist approach, but a negotiation between the two that could utilize both the critiques and positive aspects of mothering.

Poovey's call for a non-humanist subject position, for the cyborg, seems strangely out of sync with the contemporary political situation and climate. Haraway has repeatedly invoked the cyborg subject position as one in which traditionally patrolled and policed boundaries and borders have broken down in the face of late capitalism. The cyborg subject position "results from and leads to interruption, diffraction, reinvention. It is dangerous and replete with the promises of monsters."[39] "There is," further, "no drive in cyborgs to produce total theory, but there is an intimate experience of boundaries, their construction and deconstruction."[40] We are already witnessing a moment in which such constructions and deconstructions of boundaries are occurring. Heterosexual sex is no longer the prerequisite for fertilization and pregnancy. Lesbians and single women who want to bear children have taken matters into their own hands, so to speak, and have been successful in fertilizing themselves without medical or legal intervention. The proliferation of definitions of "mother" is at once a site of intensifying oppression and of potential liberation.[41]

On the other hand, it seems to me that a cyborg has arrived on the scene with a vengeance, but it is a cyborg created out of circumstances distinctly not of our choosing and a cyborg that, in what might be construed as the apex of anti-essentialist thought, threatens to completely overwhelm material female bodies, in favor of hegemonic forces. For the fetus is indeed "the illegitimate offspring of militarism and patriarchal capitalism,"[42] from the military origins of the sonogram in the SONAR (an acronym for "sound navigation and ranging") used to detect submarines in World War I, to the militaristic exploits of the embryo/fetus.

In the face of this, feminists might want to take on the long overdue question of pregnancy. The most difficult task ahead lies in disarticulating the pregnant body from the maternal body. And although feminists must insist that pregnancy is not identical with mothering, they must also insist that both are "biosocial" experiences—that pregnancy, like mothering, is something that occurs within a specific social, economic, cultural, and historical environment and that the experience of pregnancy, as such, is structured by social relations. It is work that women may not, or may, decide to undertake. What is at stake in this framework is not reducible to "choice," but inclusion in decision-making processes that affect women's health and economic circumstances. Pregnancy, thus situated, in and of itself is neither a good nor a bad thing. It only acquires a positive or negative valence within a very specific set of circumstances. A contextualization of pregnancy that functioned in this way would also enable feminists to argue vehemently for prenatal care and day care at the same time that they argued for abortion rights.

I doubt that most feminists of my generation will live to see the cyborg's utopic "elsewhere," although I sense that many of us are explicitly working toward that possibility. In the meantime, in a world where so much exploitation depends upon the erasure of the oppressed and is sustained by the illusion that the postmodern, and the borderless, realm of privilege is the real, the promise of monsters and of the cyborg should not blind us to the cyborgs being forced upon us. Perhaps the first step toward a more just social order is the exposure of the borders that continue to exclude, condemn, and execute. Only when these are visible, as well as the logic that promotes them, can the contiguities and interconnections be productively orchestrated.

Notes

I would like to thank Mary Ann Doane, Keya Ganguly, and Elizabeth Terzakis for patiently wading through several drafts of this essay. The students who participated in my "Reinscribing the Feminine" seminar at Brown University were enthusiastic and crucial collaborators in the writing of this text.

1. "Harriet," *The Black Unicorn* (New York: W. W. Norton and Company, 1978) 21.
2. *Abortion and Woman's Choice: The State, Sexuality and Reproductive Freedom* (Boston: Northeastern University Press, 1990) 286. This essay is further indebted to Petchesky's "Foetal Images: The Power of Visual Culture in the Politics of Reproduction," in *Reproductive Technologies: Gender, Motherhood and Medicine*, ed. Michelle Stanworth (Minneapolis: University of Minnesota Press, 1978) 57-80.
3. Because the term "articulation" has been used in cultural studies with an increasing lack of specificity, it seems necessary to provide a definition, as well as distinguish between the political position I want to stake out and that of post-Marxists working in the tracks of Ernesto Laclau and Chantal Mouffe's *Hegemony and Socialist Strategy: Towards a Radical Democratic Politics* (New York: Verso, 1990). In "On Postmodernism and Articulation," *Journal of Communication Inquiry* 10.2 (Summer 1986): 53, Stuart Hall speaks of articulation as "the form of the connection that *can* make a unity which is not necessary, determined, absolute and essential for all time. You have to ask, under what circumstances *can* a connection be forged or made?" Although I have found the term articulation a useful one in analyzing how connections are formed into naturalized unities, I am also concerned about the more voluntarist applications of the term. The belief that the Left can merely wander about, articulating at will and, moreover, producing articulations that are purged of their historical resonances, seems a particularly inane and impoverished version of political opposition.
4. "Containing Women: Reproductive Discourse in the 1980s," in *Technoculture*, ed. Constance Penley and Andrew Ross (Minneapolis: University of Minnesota Press, 1991) 27-30.
5. Technically, the fertilized egg is defined as an "embryo" until the end of the eighth week, when it becomes a "fetus." This distinction, reserved for mammals, is based on the formation of bone cells. However, in terms of both technical and

popular discourses, this distinction is not, as Patricia Spallone observes in *Beyond Conception: The New Politics of Reproduction* (Granby, MA: Bergin and Garvey Publishers, 1986) 50, "and never has been, fixed. Usage varies depending on the context, individual preference, or convention." In most cases, the "embryo" has disintegrated in favor of the "fetus." Where there is some ambiguity about the chronological status of the fertilized egg, however, I use the term "embryo/fetus."

6. Susan Faludi's *Backlash: The Undeclared War Against American Women* (New York: Crown Publishers, 1991) contains an extremely thorough and well-documented analysis of the development and deployment of such shifts during the eighties.

7. The film's plot devolves around the murder of the male character: a macho, sexist man who is murdered by three ex-lovers. He is given the opportunity to return to life in order to redeem himself, but he has to locate one woman who loves him. In a rather banal complication (characteristic of Blake Edwards's films), he returns as a woman.

8. Hartouni 43.

9. Faludi 433.

10. If Carder had not been a white middle-class woman, would the case have made it to the headlines (as well as the story line in an episode of *L.A. Law*)? Further research is obviously necessary around the racial and class breakdown of court-imposed caesareans and fetal neglect cases over the past decade. Because court-imposed caesareans would logically result from access to prenatal care (and the ability to pay for it), I suspect that where court-imposed caesareans will involve middle-class women, fetal neglect cases will largely be aimed at poor women, many of whom are women of color. This paradoxically underscores the convergence of the legal and medical systems as repressive state apparatuses. On the one hand, pregnant middle-class women are subjected to surveillance and intervention while under medical "supervision," while on the other hand, poor women are punished for not having, or heeding, the advice of medical providers. The extent to which this further involves racist premium placed on "white" babies should also be subjected to scrutiny.

11. Katha Pollitt, " 'Fetal Rights': A New Assault on Feminism," *The Nation* (26 March 1990): 409.

12. While the analogy might be extended to "a battle between the states," in which abortion is prohibited in one state, but available in a neighboring state, the program does not deal with the ramifications of this.

13. Hartouni 51.

14. This title derives from the *Nova* special, "The Miracle of Life" (1983), which at one point describes in great detail "the penetrating *tail* of the sperm."

15. The technology used to shoot these photographs, to represent the embryo as patient, is called "endoscopy," or "intrauterine fetal visualization." It began to be utilized in the 1950s, according to Ann Oakley in *The Captured Womb: A History of the Medical Care of Pregnant Women* (New York: Basil Blackwell, 1986) 171,

"when Westin (1954) introduced into the cervical canals of pregnant women an instrument called an endoscope." With advances in microscope technology, "fetoscopy" eventually gave way to fetal surgery in 1981. Ironically, the benign procedure represented in the *Life* essays is actually a highly invasive procedure involving not only an array of other technology, but drugs as well: "Ultrasound is used to determine placental size and fetal position and lie; and, if fetal movements obstruct the view, diazepam (valium) may be used to sedate him or her. If the fetoscopist is unable to see the desired bit of the fetus, then the fetus may be 'manipulated' into view" (Oakley 172). For more on this and related technologies, see Oakley's "Getting to Know the Fetus," in *The Captured Womb*.

16. Before the early days of ultrasound imaging, obstetricians and gynecologists designated pregnancy as "the commonest abdominal tumour in women" (Oakley 159). Ultrasound, in terms of the ideological management of motherhood, became a strategy for educating women to be better mothers:

> When a mother undergoes ultrasound scanning of the fetus, this seems a great opportunity to meet her child socially and in this way, one hopes, to view him [*sic*] as a companion rather than as a parasite. . . . Doctors and technicians scanning mothers have a great opportunity to enable mothers to form an early affectionate bond to their child by demonstrating the child to the mother. This should help mothers to behave concernedly toward the fetus. (Dewsbury 1980, 481, cited in Oakley 185.)

17. Virtually all of the intrauterine fetal visualizations circulating in popular culture have been produced by Lennart Nilsson, whose other texts include *A Child is Born* (1977) and *The Body Victorious* (1987). In a *Life* magazine interview (August 1990) with David Van Biema, entitled "Master of an 'Unbelievable, Invisible World,' " Nilsson professed amazement at the manner in which his work has been taken up in the United States and its relation to the issue of abortion. When asked when life begins, Nilsson replied, "I cannot tell you. If I told you only ten days, or two days, or forty days, it would be wrong. It would. Look at the pictures. I am not the man who shall decide when human life started. I am a reporter. I am a photographer." To this disavowal, he added, "Maybe the first moment of human life, it starts with a kiss" (46).

18. As Hartouni notes, the personification of technology—as in endoscopes that can "peer"—is characteristic of the masking of scientific interest. Endoscopes don't peer—scientists do and they do for a particular set of ideologically charged reasons and not merely out of some disinterested notion of "scientific curiosity."

19. That arousal is framed only in terms of male pleasure is another marker of the sexist ideologies at work. The program discusses and represents the process whereby the penis becomes erect in extensive and graphic detail: not only is this turgid phenomenon witnessed from within the penis itself, but the spectator is treated to a number of exterior angles. Female sexual arousal, in contrast, is men-

tioned only once, in very general terms, and the extent of its visual representation (after a throw-away reference to the multiplicity of human erogenous zones) is limited to a single close-up of a heavily made-up, blinking female eye.

20. The historical resonance of figurings of the sperm as self-contained entity and the ovum as passive oven (from Aristotle onwards) are usefully examined by Emily Martin in *The Woman in the Body* (Boston: Beacon Press, 1987), as well as in her "The Egg and the Sperm: How Science Has Constructed a Romance Based on Stereotypical Male-Female Roles," in *Signs* 16 (Spring 1991).

21. The term "fetal viability" also bears further unpacking and feminist analysis. The term implies that suddenly, miraculously, a fetus is capable of autonomous existence, which serves to obscure the vast array of technology and medical intervention required to sustain such a fetus. Obviously, this comes at quite a cost, both financially and psychologically.

22. I am grateful to Meredith Kolodner for discussions about the constructedness of the photographic layout of *Life*, as well as to Lisa Billowitz for sharing her experiences as an escort at the Broad Street Clinic in Cranston, Rhode Island.

23. October 1991.

24. Hartouni 30.

25. "Birth Pangs: Conceptive Technologies and the Threat to Motherhood," in *Conflicts in Feminism*, ed. Marianne Hirsch and Evelyn Fox Keller (New York: Routledge, 1990) 289.

26. *The Dialectic of Sex: The Case for a Feminist Revolution* (New York: William Morrow and Company, 1970) 226.

27. *The Kristeva Reader*, ed. Toril Moi (New York: Columbia University Press, 1986) 177.

28. Stanworth 296-297.

29. Oakley 183.

30. Spallone 17.

31. Donna Haraway, "The Promises of Monsters: A Regenerative Politics for Inappropriate/d Others," in *Cultural Studies*, ed. Larry Grossberg, Cary Nelson, and Paula Treichler (New York: Routledge, 1991) 323.

32. Haraway 324.

33. For an incisive and provocative reading of the manner in which such a protection scenario played out in the Persian Gulf War see Susan Jeffords's "Rape and the New World Order" in *Cultural Critique* (Fall 1991).

34. Haraway 311-312.

35. Haraway 312.

36. A version of this lecture appears in *Feminists Theorize the Political*, ed. Judith Butler (New York: Routledge, forthcoming, 1992).

37. Stanworth 291.

38. An example of the effects of basing a defense on the "natural" is the natural childbirth movement, which began in the early seventies. Its benefits resulted in an increased range of options for some women, but as Elizabeth Terzakis aptly put

it in a conversation with me, in terms of economics, availability of "natural" child-birth is rather "like organic tomatoes . . . only spottily available and costs money." Moreover, many of the premises of "natural" childbirth also connect to arguments about the "safety" and "health" of the fetus, again subsuming women's rights beneath those of the fetus. I call this the cult of macho childbirth, in which women feel pressured to undergo unnecessary pain in the interests of the fetus.

39. Haraway 333.

40. Donna Haraway, "A Manifesto for Cyborgs: Science, Technology, and Socialist Feminism in the 1980s," in *Coming to Terms: Feminism, Theory, Politics*, ed. Elizabeth Weed (New York: Routledge, 1989) 204.

41. Thomas Laqueur's "The Facts of Fatherhood" in *Conflicts in Feminism* offers not only a provocative and important call for feminist attention to the category of "fatherhood," but an excellent and detailed reading of a number of custody cases involving the proliferation of "mothers."

42. Haraway, "A Manifesto for Cyborgs," 176.

6

Fetal Exposures

Abortion Politics and Optics of Allusion

▶ Over the course of the last decade, the grammar and culture of abortion have been profoundly refigured. Although a variety of factors have converged to produce this refiguration, among the most pivotal has been the increased public presence of the fetus. The circulation of fetal images by anti-abortion forces, the routine use of ultrasonography in monitoring pregnancy and labor, the development of widely publicized, culturally valorized, medical techniques in the area of fetal therapy and repair have together worked to shift the terms in which abortion is now framed, understood, experienced, and spoken even by those who champion "choice."

In this essay, through a close reading of a 1991 video called *S'Aline's Solution*, I explore some of the ways in which the public presence of the free-floating fetal form has fundamentally reshaped both the perceptions and practices that constitute abortion, as well as the parameters of contemporary debate. Produced and directed by video artist Aline Mare, this nine-minute video offers an account of one woman's struggle to come to terms with an aborted pregnancy. It depicts a moment of refusal, and seeks a certain redemption in the longing and loss that follow that moment.

The video speaks, as we shall see, in what is a distinctly post-1980s idiom with respect to abortion, deploying many of the same visual and rhetorical strategies used by prolife activists throughout the last decade to tell its story of loss, even as it also claims to affirm in that telling a "pro-choice" position. Thus, for example, the video's primary mode of visual argumentation is rooted in the authoritative power of science and medicine. In this respect, the piece is clearly reminiscent of *The Silent Scream*, a 1984 National Right-to-Life production that claimed to show a real-time ultrasound abortion from the point of view of a 12-week-old fetus. Indeed, like *The Silent Scream*, *S'Aline's Solution* appears to present a medical event or at least the biological facts of the matter that is abortion, beginning with the penetration and occupation of the "natural body." In much the same way as any of the many PBS or National Geographic specials on the wondrous workings of the human body might begin—by bringing present but hidden processes to light—the video extends our vision, technologically, beyond the everyday apparent through the use of prosthetic imaging devices: we enter a body and subsequently witness what appears to be the initiation of a second-trimester abortion, a saline abortion. In succeeding frames, we encounter the fetus in various stages of development and, in the end, are spectators to its final expulsion. The question is whether the story of struggle this video sets out to tell can be heard in the terms in which it is told. Can what are, in effect, prolife representations, meanings, and practices be (re)appropriated and oppositionally inflected to tell precisely the kind of story their deployment has otherwise worked to silence? What social, historical, cultural, and ideological terrain does the video's narrative ultimately contain and contest as well as inhabit and produce? In what respects does the "prochoice" stance it claims and articulates make sense and what does the "sense" it "makes" in the end tell us about the contemporary grammar and culture of abortion?

With the video's opening sequence, we travel up a long canal-like aperture at a slow and deliberate pace, indeed, a pace that accentuates the drama of our presence in, and encounter with, a region only recently opened for public tours—the irreducibly natural, incontestably given, seemingly "real" body, the body in all of its irreducible, functional glory (figure 6.1). And we travel, at least initially, without being told either where we are or where we are going. Nor do we know in whose body, and by whose spon-

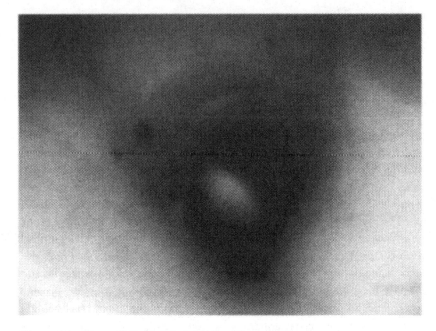

Figure 6.1   From *S'Aline's Solution* (Aline Mare, 1991).

sorship, this high-tech expedition is taking place. That we are sponsored we can be certain—for one never simply or casually crashes these borders, traverses the boundaries between inside and out, penetrates and occupies biospace on a lark. Any expedition upon which we might set out will be authorized and highly supervised—we will need an interpreter, in any event, someone or some way to decipher what it is we are and will be seeing (figure 6.2).

The video's title works, to some extent, to orient us and so too its audio, a persistent bass drone that is reminiscent of Hitchcock—foreboding, suspenseful, anxiety-inducing. Together, they establish a climate of expectation; indeed, both call into play a series of assumptions that initiate the narrative and allow this opening image to mean. Clearly, we are entering a particular social text, even as we appear only to be entering a self-evidently natural or biological one. Still, we are confidently situated within the narrative only with the next series of images and the voice-over that frames them. These images seem to establish beyond doubt in whose body this excursion of discovery has been undertaken while the voice-over

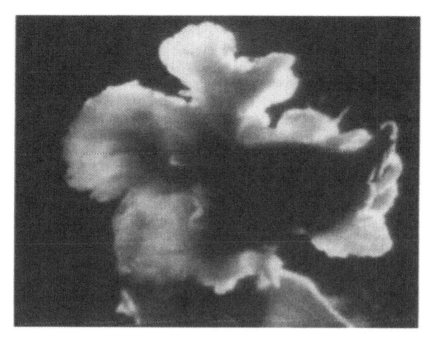

Figure 6.2   From *S'Aline's Solution* (Aline Mare, 1991).

suggests for what purposes: "*I choose, I chose, I have chosen.*" Each utterance
is set off by a woman's face, pressed against glass, wet and distorted, and
sends us tripping down the bioscape in the general vicinity of a reproductive track. Here, we witness three discrete moments in the reproductive
cycle: a follicle, hosting a ripe ovum; the ovum itself surrounded by nutri-
tive cells and water; the fimbria, or outermost fringe of the fallopian tube,
"brushing" the swollen follicle shortly before ovulation. With the assertion of a principle that has grounded feminist demands for reproductive
autonomy for over a century, but is most commonly associated with mainstream liberal struggles of the last two decades around abortion rights, this
first sequence of images is given closure: "*I choose, I chose, I have chosen*";
"*My body, my choice.*"

   The next segment of the video moves to instantiate "choice," to enact
what is an abstract value or claim through the staging of a second-
trimester abortion—a saline abortion. Rock salt falls from a hand situated
at the top of the screen in one frame, its direction reversed in the next.
This is choice reconfigured in the wake of the reproductive discourse of
the 1980s, choice that knows and speaks itself, indeed, is permitted to

speak publicly, only in the idiom of ambivalence, apprehension, and psychological perplexity. The persistent bass drone intensifies as does the sound of running water. In the event that we do not know what a saline abortion is or entails, a running text at the bottom of the screen joins with the visual text to provide us with the technical details. In fact, written text is deployed twice in this segment of the video, and serves not only to bracket a montage of images of otherwise discrete bodily processes, but to instruct us as well in their reading, even while we have been pursuing this moment since the video's opening sequence. This is its moment of truth or at least the moment when we will see revealed the truth of the matter that is abortion.

The first written text we encounter, then, initiates the abortion sequence: "*saline solution: 200 milligrams of salt and water injected into the uterus causing violent contractions within minutes*"; while the second written text closes it: "*sodium chloride . . . salt preserver . . . salt destroyer.*" Between these two moments, we find ourselves positioned once again within the body, spectators to an apparent real-time abortion from what we are encouraged to infer is the unmediated view of the victim. We see first a grainy, undulating mass of blue liquid followed by the eruption of bodily fluids: the discharge of a thick, white substance through porous tissue, muscle in spasms, the flow of what looks like the same white substance, the saline solution, through a narrow tunnel-like opening, and then once again, the mass of blue liquid. While these images are not in themselves either violent or traumatic, their organization, rapid pace of presentation, and curiously alien character foster the impression that something both violent and traumatic, alien and distinctly "unnatural," has just taken place. This impression is encouraged by both of the written texts—we are prepared to see violent contractions and salt destroy—as well as by the posture of the woman in whose body we imagine this abortion to be taking place, the same woman who appeared earlier behind glass. She is now lying on her back, eyes pinched closed, writhing in what seems to be a pain-induced dreamstate. Rock salt falls on her face like snow, while mournful groans grow in pitch and overcome the droning music. The camera closes in on her features and fixes our gaze in a studied, lingering look typically reserved for lovers. The screen then goes blank.

The uneasy intimacy into which we have been drawn is broken by the sound of a child's laughter and the image of an 18-week- old fetus floating before us, intact and presumably in utero. "In the face of th[is] portrait of fetal tranquility, the spectre of bodily dismemberment strikes an especially powerful chord";[1] indeed, we cannot help but wonder whether this is the fetus whose death it is we have just seen initiated. "*Sh, baby,*" a voice coos, "*baby sh.*"

In this third and last segment of the video, we are transported into the world of the imaginary—a world of tortured desire and festering loss, of fractured and distorted meanings. And yet, it is also a world not easily distinguished from the one produced in and through contemporary medical-scientific discourse under the sign of the real, or the one occupied by prolife advocates in public discourse and debate over the meaning of abortion. Our loss of bearings is immediate and profound. There are the images themselves: these are the work of Swedish photojournalist Lennart Nilsson and are appropriated—as is all of the video's bioscape imagery—from *Nova*'s "Miracle of Life." Under the auspices of science, this award-winning documentary purports to unveil not only the mysteries of conception, gestation, and birth, but by implication, their essential or self-evident, if also somewhat opaque, meanings, as if the camera itself were simply a vehicle for the transmission of natural truths and Nilsson, a privileged scribe.[2] And then there is the use to which these and other similar images have been put over the course of the last decade. Nilsson's "full color fetal portraits"[3] have been widely circulated by prolife activists as vivid visual evidence of what these activists regard as the biological facts of fetal life—facts that have been substantiated, or so they argue, by the new science of fetology and that reveal beyond reasonable challenge the specifically and self-evidently human quality of that life, its autonomy and identity as an innocent, vulnerable, and unique pre-formed human being, a miniature version of you or me.[4] The fetus when viewed is now heard to speak a truth about itself, indeed, in this video is heard, literally, to speak its potential or speak as it might at three or four or five through laughter. But no image is self-evidently what it is, no meaning a simple matter of natural fact brought to light, as in the case of the fetal form, by scientific advances in either fetology or fiber optics. If the fetal form speaks, it is because that form is itself a densely constructed figure of speech—a figure in and through which is condensed and articulated a full range of historically, culturally, and ideologically embedded values, assumptions, claims, and contests. As such, its meaning cannot be suspended by fiat nor easily reinflected. While the concluding segment of the video may attempt to construct the imaginary both within and against the rhetoric of the fetal image to tell a story of refusal and regret, in the end that story gives way to another, more potent, public tale of self-mutilation and murder.

In the video's last segment, then, a child's laughter, along with the image of an 18-week-old fetus raising its hand in an attempt to shield itself

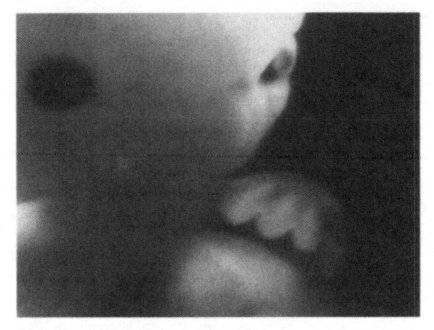

Figure 6.3   From *S'Aline's Solution* (Aline Mare, 1991).

from our peering gaze, stage our entrance into a world of condensed and contorted meanings. The image of the fetus becomes the image of a woman, again behind glass, sucking water as does fetal life in utero, her features wet and distorted. Banter begins of the sort one might hear between a mother and child—and yet, the affectionate playfulness we generally associate with such banter assumes rather sadistic overtones after what we believe we have just witnessed: "*I hear you,*" a woman's voice taunts, "*I see you. Bye-Bye, Baby*" (figure 6.3). This time, the image of a 7-week-old fetus, fifteen times its actual size, fills the screen before us, its hand moving as if to wave. "*Child of my imagination,*" the narrative continues, "*you will never be child. Flesh of my flesh, you will never be flesh.*" The image of the 7-week-old fetus is transformed into its 18-week-old counterpart, which in turn becomes the woman behind glass. We are dispatched to the moment of conception as sperm cluster about an ovum, spectators to creation and the creation story contained within it—the division of the original flesh and its subsequent corruption through an assertion of will. "*Dismember, disintegrate, dissolve*" a voice instructs, and thus is marked our fall both figuratively and literally.

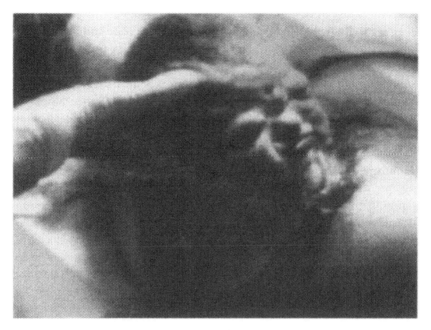

Figure 6.4   From *S'Aline's Solution* (Aline Mare, 1991).

With this imperative, we are forced downward through the passage that was our entry into the exotic interiors of biospace, expelled from the body even as we become spectators to an expulsion, a live birth that is nevertheless not one. Labored breathing attends our passage. *"These are dangerous times,"* we are told, and although we might wonder precisely for whom they are dangerous, the visual text leaves little room for question. A fetus/baby emerges into surgically gloved hands, hands which will also appear in the next several frames to reverse their action and assist as the body draws this disappearing life back into itself: *"a memory of flesh."* We see a woman lying on her back, writhing in pain and, finally, salt rock floating once again upward through water into a hand positioned at the top of the screen. With the iteration of a feminist politics now rendered parody, our excursion of discovery ends: *"My body . . . my choice . . . my childlessness"* (figure 6.4).

What makes this video make the sense it makes? What social, historical, cultural, and ideological spaces does it inhabit and produce? The program notes that accompanied at least one screening of *S'Aline's Solution* describe it as "affirm[ing] a prochoice stance while acknowledging the loss incurred in an aborted pregnancy."[5] Audiences of mixed race and gender have nevertheless found the piece both disturbing and confusing, and have tended, in post-screening discussions, to divide, more or less generationally, around one of two readings in their accounts as to why. Slightly older viewers, for example, do not recognize the stance the video adopts as "prochoice" in any substantive or meaningful sense, and point to the dissonance that is produced by the spoken, visual, and audio texts. The rhetoric of the images, along with the sense of suspense and impending doom invoked by the sound track together collide with and ultimately subvert the ostensibly prochoice rhetoric that initiates and closes the action. In addition, there is the "discourse of loss" that the piece articulates in and through the fetal form. Within the current culture of abortion, "loss" or its absence has been deployed to reframe the meaning of the practice and, in effect, function as arguments against abortion even when invoked within a prochoice context. Recall for the moment the "emergence" in the early 1980s of "post abortion stress syndrome," a condition said to afflict women, in some cases years after an abortion, and whose vast range of indications include guilt, remorse, despair, withdrawal, a sense of helplessness, a preoccupation with babies, self-destructive behavior, diminished powers of reason, diminished work capacity, anger, rage, hostility, and child abuse. Although this "condition" has thus far escaped the classificatory efforts of public and private health officials, it continues to capture the public imagination at least in part because it allays popular fears and anxieties with respect to what have been dramatic shifts in the organization of sexuality, parenthood, reproduction, and the family over the last two decades. While women may subvert their essential nature as women, the syndrome seems to suggest, nature nevertheless persists—although fetal life may be denied, maternal instincts or "the longings and aspirations of motherliness," as former Surgeon General C. Everett Koop put it, seem clearly to endure.[6] On the other hand, women who experience no sense of loss or remorse following an aborted pregnancy, while initially construed within popular discourse and debate early in the decade as callous, hard, selfish, capricious, or "unwomanly," were instead depicted by the late 1980s as maternally illiterate or simply ignorant about the true nature of fetal life.[7] This could be corrected, it was argued, through ultrasound imaging, the assumption being that after having viewed the fetus she was carrying, a woman would realize its essential or true nature as a preborn child, bond with it, and forgo her abortion.[8]

Despite authorial claims to the contrary, therefore, somewhat older viewers tended to read *S'Aline's Solution* as a prolife text. In contrast to this reading, a younger, second set of college-age viewers—viewers who came of age in Reagan's America or during a period that saw the culture of abortion profoundly transformed—tended to find the video's multi-textual renderings of both the meaning and implications of abortion unproblematic and unproblematically prochoice. What these viewers found troubling was the act of abortion itself, *given* its meaning and implications. While necessary, abortion is as the video, in their reading, accurately depicts it as being: violent and dangerous, a disruption of "natural" biological processes that naturally disturbs psychological ones and produces confusion, remorse, guilt, and despair. Curiously, however, such suffering was construed by these viewers not only or primarily as punishment, as the price women must pay, or a "residual motherliness" persisting in the absence of something to be mothered. That women might suffer the decision to terminate a pregnancy both before and after making it was read as evidence of a certain moral sensibility. Within the context of a discourse that, at least in principle, has no way of registering moral seriousness or generating moral argument—and such is the case with liberal discourse about abortion—psychological hesitation and uncertainty have come to function as their sign and substitute. Both were marshalled to counter charges heard frequently throughout the 1980s that women have abortions for reasons of convenience, and are precisely what now "legitimizes" choice in public discourse and debate. It is, then, primarily through the transposition of guilt and choice that this second, younger group of viewers apparently "resolves" what their somewhat older counterparts regard as the contradiction between the prochoice rhetoric that frames the video's visual text and the rhetoric of the text itself. The question is whether, and in what sense, such a "resolution" works to recuperate rather than reinscribe the discursive terrain prolife representations, meanings, and practices have come to dominate. Or, to put this question more generally, is it possible to reinflect signs already in circulation, as one might argue this video attempts to do, for another political end? And, with particular respect to the video, to what extent can arresting images of the fetal form floating free in space, the trope of discovery, or a particular mode of visual argumentation, rooted in the authoritative power of science and medicine, be reappropriated given that they anchor and are anchored in another set of stories having to do with the perilous plight of the prenatal iterated throughout the last decade in the streets, courts, and clinics?

Although *S'Aline's Solution* does not claim to be a "medical document," to represent the "medical reality" of abortion or the truth of natural facts as does, for example, *The Silent Scream*, an aura of medical authority, generated primarily from the images, nevertheless suffuses the text and lends it credibility. While we may query the video's politics or its broader political implications, we do not question where we have been or what we have seen, let alone how we have come to see it. We assume, and are encouraged in the assumption, that we have entered a female body and there witnessed a violent and traumatic interruption of natural processes. But, suppose it were the case, as indeed it is, that the opening sequence of the video transports us into the biospace of the genitor rather than the genetrix, and that we travel, initially, not through or along the fallopian tubes, as we might have imagined, but up the male urethra. Suppose it were the case that the sequence of images we are inclined to read as a saline abortion turn out to be ejaculation, that the white fluid we construe as the saline solution is seminal fluid, that our expulsion from the body in the concluding frames of the video is not through a birth canal, but again, through the urethra as ejaculate. Although the videomaker does not acknowledge the use of footage from *Nova*'s "Miracle of Life," all of the images of the exotic inner space of the body, as I mentioned earlier, are drawn from this production.[9] And with the exception of those images of reproductive organs unmistakably female—a swollen follicle, a ripe ovum, the outermost fringes of the fallopian tubes—it is in and through the male body that this drama of fetal life and death unfolds.

So much for the given, the unquestionable, and the self-evident. What permits us to read ejaculation as a violent, traumatic, distinctly unnatural rupture of natural processes is not only our general illiteracy with respect to the interior functioning of bodies—this is to be expected. It is our illiteracy coupled with powerful, prior notions and anxieties themselves shaped by a larger public discourse and culture of abortion about what the practice is, means, and entails. Deeply embedded assumptions about who and what women are and are for; the increased public presence of the free-floating fetal form; the construction of fetal independence and dominance, both medically, in the context of advances in the "new" science of fetology, and legally, through the aggressive implementation of fetal protection statutes; new obstetrical technologies like ultrasound, along with increasingly routinized genetic screening and subsequent shifts in the management of pregnancy and birth; the development of new reproductive technologies and their attendant discourses of female desperation and deviance; clinic bombings; the emergence of conditions like post-abortion stress syndrome; legislative and judicial struggles over abortion access; the perceived dissolution of the nuclear family; the antifeminist backlash; the production of *The Silent Scream* and such highly popular movies as *Look Who's Talking, Baby Boom, Three Men and a Baby, Alien*[3], and most recently, *The Hand That Rocks the Cradle*—all of these things together constitute the contemporary grammar and culture of abortion, and over the course of the last fifteen years have together worked a powerful restructuring of how we experience, understand, configure, and speak the practice. *S'A-line's Solution* produces, and is produced by this culture; indeed, it is this culture that allows us to connect the dots, to organize and assemble a collection of slogans and a collage of otherwise unidentifiable bodily processes in a way that creates a coherent and compelling, if also deeply disturbing, tale. It is, in the end, what enables us to tell the story we believe we are being told, what predisposes us to see in a moment of orgasmic pleasure a saline solution or final solution, genocide.

We could of course venture the telling of another story. Knowing now what the images in the video are "really" images of, that ejaculation is being deployed as the visual representation of abortion, we could embark on another excursion of discovery and attempt to rescue the narrative, force from it a certain irony, submerged logic, or set of stories perhaps more complicated, subversive, and politically clever than the story we assumed we were being told. Drawing on "subcultural" figurations of abortion as well as Old Testament allusions that riddle the narrative, we might insist that the video invites us to read against the deep structure of contemporary formulations of the dispute. It renders the female body, as much popular discourse and debate regarding abortion renders it, utterly irrelevant. In so doing, however, the video makes conspicuous the absence of this body, the gestating body, in contemporary renderings as well as its construction as both an abstraction and aberration. Within public discourse, the body that signifies and is significant, that is generative and in its generation produces both meaning and value is the (heterosexual) male body. According to biblical accounts, of course, it is the original flesh, the flesh from which all flesh originates and to which all flesh is subsequently subordinate. In the beginning there is but one flesh and it is an act of will that divides it—Eve eats from the tree of the knowledge of good and evil and is subsequently expelled from the garden along with her mate and master, Adam. Through her transgression is initiated their fall from grace and subsequent expulsion; it marks the separation of heaven and earth, the alienation of body and soul, the opposition of a flesh once one.

With the opening of the video, we enter and occupy the body of the genitor, the original flesh, only to be expelled from that body at its end as the result of choice: "*I choose, I chose, I have chosen.*" The choice that is abortion is an act of insurgence; it refuses the destiny of sperm and women's own destiny, which is derivative and dependent upon sperm for its fulfillment. It disrupts an original unity uncontaminated by sexual differentiation, disrupts the natural order of things, subverts signification, destabilizes meaning and value. It entails the dismemberment and disintegration of the generative body—indeed, mutilates the one body and produces two. In this version of the video, state-of-the-art imaging technology is deployed to tell a biblical story, the story of creation and the fall, but, shifting testaments now, also a story of possible redemption, conventionally regarded within contemporary prolife religious discourse as embodied in the figure of the fetus. While signifying women's restless agitation against a preordained natural order, the aborted fetus is also a symbol of sacrifice for prolife activists, offered for the redemption both of Man and America.[10] Recognizing her relationship with the fetus she carries, [S']Aline's solution is nevertheless to refuse its terms and thus forfeit redemption: "*my body, my choice, my childlessness.*" The sense of impending doom fostered by the auditory text both frames this refusal and tells us something about its consequences.

Now what is curious about this reading of the video is that while it remains true to the apparent truth of the images or departs from the point we assumed we were departing from originally, from the biologically given, it seems nevertheless to be more figurative, interpretive, or inferential than the drama the piece appears to present, the drama of fetal life and death. This is due, at least in part, to how conspicuous the play becomes with this alternative reading between what the images "are" and what they "mean." In order to make the visual text make sense, we are required to perform a series of translations, the obvious performance of which clearly circumscribes the persuasive force of the sense we make. Next to a story that seems simply to tell itself, to image the natural and through this imaging bring to light matters of fact, any account we might proffer, while plausible, will seem both contrived and interested, one story among many possible stories, but none of these the "real" story in some objective or self-evident sense.

The point, of course, is that both stories—the tale of innocence imperiled or of innocence lost—are densely constructed, and although the latter appears to be more obviously constructed than the former, quite the reverse is the case. Through its ostensible use of medical-scientific and visual technologies—or footage from the *Miracle of Life*—the video appears to present a biological rather than social text, the natural facts of (a saline) abortion, and acquires a certain symbolic power as a result. That we are reading the biological entirely through the lens of the social becomes obvious when we realize we have been trekking about the male reproductive track, spectators to an event we do not typically think of as either violent or traumatic. But even were this not the case, even were we "actually" situated, as we are encouraged to assume we are, in a female body, and in the general proximity of a saline abortion, we would still be mapping and reading the social. Peering technologies like ultrasound or fiber optics imaging do not simply turn the inside out, or render the opaque transparent or extend our vision to reveal the elusive secrets of nature. Technologies themselves do not peer; they are instruments and relations that facilitate or obstruct, but above all, construct "peering," indeed, instruments and relations that do not simply uncover meaning, but inscribe and enforce it.[11] Likewise "peering" is not itself a benign, impartial, disinterested, or disembodied activity, but is both mediated and situated within interpretive frameworks, points of view, and sets of purposes—how else is the body "revealed," read, or made legible to an observing eye? What we see is inseparably linked to and utterly dependent upon how we see. And, in the case of this video, how we see is, as I have been suggesting, clearly constructed in and through the contemporary discourse and culture of abortion. The issue is not what these images are "really" images of. The issue is rather "how" these images mean, what they mean, and how they have come to mean it.

Although *S'Aline's Solution* claims to represent only one woman's struggle to come to terms with an aborted pregnancy, the terms in which that struggle is figured illustrate the degree to which popular discourse and debate over the course of the last decade have profoundly transformed the perceptions and practices that together constitute abortion. In the era immediately preceding *Roe v. Wade*, "criminal prosecution, morbidity, and maternal as opposed to fetal mortality" constituted the cultural anatomy of the practice or the terms in which it was conventionally known, understood, constructed, and experienced.[12] Women struggled for control over their reproductive lives, despite legal constraints and life-threatening conditions, and many women died—indeed, women in the United States died yearly from illegal abortions in greater numbers than did U.S. soldiers in Viet Nam, and black women, eleven times more frequently than their white counterparts.[13] Throughout this era, abortion was also the privileged sign of another, always present, and constitutive, but submerged set of meanings having to do with women's sexual freedom, autonomy, and agency; notwithstanding contemporary distillations, "my body, my choice" has never been only or simply a question of protecting or expanding the procreative options of the naturally reproducing, white heterosexual body. In *Roe*, the Supreme Court chose, predictably, to circumvent the potentially more radical meanings of legalization by situating the practice within a medically defined and controlled framework. Similarly, reform groups and family planning organizations worked methodically both to contain and conceal them.[14] Clearly, however, the radical challenges potentially posed by legalized abortion to traditional gender identities and sexual relations were hardly lost on neoconservatives and their New Right and fundamentalist affiliates and, over the course of the last decade, have inflamed popular debate while themselves being recast and transformed in the process.

Thus, for example, in the presence of the fetal form and the theater of charges animating it of murder and selfishness as well as neglect and abuse, the expanded sense of freedom and power that abortion has afforded many women in allowing them to take hold of their lives is only rarely mentioned and often in a passing whisper. In the public vernacular of abortion, freedom and power have an at best pejorative resonance and function, when invoked, as a potential indictment of all women in the phantasmatic rendering of one—the casual, capricious, career-minded woman who has abandoned hearth and home and kills without conscience. Even those who champion choice have shifted registers and now speak not of freedom or power, but of dire choice and desperation. They now cast abortion as a grim and grievous practice, and the woman who has one, as either psychologically troubled and morally ambivalent, or irresponsible and promiscuous—in either case, as a victim of a regrettable if indispensable violence. Finally, within this register, "choice" too has been transfigured as the maternal body, driven by the needs and interests of others, has increasingly displaced the self-regarding sexual one as its referent. A poster at the 1989 march on Washington for abortion rights graphically depicts this shift: pictured under the boldly lettered caption "Pro-choice not Pro-abortion" and set against a black background are the lower abdomen and spread legs of a woman giving birth. An attending physician, midwife, or friend is grasping the partially emerged infant under its arms, both easing and enabling its final moments of passage. The title of the portrait is in script. It reads, "The Miracle of Birth."

Although this portrait attempts, like the video, to recuperate terrain now dominated by prolife meanings and representations by articulating what has come to be regarded as a more complex or morally textured stance with respect to "choice," in the end it reflects only their ubiquity and strength. Indeed, in the end, both video and portrait succeed only in reinscribing and fortifying these meanings, in the case of the latter, by situating the woman who is giving birth, literally, outside the frame. We see a fragment of her body, her pelvis, and only as the stage upon which a separate and determining life is enacted. She is not liberalism's bounded individual, the one who is in-divisible, who cannot be divided and, thus, the one who is able to act or exercise choice; rather, she is represented in this portrait as divided and dividing, the one who is acted upon and through.[15] Similarly, with the video, although woman and fetus are both within the visual frame, they do not share the same frame, the same body, or the same story. The fetus floats free, a discrete and separate entity, outside of, unconnected to and, by virtue of its ostensible or visual independence, in an adversarial relationship with the body and life upon which it is nevertheless inextricably dependent. It tells its own story, is an effect of power, or a figure of speech that has been both authored and authorized in the courts, clinics, and culture at large and that cannot be silenced or appropriated in the same way that women's stories and struggles are in its presence. In its presence or a context in which the image—fetus—is (mis)read and thereby constituted as the thing it signifies[16]—baby—women's stories and struggles can only be heard as thin rationalizations, "excuses," digressions, or in the case of the video, the deranged utterances of a disturbed nature.

In the end, the very terms in which this video attempts to tell its story of loss work both to indict and silence that story. For notwithstanding their general acceptance within the present culture of abortion as more scientifically informed and morally complex,[17] these terms are, nevertheless, reductive and simplifying and reflect the extent to which prolife meanings, categories, and representations have so saturated public discourse as to now seem part of the fabric of fact. For a genuinely informed and complex story of abortion to be heard, the speech that would render women speechless must be interrupted and this entails, among other things but most basically, interrupting "the visual discourse of fetal autonomy"[18]—reembodying the disembodied fetal form or resituating the gestating fetus in a uterus and the uterus in a body, thereby re-membering what is otherwise dis-membered and, as such, truly in a perilous state. Pregnancies, when they occur, occur in women's bodies; for those who champion "choice" to lose sight of this simple and obvious yet profoundly radical and consequential fact in a post-1980s struggle for reproductive freedom would be finally to surrender its possibility. If these are

dangerous times, as the narrative of the video asserts—and they are—
S'Aline's Solution could, in the end, itself be read as a striking if sobering
illustration of why.

Notes

I want to thank Roddy Reid and Gail Hershatter for reading and commenting on
early drafts of this essay. Thanks also to Lauren Crux who was an often wise and
challenging interlocutor throughout the writing of this piece on the matter and
meanings of the fetal form.

1. Sarah Franklin, "Fetal Fascinations: New Dimensions to the Medical-Scientific Construction of Fetal Personhood," *Off-Centre: Feminism and Cultural
Studies*, Sarah Franklin, Celia Lury, and Jackie Stacey, eds. (New York: Harper-
Collins, 1992) 195.
2. "The Miracle of Life," *Nova*, Swedish television production in association
with WGBH Educational Foundation (Boston: 1986).
3. The phrase is Sarah Franklin's, "Fetal Fascinations," 195.
4. For an engaging analysis of the complex rhetorical efforts entailed in generating a meaningful fetal image, see Celeste Michelle Condit, *Decoding Abortion
Rhetoric* (Chicago: University of Illinois Press, 1990) 79–92. Additional and
provocative studies include Rosalind Petchesky, "Foetal Images: The Power of
Visual Culture in the Politics of Reproduction," *Reproductive Technologies: Gender,
Motherhood, and Medicine*, Michelle Stanworth, ed. (Minneapolis: University of
Minnesota Press, 1987) 57–80; Sarah Franklin, "Fetal fascinations," 190–205;
Janelle S. Taylor, "The Public Fetus and the Family Car: From Abortion Politics to
a Volvo Advertisement," *Public Culture* 4, no. 2 (Spring 1992): 67–79; Carol Stabile,
"Shooting the Mother: Fetal Photography and the Politics of Disappearance,"
Camera Obscura, 29 (January 1992): 179–205; and Paula A. Treichler, "Medicine,
Feminism, and the Meaning of Childbirth," in *Body/Politics*, Mary Jacobus, Sally
Shuttleworth, and Evelyn Fox Keller, eds. (New York: Routledge, 1989).
5. *S'Aline's Solution* was one of six videos shown in December 1991 at the University of California, San Diego, under the auspices of a program entitled "The
Bad Body." Curated by video artist Julie Zando, and sponsored by the university's
Visual Arts department, the program featured the work of avant-garde videomak-
ers on a variety of topics within the field of body politics.
6. Cited in Rosalind Petchesky, *Abortion and Woman's Choice: The State, Sexuality, and Reproductive Freedom* (New York: Longman, 1984) 340. Koop's subsequent
report, prepared while he was U.S. Surgeon General, found no long-term psychological or physical harm.

7. For a fuller discussion of the discourse of loss and maternal illiteracy, see V. Hartouni, "Containing Women: Reproductive Discourse in the 1980's," *Technoculture*, Constance Penley and Andrew Ross, eds. (Minneapolis: University of Minnesota Press, 1991) esp. 39–47.

8. On the link between ultrasound imaging, maternal bonding, and abortion, see Joseph Fletcher and Mark Evans, "Maternal Bonding in Early Fetal Ultrasound Examinations," *New England Journal of Medicine* 308 (February 17, 1983): 392–393. I do not mean to imply in this discussion that the experience of loss some women experience following an aborted pregnancy is imagined or contrived. Rather, my point is that the public discourse of loss both simplifies and exploits the variety of women's experiences and struggles with respect to abortion—the often ambivalent and complicated feelings that attend any "serious" act—to reinscribe and enforce a narrow, ideologically biologistic understanding of gender and motherhood.

9. Or so we are led to believe. It is worth mentioning, if only in passing, that what *Nova* presents and we accept as a fantastic voyage through the exotic interiors of the natural body might be just that, "fantastic" as in phantasmagoric. Here, as with *S'Aline's Solution*, we take on faith the truth of the image and do not question where we are or what we are seeing.

10. Faye Ginsburg, "The 'Word-Made-Flesh,'" *Uncertain Terms: Negotiating Gender in American Culture*, Faye Ginsburg and Anna Lowenhaupt Tsing, eds. (Boston: Beacon Press, 1990) 68–69.

11. For especially provocative discussions of these and related issues, see Donna Haraway, "Situated Knowledges," *Simians, Cyborgs, and Women* (New York: Routledge, 1991) 183–201, and "The Promise of Monsters: A Regenerative Politics for Inappropriate/d Others," *Cultural Studies*, Lawrence Grossberg, Cary Nelson, and Paula Treichler, eds. (New York: Routledge, 1992) 295–337.

12. This point is drawn from and developed further by Rayna Rapp, "Constructing Amniocentesis: Maternal and Medical Discourses," *Uncertain Terms* 41.

13. For this statistic, see *Abortion: For Survival*, a video produced by The Fund for The Feminist Majority, 1989.

14. For a more detailed analysis of the forces and issues at play in the legalization of abortion, see Rosalind Petchesky, *Abortion and Woman's Choice*, particularly 101–133.

15. As Sarah Franklin explains, "The very term 'individual,' meaning *one who cannot be divided*, can only mean the male, as it is precisely the process of one individual becoming two which occurs through a woman's pregnancy. Pregnancy is precisely about one body becoming two bodies, two bodies becoming one, the exact antithesis of in-dividuality. This is, claims Donna Haraway, "why women have had so much trouble counting as individuals in modern western discourses. Their personal, bounded individuality is compromised by their bodies' troubling talent for making other bodies, whose individuality can take precedence over their own" (Sarah Franklin, "Fetal Fascinations," 203).

16. The recent and indiscriminate display at prolife rallies of "actual" fetal corpses alongside pictures of fetuses, both serene and gruesome, reflects and rein-

forces precisely such a misreading. Also contributing to this kind of misreading are a new series of commercials that have been aired on national television and which portray children of all ages and races—potential abortees—frolicking about in joyful play. Each commercial ends with the statement, "Life, what a beautiful choice." One particularly striking commercial in this series depicts a woman singing "Amazing Grace" in a choir. The voiceover, supposedly the woman herself, explains that she was an aborted fetus who nevertheless survived the attempt on her life. Speaking as a postnatal fetus on behalf of her prenatal counterparts, she cautions viewers about making the same mistake that was made with respect to her.

17. The argument goes something like this: since the Supreme Court handed down its ruling in *Roe v. Wade*, knowledge about the nature of fetal life as well as technological interventions to support that life have advanced dramatically, thus forcing the already complicated range of moral questions entailed in the practice of choice to be fundamentally refigured. That we increasingly treat the fetus as person/patient is generally thought to have something to do with these advances revealing its "true" or "essential" nature as such. As I have been both suggesting and implying throughout this essay, however, fetal personhood is not a "property" that can or will be "discovered" with greater scientific knowledge or increased technological capabilities, but is produced in and through the very practices that claim merely to "reveal" it.

18. The phrase is Sarah Franklin's; see "Fetal Fascinations" 196.

7

Mothers and Authors

Johnson v. Calvert and the New Children of Our Imaginations

What is a mother? Who is the mother of a child when one woman provides the ovum for fertilization and another carries the baby to term? This was the issue before the California Supreme Court in 1993 in the surrogate mother case of *Johnson v. Calvert*.[1] Faced with these conflicting biological claims, the court shifted its inquiry from the physical to the mental realm. Who had first intended to bring the child into the world? Who was the "originator of the concept" of the child? But in formulating the issue in this manner, the court was, as one justice pointed out, implicitly invoking the paradigm of intellectual property law—the owner of a creative work is the originator or author of it—and this amounted, the dissenting justice argued, to the treatment of a child as property.

Johnson v. Calvert is an extraordinarily resonant case. It echoes King Solomon's famous judgment when confronted with two women who each claimed to be the mother of a child, and it also echoes Athena's judgment in *The Eumenides* when she rules that Orestes is not related to his mother

Clytemnestra. It raises questions about our understanding of the relationship between nature and technology, and it challenges conventional
assumptions about gender and reproduction—how exactly is a woman's
role in reproduction different from a man's?—and about the nature of
kinship. Moreover, like the famous *Baby M* case in New Jersey a few years
earlier,[2] it raises questions about whether recent developments in reproductive technology are leading to a new form of the commodification of
human beings. As one jurist remarked, the case interrogates "our collective understanding of what it means to be human."[3] What principally
interests me in this essay, however, is the significance of the court's resort
to the model of intellectual property law to resolve the conflicting claims
and the implicit equation of mothers and authors.

As I have discussed elsewhere, the modern representation of the author
as the originator and proprietor of a special commodity, the work, was
formed in England in the course of the eighteenth century in part through
the blending of a Lockean discourse of property with the eighteenth-cen-
tury discourse of original genius.[4] What emerged by the early nineteenth
century was the figure of the romantic author, the notion of the author as
a creative man who by virtue of imposing the imprint of his unique personality on his original works makes them his own. This notion provides
the paradigm and reference point for intellectual property law. Historically, copyright has been an expansive, imperial doctrine, forever conquering new territory in the name of the author. Very early in its history
protection was extended from printed texts to engravings and to printed
music. In the nineteenth century, in a decisive moment, protection was
extended to photography. By today the flag of authorship has been raised
over pictorial and graphic works of most kinds, including architectural
plans and buildings, commercial advertisements, labels, and fabric designs;
over sculptural works, including dolls, toys, and jewelry; and over all sorts
of dramatic works, including pantomimes and choreographed dances.
Sound recordings are protected, as are musical works; game and contest
rules are copyrightable; and so are computer programs, which have been
called "silicon epics" and which are regarded by the law as no less works of
authorship than poems or novels. Characters such as Superman or Donald
Duck are protected, too, even apart from the contexts in which they
appear; and in some jurisdictions the public image or persona of an individual such as Groucho Marx or Vanna White is also a property that is
protectable and that can be willed to one's heirs.[5] Likewise, under patent
law it is possible to establish property rights in biological materials such as
cell lines—in a famous recent case the Regents of the University of Cali-

fornia established ownership in a cell line derived from a medical patient's spleen without his consent[6]—or even in genetically engineered plants and animals such as Du Pont's transgenic OncoMouse, a laboratory mouse designed to develop cancer.[7] There are, then, precedents for the extension of intellectual property rights to aspects of personhood and even to living materials; nonetheless, the California court's extension of the intellectual property paradigm to the determination of motherhood in *Johnson v. Calvert* represents a remarkable moment in the history of authorship.

The facts in the case were as follows. Mark and Crispina Calvert—a white man and a Filipina woman—were a married couple who wanted to have a baby. Although Crispina had had a hysterectomy, nevertheless, her ovaries remained capable of producing eggs, and the couple was considering employing a surrogate when they were approached by Anna Johnson, an African American woman, who offered to bear their child. The Calverts and Johnson signed a standardized surrogacy contract, which provided that a zygote created from Mark's sperm and Crispina's egg would be implanted in Anna, who would bear the baby to term for the Calverts. In return the Calverts would provide Anna with a life insurance policy and with $10,000 for her services, the final portion of the fee to be paid after the birth. The contract was signed on 15 January 1990, and the next day Crispina's eggs were surgically removed and combined with Mark's sperm in a petri dish. Three days later the implantation in Anna's womb took place. Unfortunately, in the course of the pregnancy relations between Mark and Crispina and Anna deteriorated. The Calverts learned that Anna had had a history of stillbirths and miscarriages, and Anna, for her part, felt that the Calverts were not emotionally supportive of her and had not fully complied with the contract on the matter of the life insurance policy. In the seventh month, finding herself in financial difficulties, Anna sent the Calverts a letter demanding immediate payment of the $5,000 due her after the birth; otherwise, she threatened, she would not give up the baby. The Calverts responded with a lawsuit seeking a declaration that they were the legal parents of the unborn child; Anna countered with her own suit asking that she be declared the child's mother. The child, a baby boy, was born on 19 September 1990, and shortly thereafter the case came to trial in Orange County Superior Court.

The facts in *Johnson v. Calvert* were thus significantly different from those in the *Baby M* case decided by the New Jersey Supreme Court in 1988. In that case, too, there was a contract between a childless couple, William and Elizabeth Stern, and a surrogate, Mary Beth Whitehead, in which a $10,000 payment was provided for the surrogate to carry a baby to term and deliver it to the couple. In the *Baby M* case, however, Mary Beth Whitehead was both the child's genetic and gestational mother, and therefore the New Jersey court was not faced with a decision about which woman was the "natural" mother. Rather, at the heart of the *Baby M* case was the question of the enforceability of the contract. The New Jersey Supreme Court ruled that, because money was involved, the contract amounted to child selling and was illegal.

The status of the contract figured in *Johnson v. Calvert* as well, but the principal issue in this case was framed as the question of gestation versus genetics. Johnson's lawyers argued the uniqueness of childbearing and the fact that from time immemorial the woman who bears a child has been regarded as the mother of that child. The Calverts' lawyers argued that genetics should determine the issue. For Judge Richard N. Parslow, Jr., the trial judge, the claims of genetics greatly outweighed those of gestation:

> Who we are and what we are and identity problems particularly with young children and teenagers are extremely important. We know that there is a combination of genetic factors. We know more and more about traits now, how you walk, talk and everything else, all sorts of things that develop out of your genes, how long you're going to live, all things being equal, when your immune system is going to break down, what diseases you may be susceptible to. They have upped the intelligence ratio of genetics to 70 percent now.[8]

Judge Parslow called Anna Johnson a "genetic hereditary stranger" to the child, saying that her relationship to the boy, if indeed she had any, was analogous to that of a foster parent.[9] The appeals court took a slightly different tack—to reach its decision it invoked a complex reading of the California Uniform Parentage Act of 1975, a statute designed to end the distinction between legitimate and illegitimate children—but finally it affirmed the trial court's decision and reinforced its emphasis on genetics:

> As evidence at trial showed, the whole process of human development is "set in motion by the genes." There is not a single organic system of the human body not influenced by an individual's underlying genetic makeup. Genes determine the way physiological components of the human body, such as the heart, liver, or blood vessels operate. Also, according to the expert testimony received at trial, it is now thought that genes influence tastes, preferences, personality styles, manners of speech and mannerisms.[10]

The California Supreme Court, however, read the Parentage Act differently, concluding that the Act equally supported the biological claims of *both* the genetic and gestational mothers. Under these circumstances, the court ruled, motherhood was ultimately a matter of intention. Even though Crispina Calvert had not borne the child, nevertheless, as the surrogacy contract demonstrated, it was Crispina who had "intended to bring about the birth of a child that she intended to raise as her own"[11] and therefore she was the natural mother. The court thus affirmed the previous rulings in favor of the Calverts.

The supreme court's decision was not unanimous. Justice Armand Arabian concurred in the majority's finding that Crispina Calvert was the natural mother, but he disapproved of the majority's taking a position on the issue of the surrogacy contract. As a matter of law, he suggested, it was unnecessary for the court to express any opinion about the contract; and, as a matter of policy, it was unwise to venture without legislative guidance into so "vast and profound" an issue.[12] The objections of Justice Joyce Kennard, the only woman on the court at the time, went further. In a long and closely reasoned dissent, Justice Kennard noted that the "originators of the concept" rationale on which the majority relied was derived from intellectual property law and that the majority opinion was thus based on an analogy between childbearing and authorship. "Just as a song or invention is protected as the property of the 'originator of the concept,' so too a child should be regarded as belonging to the originator of the concept of the child." This was, in effect, the argument that the majority had made. But the analogy was inappropriate, Kennard argued, because children are not property: "Unlike songs or inventions, rights in children cannot be sold for consideration, or made freely available to the general public. Our most fundamental notions of personhood tell us it is inappropriate to treat children as property." Therefore, Kennard said, the notion that the principles of contract law might be applied to determine the life of a child was inappropriate: "Just as children are not the intellectual property of their parents, neither are they the personal property of anyone, and their delivery cannot be ordered as a contract remedy on the same terms that a court would, for example, order a breaching party to deliver a truckload of nuts and bolts." Furthermore, she charged the majority with failing to appreciate the dignity of childbearing: "A pregnant woman intending to bring a child into the world is more than a mere container or breeding animal; she is a conscious agent of creation no less than the genetic mother, and her humanity is implicated on a deep level. Her role should not be devalued."[13] Instead of relying on principles derived from intellectual property and contract law, she argued, the court should have looked to family law and grounded its decision on the principle of the best interests of the child. She would have remanded the present case to the trial court for a determination of parentage on that basis. But in general, Kennard said, a gestational surrogacy arrangement should only be permitted under the supervision of the courts. In this way there would be assurances that no party was being exploited, that the surrogacy arrangement was a matter of medical necessity, and that all the parties met standards of fitness.

In developing intentionality as the test for motherhood, the majority opinion, written by Justice Edward Panelli, cited for support a series of three recent commentaries dealing with the determination of parentage in the context of surrogacy arrangements. The earliest, and in some ways the most interesting, was a 1986 note, "Redefining Mother: A Legal Matrix for New Reproductive Technologies," in which Andrea E. Stumpf, then a law student, first made the argument for regarding "mental concept" as the crucial issue.[14] "Prior to physical conception of a child," Stumpf wrote,

> The beginnings of a normal parent-child relationship can come from mental conception, the desire to create a child. When the child's existence begins in the minds of the desiring parents, biological conception of the child declines in importance relative to psychological conception with respect to the full life of the child. The mental concept of the child is a controlling factor of its creation, and the originators of that concept merit full credit as conceivers.[15]

Stumpf explicitly invoked the intellectual property paradigm in a note in which she remarked that the "thoughts of initiating parents which become embodied in the creation of a child parallel the mental element at the root of intellectual property protection." And she went on to cite in support of the analogy between bodily and mental creation the old fable, sometimes considered a precedent for copyright, of the sixth-century Irish King Diarmud who supposedly settled a controversy over whether the owner of a manuscript had the right to control its transcription by remarking, "To every cow her calf." "It is ironic," Stumpf noted, "that the notion of literary property should have been birthed by a notion of motherhood as construed by biology."[16] The pun on "birthed" that Stumpf allows herself reinforces the point that she is making, as does the pun on "matrix" in her title.

A few years after Stumpf's piece, Marjorie Maguire Shultz, writing in the wake of the *Baby M* decision, proposed intentionality as the appropriate basis for making decisions about legal parenthood in the context of advanced reproductive technology. She pointed out that one of the advantages of adopting the criterion of intention would be its gender neutrality, remarking that such a regime would encourage male nurturing of children no less than female.[17] Likewise, John Lawrence Hill argued for intentionality rather than biology as the essential element in parenthood, giving the position an Aristotelian color by speaking of the intending parents as the "first cause" or "prime movers" of the procreative relationship.[18] Neither Shultz nor Hill explicitly invoked intellectual property law, but Hill observed that in the context of considerations of sperm and ova as objects of property, the analogy of copyright might be employed. The publisher of copyrighted material may sell the right to use the material but the right to duplicate or alter it is not included. Analogously, the source of genetic material might be understood to retain an interest in preventing certain uses, for example, to develop an interspecies hybrid. But this copyright-like interest would not, Hill argued, necessarily give the genetic donor the right to be considered a parent, "just as a publisher has no right to reclaim a book purchased for a legitimate purpose by another."[19]

The line of thought that the majority employed had thus been developing for some years in the law journals in response to the dispersal of biological roles that results from advances in reproductive technology and the consequent abstraction of the notion of biological conception. In what sense can one speak of a baby being "conceived" in the sterile, technological environment of a petri dish? There is an understandable tendency in these circumstance to relocate begetting from the physical specificity of an individual female body to the free-floating and, as Shultz in particular emphasizes, potentially genderless sphere of intellectual conception. Furthermore, the widely disseminated popular discourse of molecular genetics, the notion of DNA as a "master molecule" that incorporates the secrets of identity, likewise involves a process of abstraction in which the physical specificity of the organism is effaced. In this discourse the genome is first essentialized as equivalent to life itself and then metaphorized as a "code." The process by which the code becomes flesh is treated as a form of "translation" in which the DNA produces the "words" of RNA and finally "expresses" itself in a protein.[20] Thus the discourse of genetics specifically invokes the metaphor of textuality—as many have noted, this discourse is the latest version of the ancient trope of the "book of nature"—and consequently, too, it generates issues of intellectual property. Can a human genetic sequence be copyrighted? Can an artificially created gene be patented? These are the kinds of legal questions that the reconceptualization of life as "information" involves.

Let us note, too, that there is a long history of reciprocity between ideas of biological and ideas of intellectual generation, a history that is implicit even in the way the term "conception" moves readily between physical and mental referents. Aristotle, whose "form and matter" theory of generation was dominant for some two thousand years, employed the analogy of the human arts in order to explain procreation. The male, he suggested, is like a carpenter whose intellect shapes the matter according to his idea of what it should be; the female merely provides the physical substance. No material part of the carpenter enters his work. Likewise, no material part of the male is incorporated in the embryo; nevertheless, the male provides the active principle that forms the child in the father's image.[21] The analogy between intellectual and physical generation implicit in Aristotle's theory was elaborated in medieval and early modern thought in the theory that mental activity takes place not within the tissues of the brain—tissue of any kind was regarded as too material to be the site of mentation—but within the ventricles or cavities.[22] In this way the brain was understood to be a kind of womb of thought, as it is, for instance, in the pedant Holofernes's representation in *Love's Labor's Lost* when he brags about his fertile invention, explaining that his wonderful ideas "are begot in the ventricle of memory, nourish'd in the womb of pia mater, and delivered upon the mellowing of occasion."[23] This was certainly how the seventeenth-century experimentalist William Harvey, the discoverer of the circulation of the blood, understood the matter. From his dissections of female deer prepared for coition Harvey concluded that the uterus and the brain were indeed alike and that this was the secret of generation: conception in the womb occurred in a manner similar to conception in the brain.[24]

Harvey's understanding of procreation was perhaps influenced by the common metaphor of a book as a child, a trope that, as Ernst Curtius reports, goes back to Plato.[25] In the "Symposium" Diotima explains that what men desire is immortality. Some seek to immortalize themselves by begetting children, others by begetting intellectual works. "Who, when he thinks of Homer and Hesiod and other great poets, would not rather have their children than any ordinary human ones?" Diotima asks. "Who would not emulate them in the creation of children such as theirs, which have preserved their memory and given them everlasting glory?"[26] A number of Latin writers followed Plato in referring to writings as children, and there are scattered examples of the trope in the middle ages as well; nonetheless, it was not until the early modern period when the systematic individuation of authorship encouraged the notion that a book might incorporate a writer's self that the trope became ubiquitous. Sir Philip Sidney, for example, opens his sonnet sequence *Astrophil and Stella* by representing himself as "great with child to speake," in this manner playing with the incongruity of a male pregnancy.[27] Likewise, in the preface to *Don Quixote* Cervantes explains that although his book is not "the handsomest, the liveliest, and the wisest" child that might be, nevertheless as an author he "could not violate Nature's ordinance whereby like engenders like." Thus, he continues, "what could my sterile and uncouth genius beget but the tale of a dry, shriveled, whimsical offspring, full of odd fancies such as never entered another's brain."[28] And the notion of authorship as a form of procreation continues to be invoked to the present day both in general discourse—though no longer, I suppose, with the sense that a mental conception might literally be analogous to an embryo in the womb—and in the context of discussions of intellectual property. James Joyce, for example, in a letter of 21 August 1912 to his wife Nora speaks of the still-unpublished *Dubliners* as this "child which I have carried for years and years in the womb of the imagination as you carried in your womb the children you love."[29] Similarly, Nathaniel Shaler, like many other apologists for intellectual property rights, defends copyright by employing the trope of procreation: "The man who brings out of the nothingness some child of his thought has rights therein which cannot belong to any other sort of property."[30]

As even a cursory invocation of the representation of authorship as analogous to procreation suggests, authorship is a gendered category.[31] Indeed, even today the principle that an author has a right to have his name attached to a work he has created is known as the "right of paternity."[32] Moreover, as a category, authorship incorporates not only the mind-body dichotomy characteristic of the Western cultural tradition but also the gendering of the mind-body opposition. Matter—the term is related to both *mater* and *matrix*—is female; intellect is male. And both the dichotomy and the hierarchical arrangement of the terms of the dichotomy, the inferiority of body to mind in the mainstream of Western thought, reflect the patriarchal structures that have been characteristic of Western societies since the classical period. Enlightened as we might suppose ourselves to be in these last years of the twentieth century, these associations and meanings still play through our language and thought. Thus even today there is, I believe, a slight sense of disjunction, a hint of the oxymoronic, about the yoking of "mothers and authors" in a single phrase.

In her dissent Justice Kennard vigorously protests the majority's devaluation of the physical contribution that the woman who bears a child to term makes to the process of reproduction. "The majority's approach entirely devalues the substantial claims of motherhood by a gestational mother such as Anna," she writes using a phrase in which "substantial" can perhaps be read in several senses at once. She goes on to note that in a previous decision the California Supreme Court acknowledged that "a pregnant woman and her unborn child comprise a 'unique physical unit' and that the welfare of each is 'intertwined and inseparable.' Indeed, a fetus would never develop into a living child absent its nurturing by the pregnant woman."[33] It seems to me that Justice Kennard can be understood to be protesting against the long history of abstraction in the contemplation of reproduction, one that reemerges in her colleagues' "originator of the concept" rationale. To be pregnant is not simply to have an idea. Authorship may be represented as a form of childbearing but childbearing is not equivalent to authorship. Perhaps, too, her reassertion of the "substantial claims" of the physical and the organic—and what I take to be her distaste for the "gender neutral" principles proposed by Shultz—can be understood as an objection to the masculine appropriation of childbearing implicit in making intellectual conception the essential act in procreation.

To refuse to acknowledge that the woman who gives birth to a child is related to the child is to repudiate the testimony of the eyes and the materiality of the body. It is, in effect, to repudiate nature—as Aeschylus's Athena can be understood to repudiate nature, and her own female gender to boot, when she accepts Apollo's argument that Clytemnestra was not Orestes's kin. The woman, Apollo says, merely nurses the man's seed, preserving it as a "stranger"—had Apollo testified in *Johnson v. Calvert* he surely would have said "genetic hereditary stranger"—in her womb.[34] This notion of procreation as essentially parthenogenic is of course nothing more than the orthodox doctrine of a patrilineal society; nonetheless, baldly stated as in Apollo's argument, the position is scandalous. This point is comically made in the episode in *Tristram Shandy* in which the pedantic Doctor Kysarcius, like Apollo, undertakes to prove that Mrs. Shandy is no relation to her son. Kysarcius cites "The Duke of Suffolk's Case," a ruling in which, as Kysarcius puts it, "not only the temporal lawyers—but the church-lawyers—the juris-consulti—the juris-prudentes—the civilians—the advocates—the commissaries—the judges of the consistory and prerogative courts of *Canterbury* and *York*, with the master of the faculties, were all unanimously of opinion, That the mother was not of kin to her child." To which Uncle Toby, implicitly citing another authority, responds, "And what said the duchess of *Suffolk* to it?" Thus Sterne mocks the pedantry that would deny a patent fact of nature.[35]

Justice Kennard's protest against the majority's devaluation of the gestational mother's contribution suggests her discomfort with this kind of repudiation of nature. It also may seem to align her with those feminists who, made uneasy by the abstractions of post-modern theory, call for the retrieval of the physical specificity of the female body.[36] Let us note that Johnson's lawyers made a similar claim for the woman's distinctive bodily contribution to procreation. In their brief to the appeals court they argued that Judge Parslow had erred in comparing Johnson to a foster parent:

> Both men and women must contribute genetic material to create a child, but it is only the women who use their entire bodies to gestate and give birth to children. . . . It was Appellant who gave birth to Baby Boy Johnson and it was Appellant's physical human relationship with the child that caused the child's existence to come into being. While millions of human sperms and eggs can join together, human nature requires a human woman to gestate the child into its very existence and natural human reproduction proceeds only on the basis that a woman will give birth to a child. . . . The court fundamentally erred in its logic by comparing Appellant's legal relationship to the child as one of a "foster parent" or a "wet nurse," as both analogies presuppose a child in existence. Nor can it be logically concluded that Appellant is merely a "carrier" of a child, as Appellant initially is inseminated with human reproductive cells and then Appellant procreates the child into its very existence.[37]

This argument attempts to retrieve a sense of the natural by representing Johnson as a mother not essentially different from any other. But the rhetoric collapses under the weight of the facts. As the Calverts' lawyers pointed out in response, Anna Johnson was never "inseminated," rather, a zygote was implanted. Nor could she be said to have "procreated" the child, for the zygote was formed in a petri dish.[38] Indeed, the conspicuous awkwardness of Johnson's lawyers' phrasing—"and then Appellant procreates the child into its very existence"—is an index of their attempt to naturalize a procreative process that was never in fact an instance of "natural human reproduction."

The Calverts' alternative insistence on genetics, ratified by both the trial and the appeals courts, was also an attempt to naturalize the birth, in this case by appealing to the principle of biological continuity and the maxim that like engenders like. "As evidence at trial showed," the appeals court remarked, "the whole process of human development is 'set in motion by the genes.' "[39] Interestingly, this popular discourse of genetics, the representation of the genes as the active force in procreation, can be understood as a successor to the ancient representation of procreation. According to Aristotle, the active but immaterial male principle was received and nurtured by the female who supplied the matter and brought the resulting child into the world. According to the current popular representation of procreation, the active principle is DNA, the bearer of the genetic "code" and the master molecule that represents the ultimate "secret of life." Figured as a code, DNA is a kind of text. But figured as an active force, DNA becomes a kind of author.[40]

Johnson's lawyers rejected this kind of genetic essentialism. "There is a misconception that a baby is made from DNA," they said, citing the words of an expert who testified at the trial. Perhaps a genetic relationship might be regarded as equivalent to parenthood in an ordinary birth, but the genetic argument failed to take into account the unusual circumstances of the present case. In the case of a "nongenetic pregnancy it can no longer be said that the genetic link is so unique or weighty as in a traditional pregnancy." Whether or not she is genetically related to the child, the birth mother "has a profound influence on the genes and every aspect of creation." As a particular example, they cited testimony to the effect that "the size and shape of the human brain is predominantly determined by the gestational mother, more so than a genetic contributor." The gestational mother had been represented as merely the passive carrier of a baby that was not hers, but this was not the case: "Baby Boy Johnson is not the same baby that would have emerged from any other birth mother's womb."[41]

Justice Kennard also implicitly rejected genetic essentialism, but neither would she have awarded the baby to Johnson on the basis of gestation. Her preferred resolution involved no dubious naturalizations but instead was concrete and pragmatic. The majority responded that she was confusing custody with parentage:

> The dissent would decide *parentage* based on the best interests of the child. Such an approach raises the repugnant specter of governmental interference in matters implicating our most fundamental notions of privacy, and confuses concepts of parentage and custody. Logically the determination of parentage must precede, and should not be dictated by, eventual custody decisions.[42]

Under a "best interests" standard parentage would be determined by the courts; under the "originators of the concept" standard, the private arrangements made by the contracting parents would prevail. But this, as Justice Kennard pointed out, was to treat a child as property.

Another possible resolution had been proposed, one that also avoided both essentialism and abstraction. The ACLU had submitted an *amicus curiae* brief arguing that the court should find that the child had two mothers, a gestational mother and a genetic mother. But the court rejected this proposal. It acknowledged that advances in reproductive technology had made more than two parents biologically possible, and it further acknowledged that as a result of rising divorce rates multiple parent arrangements had become common. Nevertheless, the court dismissed the ACLU proposal more or less out of hand, saying "we see no compelling reason to recognize such a situation here."

> The Calverts are the genetic and intending parents of their son and have provided him, by all accounts, with a stable, intact, and nurturing home. To recognize parental rights in a third party with whom the Calvert family has had little contact since shortly after the child's birth would diminish Crispina's role as mother.[43]

Let us note that in this statement the argument from genetics returns: the opinion reminds us that the Calverts are both the intending and the genetic parents. What the court is attempting to do is to preserve, as nearly as possible, the traditional nuclear family. It, too, in its own way, is seeking to naturalize the birth.[44]

As a number of commentators have observed, race was an unspoken but significant element in the case from the beginning.[45] That Johnson was black and the baby was not perhaps added urgency to the genetic claims and the principle of like engenders like. Indeed, after the trial, Richard C. Gilbert, one of Johnson's lawyers, remarked bitterly that Judge Parslow had "wanted to give the white couple the white baby."[46] Of course, Crispina Calvert, a Filipina, was not exactly white, but in the binary mode of American racial discourse she became white; and so did the child, though journalistic reports might note, implicitly making an argument for the Calverts, that the baby "has his genetic mother's dark shiny hair and wide eyes."[47] Nor was Anna Johnson, who claimed American Indian descent, simply black. But the prospect of a finding that would allow a "black" woman to be declared the natural mother of a "white" baby was clearly unsettling. And yet what aspect of this case was *not* unsettling? Sterne's Uncle Toby might mock the pedantic doctor's claim that Mrs. Shandy was not kin to her son Tristram, but what would he say about a child born from a zygote created in vitro and then implanted in a surrogate? The various attempts to naturalize this birth collapse under their own weight because the facts themselves repudiate any simple or received idea of "nature."

Valerie Hartouni has recently observed that the challenge to the courts in *Johnson v. Calvert* "was to restabilize conventional understandings of motherhood and family and thereby to recontain the proliferation of meanings, identities, and relationships generated by the panoply of new reproductive practices and, in particular, by the practice of gestational surrogacy."[48] Who is related to whom and how in a world where a child may have more than two biological parents—or, for that matter, in the world of the near future in which artificially produced embryos may be gestated in artificial wombs? But the proliferation of meanings, identities, and relationships generated by new reproductive technologies represents only one of the many unsettling social changes that have occurred in the United States in recent years. The majority opinion in *Johnson v. Calvert* noted the proliferation of multiple parent arrangements attendant on the increasing divorce rate. One might point as well to changing medical and legal attitudes toward homosexuality—a significant number of states now allow same sex partners to adopt each other's children—and, of course, to changes in the roles of women and ethnic and racial minorities in American society. As Thomas Laqueur has suggested, perhaps the great public interest that cases such as *Baby M* and *Johnson v. Calvert* have evoked, an interest quite incommensurate with the number of people who might be affected by the decisions, may be related to the way these cases function as "representative anecdotes" that serve to focus broad social anxieties.[49] Furthermore, let us note that the proliferation of social meanings merges with, and in some respects is indistinguishable from, the proliferation of cultural meanings that can be invoked by such coded terms as "multiculturalism" and "deconstruction," and that is evident in, among other phenomena, the many challenges to the received canons of art, music, literature, and history; the challenges to aestheticism and the notion that cultural productions are disinterested practices that are separable from political, ideological, and economic concerns; and the challenges to the romantic conception of the author as the unitary, creative source of meaning.

As Michel Foucault points out in "What is an Author?" the familiar representation of the author as a genial creative force, the source of proliferating meanings, disguises the fact that in practice the figure of the author has often functioned to limit and restrict meaning. We deny, for example, that such and such an author could have intended such and such a meaning, and therefore we rule that meaning out. "The author," as Foucault puts it with characteristic drama, "allows a limitation of the cancerous and dangerous proliferation of significations within a world where one is thrifty not only with one's resources and riches, but also with one's discourses and their significations. The author is the principle of thrift in the proliferation of meaning."[50] But if authorship has become a subject rather than an assumption of inquiry in academic circles, the author has remained the paradigmatic figure of intellectual property law. Thus, for example, the U.S. Supreme Court has recently reaffirmed the principle of "originality" as the "sine qua non of copyright,"[51] and in a recent book Paul Goldstein, one of the leading contemporary scholars of copyright, remarks that "[C]opyright is, after all, about authorship, about sustaining the conditions for creativity that enable an artist to create out of thin air and intense, devouring labor an *Appalachian Spring*, a *Sun Also Rises*, a *Citizen Kane*."[52] Given the long history of exchange between ideas of physical and ideas of intellectual generation, and given the continuing vitality of the figure of the author in legal discourse, it does not seem arbitrary that the California Supreme Court should have employed the authorship paradigm in its attempt to reconstruct the image of the nuclear family from an unsettling proliferation of significations.

Does *Johnson v. Calvert* represent a lasting advance of the banner of authorship or is the California Supreme Court's decision merely an aberrant ruling that will eventually find its way into the cabinet of legal curiosities? The U.S. Supreme Court declined to review the case. In New York State, however, a somewhat similar matter of disputed motherhood came before a court of appeals the year after *Johnson v. Calvert* was decided in California. The New York case, *McDonald v. McDonald*,[53] involved a divorce action in which a husband argued for custody of twin girls on the grounds that his wife was not their natural mother and that he was the only natural parent available. In this case the husband's sperm had been mixed with the eggs of an anonymous female donor and the resulting zygotes implanted in the wife's uterus and carried to term. To support his argument that his wife was not related to the children, the husband relied on Judge Parslow's decision in the trial court phase of *Johnson v. Calvert* and his finding that genetics were more important than gestation in the formation of a child. The New York court observed, however, that Judge Parslow's reasoning was not accepted by the state supreme court, which had found that either the genetic or the gestational mother could arguably be considered the child's natural mother. The New York court further noted that the California Supreme Court had anticipated precisely the circumstances involved in *McDonald v. McDonald* when it hypothesized a true "egg donation" situation—one in which a woman gestates a donated egg with the intent to raise the child as her own—and said that in such a case the birth mother would, as the woman whose intentions had brought the child into being, be the natural mother. The court took account of Justice Kennard's dissent, but said that it found the majority's reasoning to be persuasive and therefore held that Mrs. McDonald was the natural mother of the children.

But in a second case subsequent to *Johnson v. Calvert* an Ohio court rejected the California court's reasoning. In *Belsito v. Clark*[54] the issue was technical not adversarial. The case arose because according to Ohio law the gestational mother, who in this case was the genetic mother's sister, would be listed on the baby's birth certificate as the mother and the child would be treated as illegitimate. The genetic parents went to law seeking a judgment that they and not the gestational mother were the child's natural and legal parents. The Ohio court took note of both *Johnson v. Calvert* and *McDonald v. McDonald* but found fault with the intentionality test on a number of grounds including the fact that, in the Ohio court's opinion, such a test might bring about unacceptable results. For example, the court hypothesized, what if two women decide to procreate and raise a child together with one providing the egg and the other gestating the embryo? Under the *Johnson* test both would be declared natural mothers. Thus meanings and relationships would continue to proliferate. The proper test for parenthood, the court said, should be genetic. Citing Blackstone, case law, and *Black's Law Dictionary*, the Ohio court observed that kindred was a matter of "blood relations" and that this in modern terminology meant "shared DNA or genetics."[55] When gestational surrogacy techniques are employed in the procreation of a child, the court said, "the natural parents of the child shall be identified by a determination as to which individuals have provided the genetic imprint for that child."[56] Thus the court ruled that the baby was legitimate.

On the basis of these two subsequent cases it is impossible to predict how the law will develop, but it appears likely that if the *Johnson* test is not followed the courts will resort to genetics in gestational surrogacy cases. Genetics conveys both a reassuring aura of scientific certainty and a sense of continuity with traditional discourses of "blood." Even in *Johnson v. Calvert*, after all, both the trial court and the appeals court based their rulings on genetics, and the supreme court, while adopting a different reasoning, nonetheless awarded the child to the genetic parents.[57] But let us pay attention for a moment to the phrase "genetic imprint" which the Ohio court repeatedly uses in its ruling. On the one hand, the phrase perhaps evokes fingerprinting, also a technique for establishing identity in legal context; on the other, it incorporates a printing metaphor. A child bears its parents' genes as a book bears the imprint of its source. This may be understood as the publisher, who stamps the title page with his mark, or alternatively as the figure who authorizes the publisher, the writer, who also stamps the title page with his mark and who possesses, as I mentioned earlier, a legal "right of paternity." In any case, the imprint is the sign of identity, of personality, and therefore of possession.

The phrase "genetic imprint" returns us to the analogy between babies and books, parents and authors. Indeed, as we have already seen, the discourse of genetics incorporates the language of textuality and something like the idea of authorship. Perhaps in some ways, then, the genetic test can be understood as not altogether different from the intentionality test with its underlying paradigm of authorship. The point of commonality is the distinctly modern notion of the unique, autonomous individual. Though we may speak casually of "the human genome," we are equally fond of asserting that each of us has "a unique genetic makeup." Moreover, though we know that human procreation is never in fact reproduction, we nevertheless imagine that each of us has a "natural desire" to pass on his genes to the next generation, a natural desire to achieve a kind of genetic immortality. I use the masculine "his" advisedly here, for it is apparent that this pattern of thought, inflected as it might be by modern ideas of individuality and autonomy, nonetheless descends from ancient notions about the desire for immortality such as those expressed by Plato in the "Symposium." And it is apparent too how difficult it is to extract ourselves from the gendered structure of the thought patterns we have inherited, the association of the active principle of creativity with the mind and the male, and the association of the passive principle of nurturing with the body and the female.

What is striking to me is the poverty of our paradigms for explaining ourselves to ourselves. Authorship is one such paradigm. The notion of authorship is implicit in the way we explain a vast range of generative activities from the way game shows are created to the way babies are made. Perhaps this is to be expected. As Carol Delaney has shown, the way in which a culture thinks about procreation intersects with the way it imagines divine creation, and both are related to forms of social organization.[58] The romantic notion of authorship—the idea that an author creates something, as Paul Goldstein puts it, "out of thin air"—is of course a transformation of religious doctrine. And the notion that what the author creates is at once an expression of his unique personality, a kind of brain child, and an object of property is commensurate with the social ideology of democratic individualism and free market capitalism.

The intensity of Justice Kennard's uneasiness with anything that might smack of baby selling is related, I suspect, to the thinness of the partitions that separate children from property in our society, as of course in many others as well. When is an infant sold and when is it adopted? In principle baby selling is illegal. Nonetheless, in practice there is a thriving American market in babies for adoption, as Elisabeth M. Landes and Richard A. Posner, among others, point out in the famous and scandalous essay in which they propose to legalize baby selling in order to alleviate the shortage of "first quality" children available for adoption. "The antipathy to an explicit market in babies," Landes and Posner write, "may be part of a broader wish to disguise facts that might be acutely uncomfortable if widely known. Were baby prices quoted as the prices of soybean futures are quoted, a racial ranking of these prices would be evident, with white baby prices higher than nonwhite baby prices."[59] Like the *Baby M* case, then, *Johnson v. Calvert* points to the fragility of our belief that we do not treat people as commodities.

But at the same time it points to the vigor of the authorship paradigm. Romantic notions of authorship do not really fit our best understandings of how cultural production works. Even copyright lawyers realize perfectly well that texts are not created out of thin air and that most cultural productions are in one sense or another collaborative. But although we may speak vaguely—and often more with wishful thinking than with real conviction—about the death of the author, we don't yet have a really compelling alternative model to propose. And now the invention of new reproductive technologies has destabilized our understanding of human procreation as well, opening up such unnatural prospects as that of a child with multiple mothers. Do we really wish to re-naturalize these unnatural births by imposing on them a fetishizing discourse of genetic essentialism? Isn't the purpose of these technologies precisely to free people from the limitations of their merely natural capacities? What implications do fetishized essentialisms have for other reproductive issues such as abortion? The author paradigm at least recommends itself in this way, that it empowers the individual to negotiate his or her wishes with maximum personal freedom in relation to the state. But, on the other hand, do we really wish to endorse the production of children by free contract? What implications would this practice have for our sense of personhood and human dignity? Perhaps the best we can do is, as Justice Kennard suggests, to insist upon the supervision of the courts at every step in the process of a surrogacy arrangement. But can the courts really function well as the final authority in such matters? Moreover, doesn't such a prospect indeed raise, as the majority in *Johnson v. Calvert* put it, a repugnant specter of governmental interference? Doesn't it in effect constitute the courts as licensers and censors in relation to our most intimate expressions of ourselves? At the conclusion of "What is an Author?" the only

alternative to authorship that Foucault can muster is the vision of proliferating discourses developing in "the anonymity of a murmur."[60] But what is
this utopia, really, beyond the negation of romantic authorship? Likewise,
here too in the contemplation of these new children of our imaginations
what is apparent is the difficulty that we have in thinking our way toward
models that are adequate to the circumstances in which we find ourselves.

Notes

For generous assistance of various kinds while writing this essay I am grateful to
many friends and colleagues including Ann Bermingham, Robert Burt, Rowland
Davis, Sarah Fenstermaker, Patricia Fumerton, Donna Haraway, Valerie Hartouni, Thomas Laqueur, Corynne McSherry, Robert Rotstein, Patricia Shepard,
and Everett Zimmerman.

1. 19 Cal. Rptr. 2d 494 (Cal. 1993), cert. denied, 114 S. Ct. 206 (1993); hereafter abbreviated *Johnson.*

2. *In Re Baby M,* 109 N J 396 (N.J. 1988) 537 A. 2d 1227.

3. *Johnson,* 506.

4. Mark Rose, *Authors and Owners: The Invention of Copyright* (Cambridge, MA:
Harvard UP, 1993). See also Martha Woodmansee, *The Author, Art, and the Market*
(New York: Columbia UP, 1994).

5. On the extension of copyright see Peter Jaszi, "Toward a Theory of Copy-
right: The Metamorphoses of 'Authorship,'" *Duke Law Journal* 1991 (1991):
455–502. Section 102 of the U.S. Copyright Act of 1976 lists the current subject
matter of copyright in general. See the discussion in Paul Goldstein, *Copyright:
Principles, Law and Practice,* 3 vols. (Boston: Little Brown and Co., 1989) 1: 57–226.
Public images are protected under the right of publicity doctrine; see Goldstein,
Copyright, 2: 601–607. The term "silicon epics" comes from Anthony L. Clapes,
Patrick Lynch, and Mark R. Steinberg, "Silicon Epics and Binary Bards: Deter-
mining the Proper Scope of Copyright Protection for Computer Programs,"
UCLA Law Review 34 (1987): 1493–1594.

6. *Moore v. Regents of the Univ. of Cal.,* 793 P.2d 479 (Cal. 1990), cert. denied,
111 S. Ct. 1388 (1991).

7. For OncoMouse see Donna J. Haraway, "Universal Donors in a Vampire
Culture: It's All in the Family: Biological Kinship Categories in the Twentieth-
century United States," in *Uncommon Ground,* ed. William Cronon (New York:
Norton, 1995) 321–366.

8. Quoted by Janet L. Dolgin, "Just a Gene: Judicial Assumptions About Parenthood," *UCLA Law Review* 40 (1993): 685.

9. Quoted by Dolgin, 684.

10. *Anna J. v. Marc C. et al.*, 286 Cal. Rptr. 369 (Cal. App. 4 Dist. 1991), 380; hereafter *Anna J.*

11. *Johnson*, 500.

12. *Johnson*, 506.

13. *Johnson*, 514–516.

14. Andrea E. Stumpf, "Redefining Mother: A Legal Matrix for New Reproductive Technologies," *Yale Law Journal* 96 (1986): 187–208.

15. Stumpf, 195–196.

16. Stumpf, 195 n. 33.

17. Marjorie Maguire Shultz, "Reproductive Technology and Intent-based Parenthood: An Opportunity for Gender Neutrality," *Wisconsin Law Review* 1990 (1990): 297–398.

18. John Lawrence Hill, " 'What Does It Mean to Be a Parent?' The Claims of Biology as the Basis for Parental Rights," *New York University Law Review* 66 (1991): 353–420.

19. Hill, 393.

20. See Richard Doyle, "Vital Language," in *Are Genes Us?* ed. Carl F. Cranor (New Brunswick, NJ: Rutgers UP, 1994) 52–68; Evelyn Fox Keller, "Master Molecules," in *Are Genes Us?* 89–98; and Keller's, *Refiguring Life: Metaphors of Twentieth-Century Biology* (New York: Columbia UP, 1995).

21. "De Generatione Animalium," trans. Arthur Platt, in *The Basic Works of Aristotle*, ed. Richard McKeon (New York: Random House, 1941) 678.

22. See Walter Pagel, "Medieval and Renaissance Contributions to Knowledge of the Brain and Its Functions," in *The Brain and Its Functions* (Springfield, Il: Charles C. Thomas, 1958) 95–114. The Latin term *venter* may refer either to the belly or the womb. "Venter" is still current in legal usage to designate a maternal parent.

23. IV.ii.68–70; *The Riverside Shakespeare*, ed. G. B. Evans et al. (Boston: Houghton Mifflin Co., 1974) 193. In *Peri Bathous* Alexander Pope represents poetry as either "a natural or morbid secretion from the Brain," adding:

> Therefore is the Desire of Writing properly term'd *Puritus*, the "Titilation of the Generative Faculty of the Brain," and the Person is said to conceive; now such as conceive must bring forth. I have known a man thoughtful, melancholy and raving for divers days, who forthwith grew wonderfully easy, lightsome and cheerful, upon a discharge of the peccant humour, in exceeding purulent Metre;

The Prose Works of Alexander Pope: The Major Works, 1725–1744, ed. Rosemary Cowler (Hamden, CT: Archon Books, 1986) 189.

24. In a female deer prepared for coition, Harvey noted, the outer surface of the uterus "appears thicker and more fleshly" than at other times, while the inner surface "becomes more tender and corresponds in smoothness and softness to the inner parts of the ventricles of the brain." He continued:

Seeing that the substance of the uterus that has been made ready for the conception is so very like the constitution of the brain, why may we not justly surmise that the function of each of them is also alike, and that what imagination and appetitive are to the brain, that same thing, or at least something analogous to it, is awakened in the uterus by coitus and from this proceeds the generation or procreation of the egg?

William Harvey, "Of Conception," trans. Gweneth Witteridge, in *Disputations Touching the Generation of Animals* (Oxford: Blackwell Scientific Publications, 1981) 445.

25. Ernst R. Curtius, *European Literature and the Latin Middle Ages*, trans. Willard R. Trask (London: Routledge and Kegan Paul, 1953) 132–134. On the trope of the book as a child see also Terry J. Castle, "Lab'Ring Bards: Birth Topoi and English Poetics 1660–1820," *Journal of English and Germanic Philology* 78 (1979): 193–208; Elizabeth Sacks, *Shakespeare's Images of Pregnancy* (New York: St. Martin's Press, 1980); Susan Stanford Friedman, "Creativity and the Childbirth Metaphor: Gender Difference in Literary Discourse," in *Speaking of Gender*, ed. Elaine Showalter (New York and London: Routledge, 1989) 73–100; and [Mark Rose,] "From Paternity to Property: The Remetaphorization of Writing," in *Cultural Agency/Cultural Authority*, ed. Martha Woodmansee and Peter Jaszi (Durham, NC: Duke UP forthcoming). Barbara Stafford has much interesting material in her chapter entitled "Conceiving," *Body Criticism: Imaging the Unseen in Enlightenment Art and Medicine* (Cambridge, MA: MIT Press, 1991) 211–279.

26. "Symposium," trans. B. Jowett, *The Dialogues of Plato*, 2 vols. (New York: Random House, 1937) 1: 33.

27. *The Poems of Sir Philip Sidney*, ed. William A. Ringler (Oxford: Clarendon Press, 1962) 165.

28. Miguel de Cervantes, *Don Quixote*, trans. Walter Starkie (New York: Signet, 1964) 41.

29. *Letters of James Joyce*, ed. Stuart Gilbert and Richard Ellmann, 3 vols. (New York: Viking, 1957–1966) 2: 308.

30. Quoted by David Ladd, "The Harm of the Concept of Harm in Copyright," *Journal of the Copyright Society of the U.S.A.* 30 (1983): 426.

31. For a well-known treatment of authorship as a gendered category see Christine Battersby, *Gender and Genius: Towards a Feminist Aesthetics* (London: Women's Press, 1989).

32. The "right of paternity" is one of the crucial elements of the doctrine of the author's "moral right" as ratified by the Berne Convention.

33. *Johnson*, 515.

34. "The mother is no parent of that which is called/her child, but only nurse of the new-planted seed/that grows. The parent is he who mounts. A stranger she/preserves a stranger's seed, if no god interfere." *The Eumenides*, ll. 658–661, trans. Richmond Lattimore, *The Complete Greek Tragedies*, ed. David Grene and Richmond Lattimore, 3 vols. (Chicago: U of Chicago P, 1956) 1: 158. Apollo

clinches his argument by pointing to the presiding judge herself, Athena, who sprung directly from her father Zeus's head.

35. Laurence Sterne, *Tristram Shandy*, ed. J. A. Work (Indianapolis and New York: Odyssey Press, 1940) 328–330.

36. For an analysis of this position see Judith Butler, *Bodies That Matter: On the Discursive Limits of "Sex"* (New York and London: Routledge, 1993), esp. 27–55.

37. "Opening Brief for Appellant," 34–35, *Anna J.*, on file at Los Angeles County Law Library.

38. "Respondents' Brief," 22, *Anna J.*, on file at Los Angeles County Law Library.

39. *Anna J.*, 380.

40. Evelyn Fox Keller suggests that at least until World War II nucleus and cytoplasm were tropes for male and female in biological discourse and she relates this gendering of cell components to the representation of the nucleus (DNA) as active and the cytoplasm as passive. See *Refiguring Life*, esp. 38–40.

41. "Appellant's Reply," 2–4, *Johnson*, on file at Los Angeles County Law Library.

42. *Johnson*, 500 n. 10.

43. *Johnson*, 499 n. 8.

44. Randy Francis Kandel, "Which Came First: The Mother or the Egg? A Kinship Solution to Gestational Surrogacy," *Rutgers Law Review* 47 (1994): 165–239, challenges the California Supreme Court's insistence that a child can only have one mother. Kandel points out that "when it used the metaphor of naturalness, the court was also culturally constructing the nuclear family as a natural family form" (187); instead of searching for a rule to find the most "natural" mother, the court should have adopted a broader view which acknowledged the possibility of other forms of kinship relations.

45. See esp. Valerie Hartouni, "Breached Birth: Reflections on Race, Gender, and Reproductive Discourse in the 1980's," *Configurations* 1 (1994): 73–88.

46. Quoted by Dolgin, 687 n. 212.

47. Catherine Gewertz, "Parents of Child Born to Surrogate Face Final Challenge," *Los Angeles Times* 17 April 1992: A29.

48. Hartouni, 76.

49. Thomas W. Laqueur, " 'From Generation to Generation': Imagining Connectedness in the Age of Reproductive Technologies," forthcoming.

50. "What is an Author?" trans. J. V. Harari, in *The Foucault Reader*, ed. Paul Rabinow (New York: Pantheon, 1984) 101–120.

51. *Feist Publications, Inc. v. Rural Telephone Service Company*, 111 Sup. Ct. 1282 (1991).

52. Paul Goldstein, *Copyright's Highway: The Law and Lore of Copyright from Gutenberg to the Celestial Jukebox* (New York: Hill and Wang, 1994) 76.

53. 608 N.Y.S. 2d 477 (New York 1994), 196 A.D. 2d 7.

54. 67 Ohio Misc. 2d 54 (Ohio 1994).

55. Ohio Misc., 59.

56. Ohio Misc., 66.

57. Jeffrey M. Place, "Gestational Surrogacy and the Meaning of 'Mother,' " *Harvard Journal of Law and Public Policy* 17 (1994): 907–917, argues that the California Supreme Court reached the right conclusion for the wrong reasons; it should have decided the case on the basis of genetics.

58. Delaney, *The Seed and the Soil: Gender and Cosmology in Turkish Village Society* (Berkeley: U of California P, 1991).

59. Elisabeth M. Landes and Richard A. Posner, "The Economics of the Baby Shortage," *Journal of Legal Studies* 7 (1978): 344.

60. Foucault, 119.

"Lasers for Ladies"

Endo Discourse and the Inscriptions of Science

Feminist theory has produced an impressive corpus of texts on the imaging of the female body in the arts, photography, cinema, and the media.[1] This discussion of the visual has privileged the surface body, while the notion of the gaze has been premised on desire and pleasure. But what happens when feminist cultural critics delve into the taboo territory of studying the imaging of the pathological interior body? How do we then speak of text and reader, of representation and spectatorship, of producers and consumers of images? In an era when X-ray, ultrasound, and video laparoscopy have thoroughly charted the terra incognita of bones, chromosomes, and reproductive organs, feminist critique cannot afford to surrender the interior body to the curtained authority of the medical office. To unlearn the censorship of the living body's visualized organs—particularly in a context where women critics can be *subjects* of these imaging technologies—is a prerequisite for reclaiming the body from the monopoly of scientific disciplining, and for democratizing access to the medicalized body.

As part of my argument for a cultural studies intervention in medical discourses of the interior body, I will focus on a generally nonlethal female disease, endometriosis, as a site of tension between the hegemonic scientific inscription of the female body and a critical feminist voicing of women's agency. Precisely because of its gendered character and public invisibility, endometriosis illuminates the coexistence of an up-to-date endoscopic panopticon (laparoscopy, laser laparoscopy, video laparoscopy) with an old, myopic discourse concerning femaleness. My discussion here of endo discourse[2] forms part of an ongoing, resistant postmodern argument for a possible dialogue between, on the one hand, scientific research and medical technologies, and, on the other, feminist critique and community-based empowerment. Equally emphasizing discourse, institution, text, spectatorship and reception, my article interweaves an investigation into a range of writings and practices around endometriosis—from academic scientific journals and mass-media health magazines to self-help newsletters and alternative publications—with almost a decade of conversations carried out with women participating in endo support groups, with some emphasis placed on the implications of video-laparoscopic spectatorship.

A Question of Enigma and the Discourse of Hysteria

Familiarly referred to as "endo" among its bearers, endometriosis is a chronic women's disease characterized by the presence of functioning endometrial[3] tissue—the tissue of the uterine lining—in places where it is not usually found. In the case of endometriosis, the endometrium—often described as the support system of a "wasted," potential embryo, for which it regularly builds up, then sheds each month in the absence of an embryo to use it—migrates to other parts of the body and begins to grow in the form of scar tissue, cysts, and benign tumors, mostly in reproductive sites (ovaries, cul-de-sac, fallopian tubes), gastrointestinal sites (rectosigmoid colon, rectum, small bowel), urinary-tract sites (bladder, ureter, kidney), and lower genital sites (cervix, vagina, vulva).[4] These "islands" of tissue remain responsive to the body's monthly releases of reproductive hormones, which can exact from them an excruciatingly painful inflammatory response during menstruation and intercourse. They may also cause infertility, ruptured endometrioma, and ectopic pregnancy. Other symptoms include vomiting, fatigue, low back pain, rectal pain, blood in the stool, blood in the urine, fever, and tenderness around the kidneys.

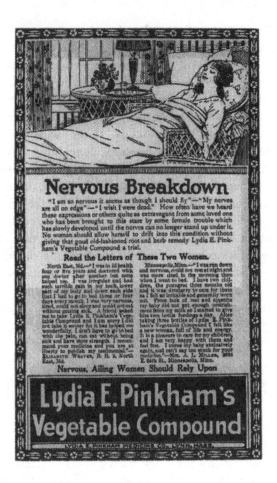

Figure 8.1

Endometriosis was not recognized as a disease for a long time. It was first described in the medical literature in 1896,[5] but was not named until 1925 by Dr. John Sampson. The submerged presence of endometriosis can be detected in a nineteenth-century ad for Lydia E. Pinkham's Vegetable Compound: below an image of a sick white woman in bed, surrounded by feminine cushions and flowers, appear the words "Nervous Breakdown" (figure 8.1). The testimonials that follow describe "female trouble," and are clearly symptomatic of endometriosis, but the convoluted language of "nervous, ailing women" inscribe a hysterical female figure.[6] Almost a century later, the ad for the Endometriosis Association used the image of a sick woman to promote endo consciousness by clearly

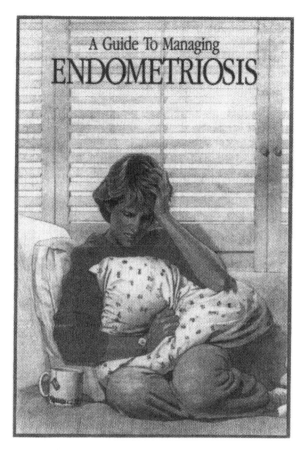

Figure 8.2 Endometriosis ad, reprinted from Mary Lou Ballweg and the Endometriosis Association's *Overcoming Endometriosis: New Help from the Endometriosis Association* (New York: Congdon & Weed, 1987).

asserting the materiality of a disease: a woman in bed, who has just rushed back home from work—the shoes and the briefcase are still by her bedside—holding a bottle of hot water on her abdomen. In marked contrast to the dreamy look of Lydia Pinkham's woman, the facial expression of pain in the Endometriosis Association woman, or in that of an 1987 Krames Communications booklet, "A Guide Managing to Endometriosis," illustrate the everyday experience of illness (figure 8.2). The texts, meanwhile, call attention to symptoms such as severe menstrual pain and heavy menstrual flow as signs of pathology, rather than of female (ab)nor-

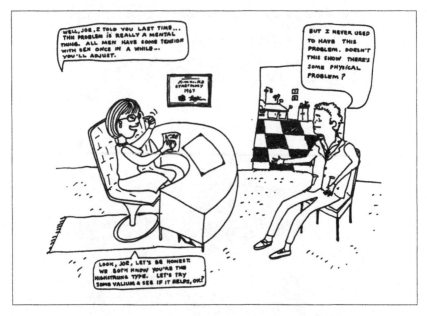

Figure 8.3   From Mary Lou Ballweg and Meri Lau's "Joe with Endo" cartoon series, reprinted from *Overcoming Endometriosis*.

mality, showing women of diverse racial backgrounds taking charge of their bodies and lives despite endometriosis.

An estimated five to ten million women in the United States today suffer pain and disability from endometriosis, yet little is known about the causes of what is still referred to in medical circles as "the female plague."[7] The enigma around the disease is accompanied by frequent ignorance and misdiagnosis in medical clinics, where women are prescribed tranquilizers to cure what doctors commonly describe as "a problem in the head." Women's pain, particularly in the area of their reproductive organs, tends to be attributed to fantasy, to signs of a neurotic personality, or just to the melancholic fate of being a woman. As Nancy Peterson, the director of the Endometriosis Treatment Program in Bend, Oregon, ironically comments: "If a man had a disease that causes him to be unable to father a child, to have unbearable pain during sex and unbearable pain during bowel movements, [which was] treated by feminizing hormones and surgery, endo would be declared a national emergency in this country."[8]

As part of the struggle to empower endo women, Mary Lou Ballweg, cofounder and president of the U.S.-Canada Endometriosis Association, has produced a series of cartoons, "Joe with Endo," in collaboration with the artist Meri Lau, in which a reversal of gender roles points to the role of institutional power in rendering endometriosis as female hysteria. In one cartoon a woman gynecologist paternalistically tells her ailing patient: "Well, Joe, I told you last time . . . this problem is really a mental thing. All men have some tension with sex once in a while . . . you'll adjust." And when Joe argues that he has never had this problem before, suggesting that it may actually be a physiological problem rather than psychological, she replies, "Look, Joe, let's be honest. We both know you're the high-strung type. Let's try some valium and see if it helps, o.k.?"[9] (figure 8.3).

The frequency of words like "enigma," "conundrum," "unknown," "perplexing," "mystery," and "puzzling"[10] in endo medical texts clearly recalls the discursive history that links female anatomy, sexuality, and psyche to the uncanny. Indeed the medical investigation of endometriosis perpetuates the "gendering" scientific ritual of measuring the unruly body against the norms of the observing scientist. Medical writing has clearly theorized endometriosis in terms of disorderly female biology, behavior, and personality, at times measuring women's reproductive physiology against a primate model. As Dr. Joe Vincent Meigs wrote in 1940:

> The monkey mates as soon as she becomes of age, and has offspring until she can no longer have any or until she dies. Menstruation in this animal must be rare. As women have the same physiology it must be wrong to put off childbearing until 14 to 20 years of menstrual life have passed.[11]

Apart from the dubious notion of erecting primate behavior as a model for women's choices, one notes in this passage that social expectations of women as mothers are still haunted by the masculinist mythology of the bleeding woman.[12] Menstruation is perceived as abnormal; its presence must be minimized. If the female cycle is extolled "as a productive enterprise," Emily Martin points out, "menstruation must necessarily be viewed as a failure."[13] Considering the theory that endometriosis is caused by a retrograde menstruation,[14] Meigs argued that "nature certainly did not intend that refluxed bleeding should be responsible for the growth of invasive tissue in the pelvis. Menstruation itself may be a kind of abnormality, for it occurs only infrequently in monkeys in their natural habitat."[15] Beneath such attempts to suppress "female" blood lies the suggestion that female physiology is a priori unnatural, even prior to the a posteriori deviance of delaying pregnancy. The submerged anxiety over the menstruating woman historically inscribed in masculinist popular culture, and notably in medical writing, is exacerbated in the case of menstrual "endo women," whose blood tends to be "thicker" and flows "excessively."

The biological "abnormalities" of 1940s medical discourse have now, to some extent, given way to other terms, focusing on psychological disorders. A recent study of chronic pelvic pain found no association between affective disorder and endometriosis.[16] Nevertheless, most studies since the 1950s have attempted to establish such links. In the 1980s, in academic publications such as the *American Journal of Psychiatry* and the *Western Journal of Medicine*, scientists argued for the relationship between endometriosis and "bipolar mood disorder," "affective disorder," and other mental illnesses. By positing a necessary "interaction of body type and psychic demeanor,"[17] these scientists associate endometriosis with a deviant personality: "The main characteristics involve being mesomorphic but underweight, having above-average intelligence, a higher than normal anxiety level, egocentrism, and a need for perfection."[18] These scholarly articles argue that endometriosis and bipolar mood disorders are "two poorly understood clinical syndromes," and since "hormonal fluctuations have been studied in relation to both, there could be a possible relationship."[19] The logic behind such studies, it seems, is that the addition of one female enigma to another may lead to an unveiling of the mysteries of the female organism. However, it is precisely the unresolved status of endometriosis that allows for this explanation of one enigma by another, ultimately positing femininity as overflowing the boundaries of rationalist discourse.[20]

Race, Class, and the "Career Woman's Disease"

The attempt to establish links between women's behavior and endometriosis is imbricated in the social construction of gender. In his 1940 article in *Annals of Surgery*, Meigs writes:

> In August, 1938, in an editorial, attention was drawn to the fact that endometriosis was increasing in frequency and that there was probably some reason for it. It was felt that the increase might be due to delayed marriages and the lack of early and frequent child-bearing, and suggested that the economic difficulties of the day were responsible for the increased frequency. . . . The real reason for the frequency [of endometriosis] is that endometriomata are not tumors but represent abnormal physiology due to the late marriage and delayed and infrequent child-bearing. The latter is due to the economic times we live in, and my plea is that patients with apparent infertility, evidences of underdevelopment, and older girls about to be married, be taught how to become pregnant and not how to avoid pregnancy, even though their finances are limited.[21]

Medical texts have often attributed endo-related infertility to lack of reproductivity: "If girls would learn to follow nature and have children early," doctors have warned, "neither endometriosis nor the resulting infertility would exist."[22] The anxiety that medical texts manifest around the non(re)productive vessel is sometimes displayed in a rhetoric that weaves the scientific and the metaphysical in a way unusual for the post-Enlightenment. As Dr. Roger Scott and Dr. Richard Te Linde write in their *Annals of Surgery* 1950s article, "External Endometriosis: The Scourge of the Private Patient," "a large number of women must accept this childless state as God's will or fate's bidding until the element of pain presents itself."[23] Their study reverberates with quasi-Biblical castigation, implying that women who postpone or forgo childbearing betray the telos of their natural role. But women's misguided conduct, it is suggested, is redeemable if they redirect themselves toward a blessed heterosexual union, which will put an end to endo—hence the article's focus on "behavioral changes." Implicit in this perspective is the suggestion that medical research into the etiology of endometriosis is almost unnecessary, for the disease is clearly an unfortunate consequence of a woman's deviant lifestyle.

Since the early 1940s, the principal hypothesis of the origins of endometriosis has revolved around late marriage and childbearing. But given that in the post-World War II era "earlier marriages and childbearing have been the rule,"[24] 1950s medical texts faced a new challenge in theorizing about endometriosis. Adding some new insights, they argued that "possibly, more than a passing consideration should be given to the dietary habits or the emotional and environmental changes incidental to the larger pocketbook."[25] The shift into a skewed version of class analysis within the brief period of one decade indicates the transition of the North American middle class into the relatively prosperous 1950s. In the context of the 1950s obsessive popular images of "the American family"—male provider in gray flannel suit coming home to playful son, daughter, dog, and beaming blonde wife, who, with perfect timing, delivers a roast turkey straight from a shining oven—scientific discourse delivered its own vision of the gendered division of labor. Lurking behind the desire to detect endometriosis in the "larger pocketbook" is an ideological subtext of benevolent equilibrium and fair exchange: in an era of multiplying magical household gadgets born of the wedding of science and capitalism, women, presumably with new "free time" to spend in leisurely consumption, must pay back with female labor, producing new human beings out of the (female) reproductive machine.

Since the 1960s, in the context of the feminist movement, endometriosis has often been referred to as the "career woman's disease," because of its enduring association with the choice not to bear children. Some recent studies have shown endometriosis to be an "equal opportunity disease," striking women of all socioeconomic, racial, and age groups,[26] but doctors are still inclined to diagnose it largely in white professionals. In December 1980, in the *Houston Chronicle*, Dr. Veasy Buttram described "the typical patient with endometriosis as an ambitious woman who delays marriage until completion of college and postpones childbearing until financial security has been attained."[27] The rhetoric of earlier decades—"modern economic trends are responsible for delayed marriage," "youth is the proper time to have children and it is right that [women] be urged to do so"[28]—echoes still in contemporary medical texts: doctors still prescribe pregnancy as a cure for endometriosis, eliding the typical scenario of the endo woman who does get pregnant, but then simply becomes a mother with endometriosis.

Despite the differences between changing historical moments, most endo theories share a structural positioning of women as the generators of their own disease. Writing from their specific sexual, class, racial, and national context, scientists have systematically closed their eyes to the startling fact that the disease has been diagnosed in girls in their early teens as well as in women who have given birth to over ten children—a contradiction of the hegemonic endo theory that "prolonged cyclic menstruation not interrupted by pregnancy constitutes a major risk factor for the disease."[29] Science's rush to search for the origins of endo in the fertile area of female deviation recalls AIDS discourses in relation to gay men: the victims are blamed for bringing the disease upon themselves. Relegated to the realm of the metaphysical, endometriosis is seen as the inevitable conclusion to the hubris of "going against nature." Just as AIDS is deemed God's revenge on "unnatural" homosexual conduct, endometriosis is deemed God's revenge on the unnatural conduct of preternaturally ambitious professional women.

Furthermore, much of the 1980s research into the condition has been dedicated to the assumed relationship between endometriosis and infertility. The authors of diverse classifications of endometriosis, for example Buttram's, are fond of the peritoneal/ovarian/tubal/cul-de-sac division. Concerned only with forms of endometriosis related to infertility, they consider other forms so insignificant as hardly to merit classification. Endometriosis of the ureter or appendix, let alone of the lungs, the muscles of the arms or legs, or the pelvic lymph nodes, is shrugged off, since endometrial symptoms in these areas "have not yet been related to infertility," and therefore "a separate classification seems impractical."[30]

Medical writings tend to categorize endometriosis patients and pre-scribe remedies according to a woman's reproductive age and her desire for fertility. Ovaries are not removed if a woman's ability to bear children can be preserved, but "patients in whom childbearing is complicated or not desired" are met with "definitive treatment by surgical excision of the endometriotic tissue and the pelvic organs."[31] The "hysterectomy treat-ment" is the standard prescription for women who express disinterest in bearing children, and for those who have already performed their repro-ductive duty. In medical texts on endometriosis, however, the conse-quences of hysterectomy for women, such as osteoporosis and heart disease, not to mention emotional trauma, are relegated to marginalia. One of the "Joe with Endo" cartoons again deploys the carnivalesque strategy of gender inversion to criticize physicians' automatic decision to use hysterectomy to "solve" endo: a female doctor casually misinforms Joe that "the definitive cure is the removal of the testicles. Then there'll be no hormones to feed this endometriosis." Shocked and alarmed by the idea of castration, Joe receives the blasé response that "we don't usually use that word . . . too frightening." And to Joe's proposal that "there *must* be some-thing else!" the doctor answers patronizingly: "You men. You get so attached to your organs. Besides, if we remove them you'll never worry about cancer."[32]

The notion of cure for endometriosis through the two extreme approaches of sterilization and childbearing is thoroughly mythologized. Similarly, other "treatments"—conservative surgery and hormonal ther-apy—are meant to enable reproduction in the future. Since endometriosis is often defined in terms of women's reproductive capacities, some gyne-cological clinics are reluctant to treat endo women unless they demon-strate a desire to conceive. Women with endometriosis may also be pressured into having babies as therapy, even when they are ambivalent about or clearly disinterested in the prospect of motherhood. The walls of expensive clinics are often decorated with the doctor's triumphant tro-phies: photographs of the scores of babies issuing from treatment, signed, as it were, with the doctor's authorial signature.[33] The medical apparatus nurtures the female organs (for women who can afford it) toward the tri-umphant resolution of reproduction. Endometriosis is treated seriously only when it interferes with conception, displacing a more conventional medical narrative of healing bodies no matter what. Thus it is difficult to imagine less reproductively oriented photos in a gynecological clinic—of women dancing without pain, for example, or performing sex in acrobatic positions. Endo discourse suggests that science has made it possible to correct nature's "fuck-ups," but in the "natural" way: by helping to strengthen the traditional heterosexual family.

It is not women's desire for heterosexual marriage and children that is being criticized here but rather the medical establishment's representation of endometriosis as merely an obstacle to the normal trajectory of motherhood.[34] In fact, the fertility approach to endometriosis often introduces a catch-22 situation: pregnancy is recommended as the cure for endo, but endo that affects fertility makes pregnancy impossible. To superimpose a teleological narrative of birth, motherhood, and heterosexual parenthood on endometriosis only hinders a serious investigation into the cure for the disease. Babies do not cure endometriosis, and fertility clinics do not cater to endo women's health needs. What about the women with endometriosis who *can* conceive children? What about the woman already having both children and endometriosis? Or the woman who continues to have endometriosis even after hysterectomy? While the in/fertile female constitutes the desired object of the scientific gaze, the endo female looms in the background as an object yet to be deciphered—a split that renders both subjectivities invisible.[35]

The erasure of women's agency in medical discourse is deeply ingrained in class and racial discourses, grounding the racialized female body differently, and even in opposite ways. In most medical studies, white upper-middle-class professional women are considered the primary risk group for pelvic endometriosis.[36] At times, class analysis of endometriosis overrides race considerations: Dr. F. P. Lloyd wrote in a 1964 issue of the *American Journal of Obstetrics and Gynecology* that the occurrence of pelvic endometriosis in blacks approaches that of whites as blacks achieve a higher socioeconomic status and standard of living.[37] It seems that African American women cannot move up the social ladder without risking a white-professional-female disease—a revealing sign that both groups of women "moved out of their place." (One wonders at exactly which step of the tax bracket the disease is likely to strike.)

Race, however, remains a major paradigm for medical researchers, at pains to prove that women of color and Third World women are endo free.[38] Many medical scholars who have "researched" Third World women have reached the astonishing conclusions that "in the Middle East and in India our colleagues seldom encounter endometriosis," that "through personal observations endometriosis is almost nonexistent among peasant women of South Vietnam and Afghanistan," and that "endometriosis was comparatively infrequent in Mexican Indian women."[39] Scientific studies that racialize endometriosis lead to the misdiagnosis of women of color, whose endo symptoms may be due to other causes, such as pelvic inflammatory disease.

Inflammatory ailments carry sexual overtones of redness and heat. While upper-middle-class white women are diagnosed with a career-related disease, black women are diagnosed with a sexually connoted one.[40] In a recent series of 190 laparoscopies performed on black women, Dr. Donald L. Chatman noted that 21 percent of his subjects, previously diagnosed as having pelvic inflammatory disease, in fact had endometriosis.[41] The real question, then, is not why endometriosis strikes the white-skinned woman, but what is at stake in the massive medical literature that persists in racially codifying a disease associated with the reproductive organs. It seems obvious that the relationship between race and the diagnosis of endo might be better explained by differential access to good medical care and health information,[42] but what, then, are the implications of positing a low rate of endometriosis for women of color and Third World women? Medical discourse, implicitly, it seems, makes the argument (for white women to hear) that Asian or African women's low rate of endometriosis and high birthrate prove that the postponement of pregnancy adds to the risk of developing the disease. "Paradoxically, white middle-class women," as Rayna Rapp points out, "are both better served by reproductive medicine, and also more controlled by it, than women of less privileged groups."[43]

Women of color and Third World women are subjected to what one might call a dis-reproductive medical apparatus: by avoiding diagnosis of endometriosis—a disease publicly linked to infertility—in women of color, the medical system excludes them from the reproduction track of presumed cure. Physicians may be more likely to diagnose pelvic inflammatory disease in women of color because the "cure" is often sterilization. The selective approach that tends to apply the hysterectomy solution to white endo women according to age and the desire to have children, takes on an entirely different accent in the case of women of color for whom hysterectomy is seen to be the one and only cure. It is difficult to avoid the conclusion of what Stuart Hall calls "inferential racism" in the treatment, knowledge, and approach to endometriosis. If white women's delayed childbearing is presented as disorderly conduct, women of color's precipitous fertility is seen as disorderly for the opposite reasons. And while one type of disorderly conduct requires coaxing into fertility as a cure, the other requires reinforcement of infertility.

That prolifers choose to remain willfully ignorant of the policies of sterilization found, for example, in Bolivia and Puerto Rico and documented, respectively, in films like Jorge Sanjiné's and the Grupo Ukamau's *Yawar mallku* ("Blood of the Condor," 1969) and Ana Maria Garcia's *La Operación* (1981) shows the hypocrisy and contradiction of their lack of concern for *these* women's bodies. With U.S. complicity, and without a single prolife silent scream, Bolivian indigenous women have been forcibly sterilized, at the same time that the former Banzer regime, as Angela Gilliam points out, agreed to resettle thirty thousand white South Africans in order to help the "racial imbalance" of a country that still has an indigenous majority.[44] The U.S. government legalized sterilization in Puerto Rico in 1937 to manage the menace of what was called "excess population."[45] Federal strategies of modernization, as Maria Milagros Lopez points out, have included population control through a massive program of public sterilization "services."[46] Since the 1950s, 35 percent of Puerto Rican women in their reproductive years have been sterilized, at times pressured by doctors' "modern" advice, at others, waking up to a reality of "tied tubes," performed without their prior knowledge or consent.

If in Puerto Rico women were the guinea pigs for contraceptive experimentation, in the United States, as Angela Davis points out, women's bodies have been the site of a historical overlapping between the movement for birth control and the ideology of eugenics.[47] And as Cheryl Johnson-Odim argues, "the fact that surgical sterilization remains free and that federal funding for abortions has been disallowed means that it is poor women to whom the *choice* to abort is denied, and their ranks are disproportionately populated by women of color."[48] This history of discriminatory sterilization policies and the medical establishment's unfounded racialization of the female body discursively constructs an endo body with a hidden demographic agenda.

Video Laparoscopy and Laser Illuminations

A key therapy for endometriosis "requires hormonal suppression of the production of estrogen by the ovaries."[49] Given the fertility dogma, articles have proliferated in medical journals on methods of hormone suppression. Strangely echoing the figure of the menstruating body as aberrant, the endo body undergoes a hormonal mimicry of either menopause or pregnancy, in what amounts to a postmodern virtual demenstrualization of the bleeding female. Hormones (Danazol and Lupron, for example), have deleterious side effects that are obscured by the triumphant narrative of hormonal progress. They produce pseudomenopause, forcing a young woman to proleptically experience a kind of flash-forward: in her early 20s she is turned into a simulacrum of youth with the physiology of a woman in her 40s or 50s trapped inside her; she may experience hot flashes, osteoporosis, and decreased sexual drive. Pseudomenopause, then, is a painful preview of aging and mortality.[50] This virtual-menopausal hybrid woman transgresses conventional concepts of pre- and postmenopausal women: she is an "in-between" woman, occupying two temporalities. (An exploration of this pre/post-hybrid might have added an interesting dimension to the discussion of female spectatorship in Yvonne Rainer's 1990 film, *Privilege*, which considers the politics of aging and menopause.) Both chemically or hormonally induced pseudomenopause and pseudopregnancy may lessen the symptoms of endometriosis, but they do little to heal endo women and much to undermine their health. Recent studies of the links between endometriosis and the immune system[51] propose a female body that ought to remain open and ready for any kind of hormonal (mis)treatment to maximize its procreativity.

Surgery as a "cure" for endometriosis encompasses a variety of procedures, from traditional laparotomy to video (laser) laparoscopy. But given the degree of specialization and practice required to use laser laparoscopy, most doctors still choose the traditional laparotomy operation. Often performed on an outpatient basis, and under general anesthesia, laparoscopy involves the insertion of a lighted periscopelike instrument through a small incision near the navel, enabling the surgeon to inspect the organs in the abdomen. Laparoscopy has been combined with laser technologies, first medically employed for eye surgery, and used in gynecology only since 1980.[52] More precise than electrocautery or cryosurgery, the powerful combination of the laser and the laparoscope reduces blood loss as well as the risk of infection from external viruses. As Dr. Camran Nezhat, the director of the Fertility and Endocrinology Center in Atlanta and an advisor to the Endometriosis Association, points out, the laser can be concentrated and its energy focused to a pinpoint, allowing the vaporization of small endometrial implants without the destruction of surrounding tissue. Moreover, the laser beam can reach sites that would be difficult to reach with the scalpel. Laser surgery can also be done more quickly than conventional laparotomy, so that the patient can be anesthetized for less time; it also reduces the possibility of scar formation. With the CO_2 laser beam, surgeons can vaporize or make an incision as small as a millimeter without touching the tissue. The energy of the carbon dioxide laser beam is absorbed almost completely at a depth of a millimeter from the tissue. It can therefore be used over vital organs without damaging underlying structures.[53]

Gradually, more surgeons are combining a video camera, video recorder, and high-resolution video monitor with laser laparoscopy. Here a view of the operating field (what the surgeon sees through the laparoscope) is projected onto the video monitor and videotaped for future reference. The surgeon views the monitor during the procedure, rather than looking through the laparoscope.[54] According to Dr. Nezhat, this is a significant advantage, for it allows the surgeon to work in a comfortable, upright posture (watching the video monitor) rather than bent over the laparoscope. Fatigue is lessened and precision is enhanced. The second major advantage is having a permanent video record of the procedure, for verification, insurance, and follow-up purposes.[55]

These meaningful advances in medical technologies have substantially improved endo women's quality of life. Like hormones, however, laser surgery removes the symptoms of endometriosis only temporarily. Laser laparoscopy is generally followed by hormone treatments that suppress the disease but often leave the woman susceptible to a "return of the repressed" in the form of myriad future side effects. Thus, while the advent of relatively noninvasive procedures such as laser laparoscopy used in tandem with video augers a technical/medical advance, the continued medical resistance to more collaborative models of treatment and healing remain a problem. Hence, I am certainly not proposing that there is something inherently wrong with the technologies or the doctors that use them. Rather, my concern is with a discursive tradition that has consistently dismissed the voices of endo women and refused any dialogue with self-help organizations that have been in the forefront of facilitating the circulation of information on endo. For example, a *Newsweek* article, "Conquering Endometriosis: Lasers Battle the 'Career Woman's Disease' " (1986), presents lasers as a panacea, offering a triumphal narrative of science coming to women's rescue.[56] Similarly, a *Science News* article of 1981, "Lasers Versus Female Complaints," sets up a classical gendered opposition, casting women as hysterical whiners and associating lasers with the male scientists who use technology to take care of "female complaints"[57] (figure 8.4).

To posit science as masculine and nature as feminine, as some of these articles implicitly do, effectively requires a narrative of heroic mastery, in which women have no investigatory role in their own bodies. This medical discourse not only excludes the voices of women scientists and patients, it paradoxically hails the advances of the technology—which is a treatment, but not necessarily a cure—while simultaneously undermining the reality of the disease. It is no surprise then that the images accompanying such articles typically show male doctors holding the video laparo-

Lasers Versus Female Complaints

Laser surgical techniques now promise increased benefits in gynecology

BY DIETRICK E. THOMSEN

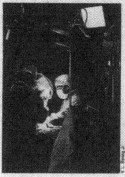

People who think of lasers in surgery are likely to think first of eye surgery. It was in that department of surgery that lasers were first employed, and in which over the years they have received a good deal of publicity. Gynecology is reputed to be one of the largest medical specialties. Whatever may be the comparative statistics between gynecological surgery and ocular surgery, it is certain that the world's hospitals see a good number of gynecological operations in a year. Thus, the extension of laser techniques to gynecological treatments, which has begun in the last couple of years, promises to add greatly to the number of those who benefit from the laser's surgical capabilities.

Among those benefits, according to J. H. Bellina of Louisiana State University School of Medicine, who was invited to review progress in the field at the recent Lasers '80 Conference in New Orleans, is a higher probability of eradication of premalignant and malignant conditions and the maintenance or restoration of fertility in cases where other techniques could not. The instrument generally used for this work, he says, is the so-called AO 100, which uses articulated mirrors to deliver a spot of laser light to the point where the surgeon wants it. This system has gotten smaller over the years since 1974, Bellina says, both in gross physical size — its electrical housing was once six feet across — and in the size of the spot of laser light it delivers, which can now be as small as 125 micrometers under certain conditions.

One purpose of these tiny pinpoints of light is to destroy the abnormal growths in the lining of the cervix, known as dysplastic cells, and the carcinoma *in situ* or superficial cancer that sometimes develops from the dysplastic lesions.

Dysplasia is not a rare disease. Bellina says it is reaching epidemic proportions in the United States, not to mention other parts of the world. Furthermore, the age of onset has been dropping. Years ago dysplasia was seen usually in mature women, women in their thirties and older. Now the average age of incidence is in the 14- to 25-year range, Bellina says, and pushing toward the pre-teen years. The carcinoma that may develop from it is not far behind. Bellina says the earliest carcinoma *in situ* in his experience was in a 14-year-old. "And I've had a 21-year-old already dead from it," he adds.

Not all appearances of dysplasia — which is sometimes called precancerous tissue — develop into malignancies. The figure is about 30 percent. The rest tend to regress and disappear. "But we don't have a good model to tell us which will and which won't," says Bellina.

So the obvious therapeutic procedure is to get rid of it all, to destroy the dysplastic cells thoroughly enough to prevent recurrences.

At the beginning of the 1970s cryosurgery was applied, but there seemed to be a hazard: the survival of a certain amount of the DNA of the dysplastic cells, which could then serve to trigger a recurrence. Lasers were brought in to see if they could do better.

One question was how deep the killing of cells and destruction of DNA had to go. The textbooks said 3 millimeters deep. Cryosurgery had gone that deep, but apparently something underneath had escaped. Textbooks to the contrary, Bellina says, "Nobody had ever sat down and measured this." The laser surgeons tried at first to develop some range finding indicators, but the effort proved costly, and the patients' heartbeats were confusing the issue because they gave the tissue pulsations with a 2-millimeter amplitude.

The researchers decided to do the job clinically, starting very shallow and going deeper and deeper till they reached a point of optimum benefit. At 3 millimeters they had a 16 percent recurrence rate. They decided, Bellina says, "We'll go wider and just go deeper." The depth went to 4, 4.5, 5 even to 7 millimeters. Below 5 millimeters they got the recurrence rate down to 4.4 percent. As of today, in 1,500 cases that they have followed for some time, there is a recurrence rate of about 5 percent.

Where there is carcinoma *in situ*, the laser technique is to try to destroy all of the tumor. The way this is done, the way the laser heat transfer vaporizes the cells and destroys the chemical bonds in their DNA and RNA material, seems particularly effective in destroying the malignancy and preventing recurrence. As an example, the 14-year-old girl mentioned above, who caught the disease from her mother, has now been followed for two years without a recurrence.

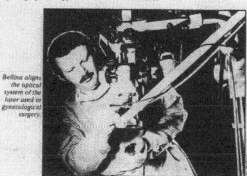

Bellina aligns the optical system of the laser used in gynecological surgery.

Figure 8.4a and b   An article with photographs of Dr. J. H. Bellina next to the lasers and video laprascope. Reprinted from *Science News*, Vol. 119, no. 6 (7 February 1981): 90–91.

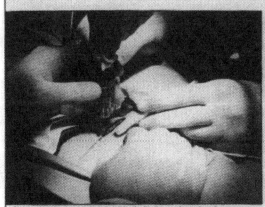

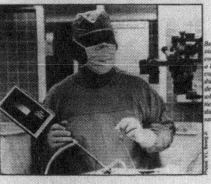

Figure 8.4b

LASERS FOR LADIES

. . . ladies with gynecological warts
and other problems

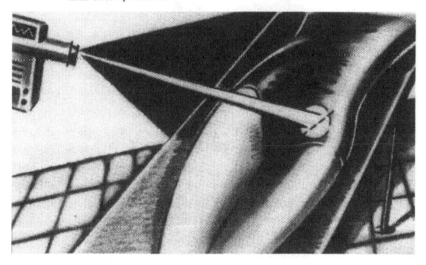

Figure 8.5   A 1983 illustration in *Health* magazine accompanying the article "Laser for Ladies."

scope, while women are represented as framed body parts. A 1983 cartoon in *Health* magazine, accompanying an article entitled "Lasers for Ladies," shows a video camera shooting a phallic laser ray which penetrates the lower abdomen of a reclining (headless) female in a bathing suit, creating a prominent hole (figure 8.5).[58] Without any apparent irony, this visualization of penetration transmutes medical scrutiny into an erotic gaze.

The erotic component of the (masculine) gaze of knowledge/power and in this instance—medicine—focused on its female object has been the subject of much feminist investigation. And in fact, a number of feminist artists have addressed this pattern in the mass-media representations of medical technologies and female patients. Sherry Millner, in a recent collage entitled *Love at First Site* (1990), juxtaposes 1950s magazine images of three male gynecologists hovering over a female patient, each facing a strategic part of her body: two have their heads in close proximity to her breasts, the third holds a camera at her vagina. The "patient" is in fact a mannequin wearing a 1950s bathing suit, thus placing the artificially con-

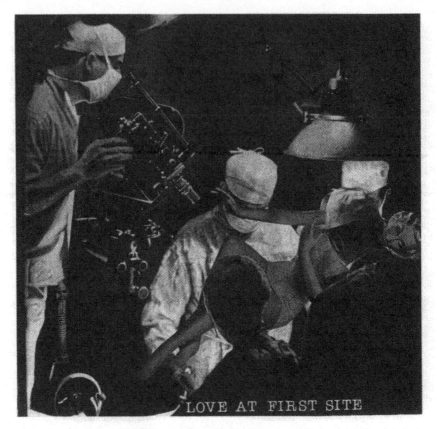

Figure 8.6   Sherry Millner, *Love at First Site* (1990).

structed woman of the fashion industry on a continuum with the woman
as constructed by the medical gaze (figure 8.6).

In sharp contrast to the feminist publications of the Endometriosis
Association, articles in scientific journals and mass-media magazines, as
well as their accompanying visuals, suppress women's narratives, women's
struggles for democratic access to new technologies and to research on
alternative healing. In other words, the scientific and mass-media discourse
on endo surgically removes women's voices from the discussion of their
own bodies. While the hormone treatment discourse focuses on the suppression of the disorderly body, the representation of laser-video gyno-
technology privileges an exploratory voyeurism into an anesthetized body,
and it is this form of voyeurism that subtly underpins the ways in which
video and laser laparoscopy lends itself to a master narrative of penetration,

exploration, and cleansing of an always and already polluted female body. (Laparoscopy's nickname is "keyhole surgery.")[59] Video laparoscopy narrates the very act of transformation from the inside out. Whereas in physiological cinema the camera, as Lisa Cartwright points out, was "incorporated as an instrument within the life of the body under study,"[60] in video laparoscopy the camera not only observes and documents the surgery, it also performs it, thus becoming an agent "acting not only on the body but in and through it."[61]

In hegemonic endo discourse the video camera renders the interior body accessible, while also transforming the doctor into the author of a videotape of a newly fashioned body. The combination of video and laser laparoscopy can also record the surgical procedure; the doctor becomes filmmaker, or, more precisely, videomaker. The hand that wields the scalpel triggers the camera. Although this transformation of the act of looking into the act of visual recording results in the patient having access to a video-laparoscopic record of the surgery and the interior of her own body, the medical discourse exclusively focuses on the surgeon as the videotape auteur.

Along with the language of voyeurism and auteurship, one also finds in this discourse a rhetoric of pollution and purity. Indeed in some gynecological clinics, the term "clean up" is casually used to refer to the laser-surgery cleansing of the body. Video laparoscopy is used not only to document endometriosis but to (temporarily) cleanse the body: the silvery tube of the laser is seen cutting, burning, and separating out the malignant tissues, shooting water to rinse away the blood, and finally vacuuming away the unwanted matter. Abnormal tissue and tubal obstructions are vaporized; the smoke is suctioned out. Although the rhetoric of "clean up" pervades all surgical discourse, and is in no way restricted to women and their reproductive organs, it has special resonance and irony when applied to women, given the medical discursive legacy that figures the female body as a walking pathological laboratory. Thus in medical texts, one often encounters a subliminal image of a filth-producing female body foiled by science's laser-eye machines, which probe the interior and spit out a cleansing fire. Video images of blood, smoke, and water on the screen depict the viscera as a kind of abstract action-painting battle zone. It is an apocalyptic imagery of cleansing the landscape through fire and flood. But in spite of all the thrilling special effects of the endo surgery, only the symptoms have been eradicated; the "evil" is left to fester—the endometriosis has not been cured and can always return.

Although medical and mass-media texts show a near-fetishistic fascination with each new gyno-technological invention, most remain silent about the stagnation in endometriosis research. Endometriosis activists, however, are often much more ambivalent about novel uterus-imaging technologies. When video laparoscopy, for example, is hailed for conquering the farthest reaches of the interior, it is not the effectiveness of this technology that is in question; rather it is the scientific community's unwillingness to address endo etiology, that is, its origins, as well as its prevention and cure.

This privileging of industrial gyno-technological discoveries fails to acknowledge the perspective of the "object" under investigation. In the case of video laparoscopy, the notion of scientific discovery is grafted onto a discourse of technological expansion into the "virgin land" of the female body, hitherto untouched by such a penetrating gaze. This implicit link between the technological and the epistemological dates back to Francis Bacon's analogy between scientific and geographic discoveries. ("And as the immense regions of the West Indies had never been discovered, if the use of the compass had not first been known, it is no wonder that the discovery and the advancement of arts hath made no greater progress, when the art of inventing and discovering of the sciences remains hitherto unknown.")[62] It also evokes Sigmund Freud's analogy between psychoanalytic and archeological excavations: he compares "clearing away the pathogenic psychical material layer by layer" with "the technique of excavating a buried city."[63] An enigmatic space, the endo female body requires the "pioneering work" of voyages into unknown "dark continents," its terra incognita.[64] The visual lay of the body, spread out for exploration, promotes sonogram and video laparoscopy as the postmodern cartography of the female interior. And it is thus the language of "exploration" and "conquest" that shapes these ultrasound and video-laparoscopic visuals. With X-ray as a black and white photograph, and video laparoscopy as a color documentary film, the surgeon is positioned as a traveling image maker of the female body, whose organs s/he explores, documents, and rearranges.

In other words, video laparoscopy is more than a means of observing and recording pathological organs; it literally reconfigures the body. Whereas access to the invisible interior was formerly only possible by dissecting cadavers in autopsies and cutting the body open in surgery, recent imaging technologies permit that access with only a minimal incision. Through the camera/monitor apparatus, the surgeon can remove an ovarian cyst without having to remove the ovary, helping the patient to maintain an externally more aesthetic body, with fewer scars. Video laparoscopy, like cosmetic surgery, even allows for a "before" and "after" image. Yet the tendency of endometriosis to recur means there can never be a perfect cosmetic reconstruction; the laser's costume designing of the body is not permanent, and there may be many "befores" and many "afters."

Institutionalized endo discourse tends not to acknowledge this limitation and celebrates instead the "revolution"[65] of laser laparoscopy as a new weapon in science's video war against a self-destructive uterus. The laser, Prometheus-like, brings light into the body's dark corners. The once opaque womb is stripped of its mystery, and the light of scientific knowledge shines on the dark inner sanctum. Tropes of light and darkness, informed by Enlightenment ideas, are projected onto an out-of-control (female) nature. Superimposed on the language of exploration in endo discourse, then, is a military language of firing with precision at the target "by going into the uterus through the vagina."[66] As constructed in scientific discourse (Bacon, Freud), the enigma often requires uncovering, unveiling, and penetration. Video laparoscopy, in a sense, only literalizes the metaphor.

While the language of infiltration is on one level appropriate since there is an actual penetration in such surgery, on another it occludes women's voices and historically has been premised on a colonizing model of exploration. However, medical technologies could be alternatively conceived as a collaborative project in which women participate in scientific investigation and technological healing. In this perspective, scientific enigmas are not detached from women's bodies but are studied and remapped through a dialogical process.

Already this other story is beginning to be enacted by the few scientists who have worked with self-help organizations. In his forward to Mary Lou Ballweg and the Endometriosis Association's *Overcoming Endometriosis*, Dr. Camran Nezhat, for example, speaks in language rooted in community ("sharing," "partnership," "working together"). The only time the word "conquering" is evoked, it is used instead to suggest a notion of community, of "conquering together" the disease. Working closely with the Endometriosis Association, doctors such as Maria Menna Perper and Camran Nezhat, who conceive of making the "doctor-patient relationship truly a partnership,"[67] disrupt science's institutional authority. These few pockets of disruption represent the possibility of shifting from a science constituted by knowledge and power to a science shaped by community values and needs.

Part of the new endo story being told involves accepting endometriosis as a disease worthy of research and funding. The point is to argue that medical texts' celebration of laser surgery often displaces the issue of research into endometriosis—research not profitable to the multimillion-dollar medical-technology industry. Critical endo discourse, in other words, promotes the aim of raising awareness about preventive and holistic care and funding research over the special effects of gyno-technology.

Self-Spectatorship and Healing Strategies

In the fertility clinic, where the surgeon tends to be represented as both a scientist and a videomaker documenting "science's war against nature," video laparoscopy becomes a tool to plumb the "inherent" mysteries of the female body and female sexuality. Although a surgical procedure, video laparoscopy must also be understood as a form of cinematic representation of the female body, taking into account the complex relations among looks, spectatorship, and gendered/racialized identities found there. The ways that endo women view video-laparoscopic images pose a challenge to models of spectatorship premised on desire and pleasure. For example, the eroticism associated with the scientific gaze, as vividly illustrated in the lasers-for-ladies cartoon, is radically undermined in video laparoscopy by the endo spectacle itself. The interior inscribed on the video screen is more emetic than erotic: pinkish, reddish, and brownish organs and viscera, which recall those of poultry,[68] confront most viewers with a sense of dizzying mortality, only heightened by the fact that these images give visual form to the fighting of a disease. This suggests a model of spectatorship in which endo women are agents in a healing gaze—a kind of spectatorship that has not been addressed in film theory.

Insofar as the video screen is transmuted into a specular image of the interior body, which cannot ordinarily be reflected in the mirror, binaries of beautiful/ugly and black/white are temporarily erased. Going beyond the epidermis appears to erase the markers of racial difference. Video laparoscopy not only allows one to look into a previously invisible interior of the body but also to create a narrative of bodily transformation and healing. Video laparoscopy, then, raises questions about narrative structure and spectatorial identification, specifically bringing up the issue of what one might call *self-spectatorship*. How can feminist cultural criticism address the particular experiences of women watching their own surgery post facto? And what is the nature of identification for a female spectator watching a body on the screen that is her own?

Conversations with endo women who have watched their own video laparoscopy tapes[69] reveal certain spectatorial tendencies, ranging from an anxious refusal to watch something that brings back a traumatic moment, to a more confident hope that watching these images will contribute to healing through the process of "getting back in touch with our bodies."[70] The refusal to watch is not solely limited to women who experienced unsuccessful surgeries. Post-video-laparoscopic spectatorship is ambivalently implicated in unconscious body memory. In this rendezvous between conscious spectator and unconscious patient, who happen to be one and the same person, video-laparoscopic images may trigger a relived memory of past pain, along with a prosthetic experience of the removed cyst in the form of renewed endo pain. Many endo women describe their anxiety about confronting a cinematic depiction of their own bodily fragility, along with a fear of reexperiencing consciously what they formerly experienced unconsciously: the penetration of camera-tube, laser, vaporizer, and the action of cutting, burning, and suctioning, seen in a kind of a retroactive mirror image. Women watching their video laparoscopy tapes speak of a visceral, physical reaction, of intuitively touching the previously or currently sensitive organs, particularly those in the lower abdomen. Those who cannot bear the sight are divided between their fear and their temptation to look at the video screen.

The knowledge of whether the surgery was a success or failure affects how the endo spectator responds to the images. In a "happy ending" video laparoscopy, it is not unusual for spectators to cheer the slow efforts of tweezers grabbing scar tissue, or the vaporizer suctioning out a cyst, particularly when some women feel that they have been "invaded by a sneaky unstable alien."[71] In instances of unsuccessful video laparoscopy when the surgeon was unable to excise a cyst, and had to revert to traditional laparotomy, fewer women wanted to play their videotapes. Some gave them to their endo support group to watch and study in their absence, as part of a follow-up discussion. In all cases the desire to master the details of the medical procedure, whether through viewing the tapes or discussing them in a group, is bound up in the wish to be an agent of one's own healing.

For some, it is the strange reflexivity of these images that make them difficult to view. Just as videotaped laser eye-surgery suggests, à la Buñuel, the slicing of an open eye, video laparoscopy evokes the camera obscura of the cinematic apparatus. The metaphors of cinema as dream, of regress to the womb, are here literalized by a spectator who peers into the uterus, although one that is well-lit and in living color. On the other hand, the living color of dissected organs subverts the subject-effect; here there can be no regression to protective darkness. And in any case, what does it mean for the self-spectating woman to "escape" to her own ailing womb?

Microscopic video enlargement makes the visuals strikingly dramatic by providing a magnified look at the organs and the machinery. In endo self-spectatorship—or, better, in vicarious self-spectatorship—identification with one's own organs, temporarily injured by the invasive burning/cutting machine, is inevitable, even if one often has to look away from the screen. But this identificatory impulse can be accompanied by another identification with the camera itself. Sharing the point of view of the camera, the self-spectator looks at her own body through the camera's penetrating eye that preceded her into herself. If there is a kind of anxiety at the sight of the burning laser and the vaporizer taking out chunks of her body, there is also an identification—particularly after the first viewing—with the lasers and vaporizers themselves, as the machines that battle the invasive tissues. In this sense, it is also the surgeon's perspective that the spectator internalizes, thus allowing the endo woman to vicariously transform herself into a surgeon, an agent of her own healing. Video laparoscopy can realize what a member of the Endometriosis Association expressed: "I wish I could perform the 'lap' myself so I could see the 'enemy' for myself!"[72]

Viewing these silent moving images, intended to enable the scientist to monitor the surgery, can become a kind of epistemological boomerang in which the gazed upon can return the gaze. Despite the lasers-for-ladies representation of laparoscopic technologies, these techniques cannot and should not be reduced to or equated with a voyeuristic/militarist apparatus, since they can also aid the process of partial healing, especially in the context of a dialogical interaction between endo women and scientific research. Thus video laparoscopy offers the possibility not just of a "black box" documentation of a gynecological voyage of dissection and suture, but also a collaborative study of endometriosis, where the interior arena is not restricted to the eyes of the surgeon. If pathological and anatomical dissections are premised on an immobile corpse, at the service of medical and legal institutions, in video laparoscopy the "dead" object (usually) returns to life, able to watch, critique, and participate in the ongoing struggle for healing. Thus her surgical immobility assumes her future mobility—her ability to look back and talk back.[73]

Video-laparoscopic viewing, I should point out, is not a major aspect of endo self-help meetings, which are dedicated to diverse forms of sharing information and support. In fact, more commonly, endo women first watch the Endometriosis Association production *"You're Not Alone . . . Understanding Endometriosis"* (1988). This film is a conventional documentary about the disease featuring experts in the field as well as voices of the association chapters' members who speak of their experiences—from pre-diagnostic loneliness to postoperative participation—in self-help groups. When women in the self-help groups do view the videos they do so in a context of ongoing support and a certain shared intimacy. The group often becomes a site where a range of intense emotions are expressed, including tears, frustration, and even a carnavalesque laughter at the grotesque nature of the body, caught up in chronic disease and its own mortality.

If women are to become active participants in a multidimensional project to heal female diseases, collective viewing of medical procedures such as video laparoscopy may serve to counter the ceding of the female body to medical institutions, and to shape healing-oriented spectatorship. Although a few self-help endo groups come close to video laparoscopy activism, the use of camera and monitor in video laparoscopy cannot be compared with media activism around AIDS, for example,[74] since the subject of the videos is a strictly surgical procedure, and their producer is not exactly the endo patient. Video-laparoscopic tapes are owned by a selective group of endometriosis patients who have had access to this kind of still relatively uncommon surgery, and who asked for (or were given) the tape from the surgeon. However, one might easily imagine an endo media activism that would include self-spectating women narrating their experiences and receptions of video laparoscopy, as well as using these images in the mass-media to gain political visibility for endometriosis. As a strategy for empowerment, collective self-spectatorship allows nonprofessionals to study diverse surgical performances outside the disciplinary boundaries of the medical establishment. Procedures such as video laparoscopy can play a significant role in democratizing access to our bodies, potentially turning patients, their families, and their communities into knowledgeable participants in scientific research and medical technologies.

Notes

I thank the Endometriosis Association, and particularly Mary Lou Ballweg, its cofounder and president, for its invaluable information and courageous work over the years, and Cecily Marcus for her enthusiastic assistance in my research into medical discourses about endometriosis. I am especially grateful to Robert Stam for his generous support, whether through our conversations or through his comments on the essay. I am also indebted to the supportive discussions and suggestions I have received from Mary Lawler, Ivone Margulis, Caren Kaplan, Eric Smoodin, Lynne Jackson, Faye Ginsburg, Lisa Cartwright, Paula Treichler, Con-

stance Penley, and Smadar Lavie. Special thanks to Lisa Cartwright and Ann
Kaplan for encouraging me to present sections of this article at the Pembroke
Center at Brown University and at the Humanities Institute at State University of
New York at Stony Brook. Finally, I would like to acknowledge the Society for the
Humanities at Cornell University for awarding me time, during 1991–92, to begin
writing on a topic I had contemplated for years but until then never dared broach.

1. The title "Lasers for Ladies" is borrowed from a short article by Michelle
Bekey (of the same title) that appeared in *Health*, vol. 15 (May 1983): 16.

2. I will use the phrase "endo discourse" to encompass a whole textual body
produced around endometriosis that refers both to hegemonic medical and alternative discourses. Although physicians use the official name "endometriosis," it is
at times referred to as "endo" in self-help groups.

3. The etymology of endometrium derives from the Greek "endo," the
mucous membrane lining, and "metra," uterus, which itself derives from "metr,"
mother. The endometrium tissue which lines the inside of the uterus builds up and
sheds each month in the menstrual cycle.

4. For a full account of sites, symptoms, and complications, see Mary Lou
Ballweg and the Endometriosis Association, *Overcoming Endometriosis: New Help
from the Endometriosis Association* (New York: Congdon & Weed, 1987), and Kate
Weinstein, *Living with Endometriosis: How to Cope with the Physical and Emotional
Challenges* (Reading, Mass.: Addison-Wesley Publishing Co., 1987).

5. George B. Haydon, MD, "A Study of 569 Cases of Endometriosis," *American Journal of Obstetrics and Gynecology*, vol. 43 (1942): 704–709, 704.

6. The ad is reproduced in Ballweg and the Endometriosis Association, *Overcoming Endometriosis*, 19.

7. The phrase is taken from J. H. Bellina of Louisiana State University School
of Medicine in Dietrick E. Thomsen, "Lasers Versus Female Complaints," *Science
News*, vol. 9, no. 6 (7 February 1981): 91.

8. Cited in Carolyn DeMarco, "Endometriosis: Options for Treating a Puzzling Condition," *Sojourner: The Women's Forum*, vol. 17, no. 7 (March 1992): 19H.

9. The cartoon appears in Ballweg and the Endometriosis Association, *Overcoming Endometriosis*, 72.

10. Craig A. Molgaard, PhD, Amanda L. Golbeck, PhD, and Louise Gresham,
MPH, "Current Concepts in Endometriosis," *Western Journal of Medicine*, vol. 143
(July 1985): 42–46.

11. Joe Vincent Meigs, MD, "Endometriosis: Its Significance," *Annals of
Surgery*, vol. 114 (1940): 866–874, 869.

12. On the discourses on menstruation, see Janice Delaney, Mary Jane Lupton,
and Emily Toth, *The Curse: A Cultural History of Menstruation* (Urbana: University
of Illinois Press, 1988).

13. Emily Martin, "The Egg and the Sperm: How Science has Constructed a
Romance Based on Stereotypical Male-Female Roles," *Signs*, vol. 16, no. 3 (Spring

1991): 485–501, 486; and Emily Martin, *The Woman in the Body: A Cultural Analysis of Reproduction* (Boston: Beacon Press, 1987).

14. Dr. John Sampson's theory of retrograde menstruation, formulated in 1921, is the oldest and still most widely accepted explanation for endometriosis. According to Dr. Sampson, during menstruation, a certain amount of menstrual fluid is forced backward from the uterus through the fallopian tubes and showered upon the pelvic organs and pelvic lining. See Weinstein, *Living with Endometriosis*, 23–25.

15. Meigs, "Endometriosis: Its Significance," 868.16.

16. Edward Walker, MD, Wayne Katon, MD, Lindy Michael Jones, MD, and Joan Russo, PHC, "Relationship Between Endometriosis and Affective Disorder," *American Journal of Psychiatry*, vol. 146, no. 3 (March 1989): 380–381.

17. Molgaard et al., "Current Concepts in Endometriosis," 43.18.

18. Molgaard et al., "Current Concepts in Endometriosis," 43.

19. Dorothy Otnow Lewis, MD, Florence Comite, MD, Catherine Mallouh, BA, Laura Zadunaisky, MS, Karen Hutchinson-Williams, MD, Bruce D. Cherksey, PhD, and Catherine Yeager, MA, "Bipolar Mood Disorder and Endometriosis: Preliminary Findings," *American Journal of Psychiatry*, vol. 144, no. 12 (December 1987): 1588–1591, 1588.

20. For another argument along these lines, see Hillary Allen, "At the Mercy of Her Hormones: Premenstrual Tension and the Law," *m/f*, vol. 9 (1984): 21–43.

21. Meigs, "Endometriosis: Its Significance," 866 and 869.

22. Meigs, "Endometriosis: Its Significance," 866.

23. Roger B. Scott, MD, and Richard W. Te Linde, MD, "External Endometriosis: The Scourge of the Private Patient," *Annals of Surgery*, vol. 131 (May 1950): 697–720, 701.

24. Scott and Te Linde, "External Endometriosis," 700.

25. Scott and Te Linde, "External Endometriosis," 700.

26. Two of the exceptions I have come across: Diana E. Houston, "Evidence for the Risk of Pelvic Endometriosis by Age, Race and Socioeconomic Status," *Epidemiologic Reviews*, vol. 6 (1984): 167–191; and Donald L. Chatman, MD, "Endometriosis in the Black Woman," *American Journal of Obstetrics and Gynecology*, vol. 125 (1976): 987–989.

27. Veasy C. Buttram, in an interview that appeared in the *Houston Chronicle* (December 1980), cited in Houston, "Evidence for the Risk of Pelvic Endometriosis," 182.

28. Meigs, "Endometriosis: Its Significance," 866.

29. Houston, "Evidence for the Risk of Pelvic Endometriosis," 178. Diana Houston argues, on the basis of many case studies, that the rate at which endometriosis afflicts teenaged women is unknown.

30. Veasy C. Buttram Jr., MD, "An Expanded Classification of Endometriosis," *Fertility and Sterility*, vol. 30, no. 2 (August 1978): 240–242, 241.

31. Buttram, "An Expanded Classification of Endometriosis," 242.

32. "Joe with Endo" by Ballweg and Lau, in Ballweg and the Endometriosis Association, *Overcoming Endometriosis*, 181.

33. This information is based on visits to several fertility clinics in the New York area and Atlanta.

34. For a social and discursive analysis of the desperate infertile woman, see Sarah Franklin, "Deconstructing `Desperateness': The Social Construction of Infertility in Popular Representations of New Reproductive Technologies," in *The New Reproductive Technologies*, ed. Maureen McNeil, Ian Varcoe, and Steven Yearly (New York: St. Martin Press, 1990) 200–229.

35. Similar analyses have pointed out the invisibility of women in the discourses around AIDS, abortion, and reproductive technologies. See Paula A. Treichler, "Beyond Cosmo: AIDS, Identity, and Inscriptions of Gender," *Camera Obscura*, vol. 28: 21–75; Faye D. Ginsburg, *Contested Lives: The Abortion Debate in an American Community* (Berkeley: University of California Press, 1989) 1–315; Deborah Lynn Steinberg, "The Depersonalization of Women through the Administration of In Vitro Fertilization," in *The New Reproductive Technologies*, ed. McNeil et al.; and Valerie Hartouni, "Containing Women: Reproductive Discourse in the 1980s," in *Technoculture*, ed. Constance Penley and Andrew Ross (Minneapolis: University of Minnesota Press, 1992).

36. Joe Vincent Meigs, MD, "Endometriosis: Etiologic Role of Marriage Age and Parity; Conservative Treatment," *Obstetrics and Gynecology*, vol. 2, no. 1 (July 1953): 46–53.

37. F. P. Lloyd, "Endometriosis in the Negro Woman: A Five Year Study," *American Journal of Obstetrics and Gynecology*, vol. 89 (1964): 468–469.

38. For example Stephen Corson writes that "incidence rates [of endometriosis] in England and Australia were less than those in the United States, and rates for caucasians were higher than those for blacks." Stephen L. Corson, MD, "Use of the Laparoscope in the Infertile Patient," *Fertility and Sterility*, vol. 32, no. 4 (October 1979): 359–369, 364.

39. Houston, "Evidence for the Risk of Pelvic Endometriosis," 179.

40. Houston, "Evidence for the Risk of Pelvic Endometriosis," 179.

41. Chatman, "Endometriosis in the Black Woman."

42. A recent study by Chatman challenges the view that endometriosis is uncommon in blacks after finding pelvic endometriosis in over 20 percent of his private black patients undergoing diagnostic laparoscopy. Diana Houston, meanwhile, calls for more specific studies with identified variables of race and class and a definition of the epidemiologic characteristics in order to understand the etiology of the disease.

43. Rayna Rapp, "Constructing Amniocentesis: Maternal and Medical Discourses," in *Uncertain Terms: Negotiating Gender in American Culture*, ed. Faye D. Ginsburg and Anna Lowenhaupt Tsing (Boston: Beacon Press, 1990) 40.

44. Angela Gilliam, "Women's Equality and National Liberation," in *Third World Women and the Politics of Feminism*, ed. Chandra Talpade Mohanty, Ann Russo, and Lourdes Torres (Bloomington: Indiana UP, 1991) 224.

45. For more documentation, including archival footage, see Ana Maria Garcia's *La Operación*.

46. Maria Milagros Lopez, "Sterilization and Cesarean Operations in Puerto Rico: Women's Bodies and Strategies of Development," a paper presented at "Cross Talk: A Multicultural Feminist Symposium," organized by Ella Shohat for the New Museum in New York City, June 1993. This paper is forthcoming in *Social Text* in a special issue based on the symposium, edited by Ella Shohat.

47. Angela Davis, *Women, Race, and Class* (New York: Random House, 1981) 213–216.

48. Cheryl Johnson-Odim, "Race, Identity, and Feminist Struggles," in *Third World Women and the Politics of Feminism*, ed. Mohanty et al., 323.

49. Robert L. Barbieri, "New Therapy for Endometriosis," *New England Journal of Medicine*, vol. 318, no. 8 (25 February 1988): 512–514, 512.

50. It should be pointed out that most hormonal treatment, including birth control pills, is not covered by health insurance. Drugs such as GnrH, meanwhile, are still considered experimental.

51. See the section "New Directions: Is Endometriosis What We Think It Is?" in Ballweg and the Endometriosis Association, *Overcoming Endometriosis*, 197–233.

52. Thomsen, "Lasers Versus Female Complaints."

53. Dr. Camran Nezhat, "Laser Overview and the Carbon Dioxide Laser," in Ballweg and the Endometriosis Association, *Overcoming Endometriosis*, 63–68.

54. Nezhat, "Laser Overview."

55. Nezhat, "Laser Overview."

56. Matt Clark with Ginny Caroll, "Conquering Endometriosis: Lasers Battle the 'Career Women's Disease,'" *Newsweek* (13 October 1986): 95.

57. Thomsen, "Lasers Versus Female Complaints," 90–91.

58. Michelle Bekey, "Lasers for Ladies," *Health*, vol. 15 (May 1983): 16. Cartoon by Bob Hiemstra.

59. "Laser Laparoscopy Offers New Hope for Infertility," *American Family Physician*, 27 (April 1983): 267.

60. Lisa Cartwright, "'Experiments of Destruction': Cinematic Inscriptions of Physiology," *Representations*, 40 (Fall 1992): 129–152, 138.

61. Cartwright, "'Experiments of Destruction.'"

62. Francis Bacon, *Advancement of Learning and Novom Organum* (New York: Colonial Press, 1899) 135.

63. Joseph Breuer and Sigmund Freud, *Studies on Hysteria*, trans. James Strachey in collaboration with Anna Freud (New York: Basic Books, 1957) 139.

64. For the relations between science, spectacle, and the discourses of discovery, particularly as manifested in metaphors such as the "virgin land" and the "dark continent," see Ella Shohat, "Imaging Terra Incognita: The Disciplinary Gaze of Empire," *Public Culture*, vol. 3 (Spring 1991): 41–70.

65. Thomsen, "Lasers Versus Female Complaints," 91; and "Laser Laparoscopy Offers New Hope for Infertility," 267–268.

66. "Laser Laparoscopy Offers New Hope for Infertility," 267–268.

67. Dr. Camran Nezhat, "Foreword" to Ballweg and the Endometriosis Association, *Overcoming Endometriosis*, xv.

68. One is reminded of the Spanish proverb: "*Abre tu cuerpo veras un puerco,*" which translates as "open your body, and you'll see a pig."

69. Although I did not conduct extensive research, I certainly found some clear tendencies in the reception of video laparoscopy.

70. I should emphasize that not all laser surgeons use video laparoscopy, and, when they do, not all give them to the patients. I spoke largely with self-help groups in the New York area, and read letters written to the Fertility and Endocrinology Center in Atlanta. My research, in this sense, does not attempt to represent *all* patients, or to cover a whole broad spectrum of patients' responses to their own images.

71. Ballweg, from a letter written to the Endometriosis Association, in *Overcoming Endometriosis*, 170.

72. Ballweg and the Endometriosis Association, *Overcoming Endometriosis*, 170.

73. I am using this phrase in its empowering sense as discussed by bell hooks. See bell hooks, *Talking Back: Thinking Feminist, Thinking Black* (Boston: South End Press, 1989).

74. See for example, Alexandra Juhasz, "WAVE in the Media Environment: Camcorder Activism and the Making of HIV TV," *Camera Obscura*, vol. 28 (January 1992) 135–152 and Juanita Mohammed, "WAVE in the Media Environment: Camcorder Activism in AIDS Education," vol. 28 (January 1992): 153–156.

Living on Disability

Language and Social Policy in the Wake of the ADA

Since the passage of the Americans with Disabilities Act (ADA) in 1990, there has begun to appear a literature of striking breadth and potentially great social significance.[1] Emerging from nearly every conceivable sector of the public sphere, the new literature on "disability" promises to reconfigure the relations among individuals, states, and the mechanisms of civil society—from public transportation to public education and public health administration. The immediate textual result is that if your local public library were to come up with a comprehensive Disabilities section, it would have to include everything from highly technical discussions of genetic anomaly and neuromuscular disorder, to social histories of mental retardation, to personal testimonies written by young adults with Down syndrome, to laypersons' handbooks on how to negotiate the legislative labyrinth of "disability" law. Of course, any coherent language and legal apparatus of disability, no matter how multifarious, will depend for its realization on a discursive formation in which it can be spoken; what's really interesting about the emergent discursive formation constructing disability, from this angle, is that it isn't fully formed yet.[2]

As parents of a young child with Down syndrome, we discover daily how almost every facet of our lived relationship with Jamie has already been structured by the legal and social institutions that attend "mental disability." Sometimes the connections between Jamie and the administrative apparatus of disability seem absurdly ephemeral: the tender body of our toddler doesn't feel as if it's related to the historical narratives of mental retardation in the United States; the ways he greets his friends and teachers at day care don't fit the numerous cultural roles that the "burden" (and sometimes "menace") of mental disability has played in the 150 years since "idiocy" was first pathologized. We've become aware of (and imbricated in) the legislative struggles that have shaped the funding and defunding of institutions for the management of disability, but none of these struggles seems to have anything to do with the more mundane and minute struggles by which James makes known to us his passion for pizza.

Like all parents of children with Down syndrome, we owe a great deal to the authors of books like *Count Us In*—themselves young men with Down syndrome—and their families for having transformed the social meaning of Down syndrome by helping to develop what's now called "early intervention" for infants with disabilities. But we also find ourselves the unwitting heirs of people and movements we never knew we were related to. We saunter with our Jamie publicly largely thanks to Dale Evans, who, in 1953, wrote *Angel Unaware*, a best-selling memoir of her daughter Robin, who was born with Down syndrome and died at age two. Jamie's biweekly speech therapy is state funded, thanks in part to former Governor Ronald Reagan, whose mindless slashing of millions of dollars from California's budget for state mental institutions in 1967 set off a horrified public reaction from visiting foreign professionals. (Reagan, furious, called the hellish institutions part of "the biggest hotel chain in the state" [quoted in Trent, 256].) And we have a new angle on American neo-Nazis since we now know that the Third Reich eagerly adopted hysterical American warnings from the 1910s and 1920s about the "cancerous growth of bad protoplasm" occurring among the "feebleminded" (Trent, 162).

James W. Trent, Jr.'s *Inventing the Feeble Mind: A History of Mental Retardation in the United States* details these twentieth-century highlights of mental retardation's cultural play, but at the core of his history is a quasi-Foucauldian and deeply cynical reading of the growth of U.S. institutions governing mental retardation. Trent's fascinating if cluttered narrative begins in the 1840s, with the first clinics designed solely for the treatment of "idiots," who had previously been the castabout inmates of prisons, almshouses, and orphan asylums. Under the influence of French educator Edward Seguin, American reformers took up the radical idea that idiots could be educated. Seguin had aimed to school asocial (*idios*) "idiots" for participation in public life by stimulating them physiologically and cognitively. But the superintendents of American institutions soon became less interested in educating *idio*syncratic individuals and more interested in categorizing the pathologies thought to underpin mental defectiveness. This subtle shift, Trent shows, set a trend for the control of the feeble minded that continues to this day: fledgling U.S. schools for idiots eventually became autotelic institutions, their wheels oiled by stratification and standardization. And their self-promotion was mounted in the rhetoric of efficiency. As one superintendent suggested in 1860, deadbeat idiots could be reshaped to participate in industrial capitalism: "Being consumers and not producers, [idiots] are a great pecuniary burden to the state. Educate them and they will become producers" (25).

But "producers" of what? Eventually, producers of labor within the very institutions that had once trained them for jobs out in the community. As institutional workers, "inmates" (as they were soon called) served several functions: they reduced operation costs by doing the work of attendants; instantiated and thereby validated categories of pathology (whereby "high-grades" took care of "low-grades"); and—most importantly for Trent—helped to perpetuate the institution itself, whose very existence made ever more untenable the release of "idiots" (or "morons," "imbeciles," "feeble minded," depending on the era) back into communities already grappling with economic uncertainty and nervous about "mental defectives," in part because of a new (and, sure enough, institutionally generated) focus on the "laws" of heredity.

In a predictable historical development, late Victorian heredity studies coincided with the poisonous eugenics movement of the early 1900s; both were used to justify the institutional practice of "controlling" defective heredity through sterilization. Sterilization procedures became routine for all inmates at this time: female idiots, in the language of the institution, were never anything more than vesicles of degenerate reproduction anyway, and males were castrated or sterilized in order to eliminate the sperm that threatened to contaminate the population. The only "debate" over this policy concerned whether ovarian sterilization was more effective than fallopian.

Such measures of social control can seem to emerge eerily without effort or without agents in a narrative of this kind, where all institutions mirror the culture's worst repressive fantasies as they inexorably strive for internal order and homogeneity. That's an argument often made by historians who see faceless mechanisms of social control where others see only a thousand points of institutional light. But the thrust of Trent's careful history runs in a different direction: the human agents inseparable from the "routinizing" of institutions for the mentally retarded—that is, the superintendents whom Trent tracks—are unwavering in their mission to promote social control and shockingly impervious to that early moment when Seguin saw the educational potential of "feebleminded" individuals and got the whole thing started.

Hence a real tension emerges in Trent's methodology by book's end, in the 1980s and 1990s: far from turning "presentist" and judging the past by the standards of the present, he gauges the present by the damages of the past. So, finally, Trent's last chapter begs a question: can you be Foucauldian about the past and yet retain any hope for the present, for your own children? When Trent carries his argument into his own day, he is rigorously cautious about "progress," tending to see the extension of the apparatus of social control as the inevitable outcome of social policy. It is undeniably true that our generation has seen horrors uncovered by Geraldo Rivera's pack of investigators in Willowbrook in the 1970s, fights over mainstreaming in the 1980s and inclusivity in the 1990s, and a new national hysteria over deinstitutionalized and homeless "mental deficients." But we have also seen Kennedy administration money lead the way for unprecedented federal legislation, and we know that without that money and legislation, most of the liberatory developments of the past thirty years would be just plain unthinkable. The question for Trent, of course, is whether these developments can be thought of as "liberatory" at all.

But the answer isn't clear. In the end, Trent's not sure whether institutions must always be as they have always been, or whether there's hope for those of us who live among institutions now. His is an ambivalence we confess we sometimes share, however reluctantly; we know that the mechanisms of social control can subsume any individual agent who inhabits and tries to redirect them. Nevertheless, we have no choice but to behave as if our nation's contemporary institutions and discourses can work in our child's interest, and no choice but to inform ourselves about the workings of the social apparatus responsible for governing "retardation." But we are heartened by the fact that current U.S. policies have been formed in part by the voices—and political strategies—of activist groups like the Arc (formerly the Association of Retarded Citizens) and SAFE (Schools Are For Everyone). Jamie has introduced us to a fascinating world, and it complicates our take on Trent's narrative so thoroughly that we no longer know what we make of our ambivalence about Trent's ambivalence.

Besides, since we have a child of our own to "administer," we often have to stop thinking about his historicity and focus instead on his immediate future. That means not only schlepping him from appointment to appointment, but also learning to be his "advocate" in a much broader sense. As we've found, the interdependence of Jamie's public and private worlds requires that disabled citizens and their advocates have to learn to play a highly specific language game in which federal, state, and local laws combine to produce a distinctive structure for the interpellation of individuals with disabilities. Still, however fascinating this structure seems to us, our guess is that few readers will curl up with a book like Ordover and Boundy's *Educational Rights of Children with Disabilities* unless they have good reason to. By the same token, however, any parent or friend of (or any kind of advocate for) a disabled child will surely find this handbook indispensable.

Written in lawyerese's closest approximation to English, yet studded with ample footnotes to all relevant regulations and case law, *Educational Rights* is a guide to the machinery of federal laws, state obligations, due process hearings, and local evaluative standards that makes up the civic world of the child with disabilities. The Americans with Disabilities Act (ADA) has changed that civic world in some significant respects, but the statutes on which Ordover and Boundy concentrate are the Individuals with Disabilities Education Act (IDEA) of 1975, and Section 504 of the Rehabilitation Act of 1973. Under IDEA, all "children with disabilities" are entitled to a "free appropriate public education" in the "least restrictive environment" (LRE); Section 504 covers "individuals with handicaps." We're not putting these phrases in quotes to be pedantic; every word here is freighted with ore—and contested anew in lawsuit upon lawsuit. "Individuals with handicaps," for instance, is a more capacious term than "children with disabilities" and covers adults as well as kids with epilepsy, AIDS, or "other health impairments" that affect their lives but don't necessarily affect their placement in school. The ADA amended the Rehabilitation Act to exclude drug users from the definition of "individuals with handicaps," but even this piece of Reagan-Bush war-on-drugs legislation allows civil rights protections for alcoholics and people who have completed drug rehab programs and are no longer "engaging in illegal drug use" (Ordover and Boundy, 93).

IDEA basically resurrected Special Ed (whose early days are covered by Trent) and assured that children with disabilities would go to school for free, just as every other American child can. Disabled children are now federally entitled to free transportation and all other services necessary to their schooling, including things like speech pathology, counseling, occupational and physical therapy, and "medical services . . . for diagnostic and evaluation purposes only" (quoted on 22). But whether they actually get these things in the way they need them depends on how knowledgeable and energetic their advocates are. Federal law sets the general standard, but the states and localities fill in the blanks, defining "appropriate education" and "least restrictive environment" as they see fit. The clause on medical services is particularly troublesome: it's not clear whether it applies only to services provided by medical doctors or whether "diagnostic and evaluation purposes" can be distinguished from educational purposes at all.

This is how it's all supposed to work: under IDEA, each disabled child gets, at age three and annually thereafter, a written Individualized Education Program (IEP); in September of 1994, Jamie got his first one. The IEP is devised by a multidisciplinary team of evaluators, and schools have to follow your kid's program or risk losing their IDEA funding. It's no accident, then, that the two longest chapters in *Educational Rights* are "Procedural Safeguards and Dispute Resolution" and "Discipline of Students with Disabilities"; these chapters offer vital advice on due process hearings, reviews, and (as a last resort) civil suits. The latter chapter stresses that disabled students can't be punished, expelled, or classified as truants and delinquents just because they have psychological or behavioral problems. But the case law is especially choppy in these straits—most obviously for kids whose behavioral problems are part of their diagnoses—and impossible to navigate alone.

The broadest philosophical essays in *Restructuring for Caring and Effective Education* basically deconstruct ADA and IDEA word by word. On one hand, educating the disabled in the least restrictive environment (LRE) is a radically democratic move, evoking visions of human community and compassion we don't normally associate with superintendents and vice principals; but on the other hand, as Stanley Witkin and Lise Fox point out, the concept of the least restrictive environment is not only violated in practice but flawed in theory as well. Because children's IEPs "often are written with the existing [educational] environment in mind" (327), they argue, they're geared toward the least restrictive *existing* environment; as a result, public schools have justified keeping disabled kids in Special Ed classes, busing them to separate facilities, and cutting corners on basic services on the grounds that they're only supposed to provide the *least* restrictive environment, not the "most enabling environment"

Witkin and Fox advocate. The problem here is that IDEA rights are inescapably individualized: that is, figuring out an LRE for each student leaves you with no analogy for the basic human rights concept of the "barrier-free environment," which allows access to public buildings for *all* people with disabilities. As Witkin and Fox note, "a building cannot be made barrier-free only for a particular individual" (328), but that is exactly the standard to which disabled kids' IEPs are built.

Grasping the contradiction between "basic human rights" and "individual education programs" goes a long way toward understanding the current social impasse between advocates of mainstreaming and advocates of inclusion. "Mainstreaming" refers to the policies that were undeniably progressive in the political context of the 1970s—namely, segregated Special Ed classes within "regular" schools where disabled kids could receive the "special" attention they needed. People who fought for mainstreaming are sometimes baffled by the proponents of full inclusion, who call for disabled children to be educated with their nondisabled peers in regular classes. Just as regular parents and teachers fear that inclusion will distract schools from teaching their regular students, the people who fought for mainstreaming fear that inclusion will deprive disabled students of the special services they fought for twenty years ago. In response to this impasse, the editors of *Restructuring for Caring and Effective Education* have put together nineteen essays addressed to disparate audiences (parents, legislators, principals, Educational policy wonks, and the like) that cumulatively make the case for full inclusion, which provides what in their view is the most enabling educational environment of all.

Despite the individualism built into the language of rights and disabilities, most of the thinking in this collection turns out to be generally communitarian, and for good reason. The strongest essay on this front is Norman Kunc's "The Need to Belong," which harks back to Edward Seguin's premise that individual human achievement is (or should be) predicated on a sense of human community rather than (as is currently the case throughout most of the world) the other way around. "Although the intent of segregation is to help students with disabilities learn skills and appropriate behavior," Kunc writes, "the very act of removing students with disabilities from the other students necessarily teaches them that 'they are not good enough to belong as they are' and that the privilege of belonging will be granted back to them once they have acquired an undefined number of skills" (35). Separate, for Kunc, is always unequal.

Now, you may have heard words to this effect before. But when they're hitched to a theory that says our motivation to achieve is predicated on our sense of belonging, they call into question the whole system of individual meritocracy on which our current educational practices are putatively based. That means, among other things, that the proponents of inclusion are deeply skeptical about tracking, standardized tests, and social studies curricula that require third graders to memorize their state's counties. Likewise, in these pages, "inclusive" education means full inclusion not only for kids with disabilities, but for children who are socially ostracized for any reason—race, religion, gender, national origin, or failure to hate Barney.

In the inclusive classroom, two fundamental and "holistic" things happen: disabled students emulate their nondisabled peers, and the nondisabled kids learn that the disabled are an integral part of their lives, not to be shunted off into separate rooms and programs simply because they're disabled. That doesn't mean that disabled kids don't need services or that they'll be able to keep up with every part of the academic curriculum; it only means that the socializing features of school should be paramount among our educational priorities for the disabled. A well-worn African proverb holds that it takes a whole village to raise a child; likewise, in the post-ADA American idiom, it will take a lot of teamwork to help disabled kids realize the Enlightenment ideal of individual autonomy.

Accordingly, much of the material in *Restructuring* is devoted to discussions of how to foster "collaborative teaming" among teachers and administrators, "circles of friends" among students in inclusive classrooms, and disciplinary systems in which students have a substantial say. Some of this stuff is deadly dull (we won't rehearse the discussion of whether change is a system or a process, or whether four-dimensional visionizing is crucial to improvement); some of it is meant for education theorists and professional lobbyists; and some of it is based, curiously enough, on business management techniques. The most engaging essays discuss "heterogeneous schooling" by way of local success stories about inclusion. Statistics gathered from various North American school districts demonstrate that segregated education, like its earlier institutional incarnations, may lead to a pattern of lifelong dependence (149); that after a year of full integration, the percentage of teachers in Saline, Michigan, who agreed with the proposition that inclusion is unfair to regular kids dropped from 80 to 12 (180); and that, as Richard Schattman reports, several regular teachers find "they already had children in their classes with more challenging academic, social, and behavioral needs" than the disabled kids assigned to their classrooms by inclusive policies (152).

First-person testimonies like *Count Us In* are resource books too, in a way, but they also tend to be deeply compelling and moving reading experiences. Understandably, most of the literature on inclusion doesn't give you a living picture of the people and lives at issue; *Count Us In* gives you Mitchell Levitz, 22, and his friend Jason Kingsley, 19, and their views on marriage, work, school, driving, *Life Goes On*, the Gulf War, the 1992 presidential campaign, independent living, each other, and what it's like to grow up knowing you have Down syndrome.

Jason's and Mitchell's parents were told their children could never learn, would never distinguish them from other adults, and would be better cared for in institutions; Jason's mother was told her son would never have "a single meaningful thought" (3). When you're dealing with people who started life with prognoses like these, you just can't help but be inspired and impressed that these kids (now young adults) speak so eloquently and incisively about the disability that was supposed to render them ineducable. Through adolescence, however, their growing self-awareness gave them an understanding not only of their potential but also of their limitations. Today, Mitchell dreams of being elected president, but also knows he may not be able to learn to drive, and the extraordinary emotional maturity with which he confronts this possibility is worth remarking: "it's difficult for me to face, but I'm learning to accept the fact that I may not be able to do some things that my sisters are doing" (160). Jason hopes to find a cure for AIDS, but also knows that to live alone, he'll need to find a good job. Still, both of them know very well what work they've already done in the world: as Mitchell says, they should rename Down syndrome "Change syndrome" because "we can't change the disability but we can change the way we feel" (44). Or as your friendly neighborhood theorist would say, to change our collective understanding of Down syndrome is also to change the conditions of people's lives.

Part of the point of the book, as both Jason and Mitchell remark on occasion, is precisely that they have published this book: this is the first book produced *by*, rather than *about*, people with Down syndrome, and though they're used to being trailblazers by now, Jason and Mitchell are pretty excited about being authors. "*Count Us In* makes the future better for people with disabilities," says Mitchell; adds Jason, "after people read this book, strangers will become our friends" (14).

Jason and Mitchell are media savvy for a reason: They've been famous most of their lives and don't think it strange to appear on television, to meet New York State Governor Cuomo (as Jason did), or to work for the man who wound up defeating Cuomo in 1994, former New York assemblyman George Pataki (as Mitchell did). Their fame, in turn, depends on their good fortune: not only were they born into extremely supportive families

that contested the medical wisdom of their day, but they were born to families well positioned for activism. Mitchell's mother had extensive training
in special ed; Jason's mother is a writer for *Sesame Street*, and Jason made
his TV debut at 15 months. In 1980, when he was 6, he was counting in
Spanish for the cameras. One of our Jamie's favorite pictures in the book,
indeed, is a still from *Sesame Street*, captioned by Jason: "this is . . . when
the Cookie Monster was showing everyone that I knew how to read."

A book like this is in part its own message, especially since it is an amal-
gam of recorded interviews (sometimes between the boys, their parents,
and grandparents, and sometimes just between the boys themselves), most
of which were typed directly onto the computer as the boys spoke. The
mothers, Emily Kingsley and Barbara Levitz, testify in their introduction
to the authenticity of the book: "no attempt has been made to 'correct'
their sometimes idiosyncratic syntax or expression. The boys have a developmental disability, after all, and we have no desire to hide or camouflage
that fact" (9). What's more, Jason's and Mitchell's own writings punctuate
the book throughout, from class assignments and brief autobiographies to
Jason's poem on the death of his paternal grandmother, Nina:

> I dreamt last night that you are in heaven,
> calmly relaxing angel.
> In our hands we'll be loving you forever.
> You mean so much to us.
> When you are dead or alive we need you in peace. (120)

The complexity of this beautiful little number is worth pausing over, not
only for its technique—which secures a vision of heaven with the unfor-
gettably concrete image of a "calmly relaxing angel"—but also for the
subtle sense of community that drives the movement from "I dreamt" to
"we need." Jason's lyric offers his calmly relaxing dream to an unending
number of Nina's loved ones: the I, we, and you whose hands massage the
drama of death and life into a hopeful portrait of Nina's peace are called
together in the present-and-future tense of Jason's closing line.

Curiously enough, ever since the time Blake first problematized childhood, the lyric has been thought to be the genre of unmediated individual
expression, and so it is here; but we ought to note also that while the poem
issues from an interiority that can only be Jason's, it nevertheless gives
voice to a collective grief and love. We trust, of course, that people will be
struck by the talent and intelligence to which Jason's poem testifies. But if
there's one thing that Jason and Mitchell have taught us, it's that talent—
even the most individual kind of talent, like writing poetry—needs a com-

munity, a social context, to enhance and appreciate it. Individualism and individual achievement, by themselves, do not create community; just ask any "gifted" student. On the contrary, we may do better to assume, as do Jason Kingsley, Mitchell Levitz, their families, and the advocates of inclusion, that individual achievement must be *predicated* on a sense of community, predicated on a social milieu that enables it and in which it makes (common) sense. It may be that antinomian libertarianism is so engrained in the American national imaginary that we "naturally" associate collectivity with homogeneity; what the disabled show us, however, is that if a collectivity isn't heterogeneous, and doesn't value heterogeneity, it simply isn't worthy of the name of "community."

Against the atomizing forces of tracking, categorization, and standardizing, then, we have to maintain the almost impossible faith that, as Mitchell puts it, "every single one counts because we are an important asset to the community and they need our voice" (14). Conservative individualists like to deride egalitarian social justice as a "fuzzy liberal value," but there's absolutely nothing fuzzy about it. It's among the finest ideals humans have so far come up with, and among the most difficult and arduous to achieve in practice. Or, as Mitchell says in the course of weighing Jason's plans to marry, "It is really about how much love and compassion that you have. That's what really counts about values" (98). And among the best reasons for full inclusion, we think (as parents, citizens, and humans), is that it stands a chance of bequeathing to us a set of "family values" worth fostering in any kind of family—or in any larger political body that cares about its individual members.

Notes

1. A substantially revised version of this essay appeared in the December 1994 *Village Voice Literary Supplement.*

2. This essay surveys a small sample of this literature, primarily with regard to its implications for revisionary understandings of mental retardation and educational policy. The texts we focus on are *Inventing the Feeble Mind: A History of Mental Retardation in the United States,* by James W. Trent, Jr. (Berkeley: U of California P, 1994); *Count Us In: Growing Up with Down Syndrome,* by Jason Kingsley and Mitchell Levitz (New York: Harcourt Brace, 1994); *Restructuring for Caring and Effective Education: An Administrative Guide to Creating Heterogeneous Schools,* edited by Richard A. Villa, Jacqueline S. Thousand, William Stainback, and Susan Stainback (Baltimore: Paul H. Brookes, 1992); *Educational Rights of Children with Disabilities: A Primer for Advocates,* by Eileen L. Ordover and Kathleen B. Boundy

(Cambridge, MA: Center for Law and Education, 1991). *Restructuring* and *Educational Rights* are relatively difficult to obtain from libraries; the former can be ordered from Paul H. Brookes Publishing Co., P.O. Box 10624, Baltimore, MD 21285–0624, and the latter from the Center for Law and Education, 955 Massachusetts Avenue, Cambridge, MA 02139, (617) 876–6611. We will hereafter refer to each of these books in the text by page number.

10

The Empire *Strikes Back*

A Posttranssexual Manifesto

➤ *Frogs into Princesses*

The verdant hills of Casablanca look down on homes and shops jammed chockablock against narrow, twisted streets filled with the odors of spices and dung. Casablanca is a very old city, passed over by Lawrence Durrell perhaps only by a geographical accident as the winepress of love. In the more modern quarter, located on a broad, sunny boulevard, is a building otherwise unremarkable except for a small brass nameplate that identifies it as the clinic of Dr. Georges Burou. It is predominantly devoted to obstetrics and gynecology, but for many years has maintained another reputation quite unknown to the stream of Moroccan women who pass through its rooms.

Dr. Burou is being visited by journalist James Morris. Morris fidgets in an anteroom reading *Elle* and *Paris-Match* with something less than full attention, because he is on an errand of immense personal import. At last

the receptionist calls for him, and he is shown to the inner sanctum. He
relates:

> I was led along corridors and up staircases into the inner premises of the
> clinic. The atmosphere thickened as we proceeded. The rooms became
> more heavily curtained, more velvety, more voluptuous. Portrait busts
> appeared, I think, and there was a hint of heavy perfume. Presently I saw,
> advancing upon me through the dim alcoves of this retreat, which distinctly
> suggested to me the allure of a harem, a figure no less recognizably oda-
> lesque. It was Madame Burou. She was dressed in a long white robe, tasseled
> I think around the waist, which subtly managed to combine the luxuriance
> of a caftan with the hygiene of a nurse's uniform, and she was blonde herself,
> and carefully mysterious. . . . Powers beyond my control had brought me to
> Room 5 at the clinic in Casablanca, and I could not have run away then even
> if I had wanted to. . . . I went to say good-bye to myself in the mirror. We
> would never meet again, and I wanted to give that other self a long last look
> in the eye, and a wink for luck. As I did so a street vendor outside played a
> delicate arpeggio upon his flute, a very gentle merry sound which he
> repeated, over and over again, in sweet diminuendo down the street. Flights
> of angels, I said to myself, and so staggered . . . to my bed, and oblivion.[1]

Exit James Morris, enter Jan Morris, through the intervention of late
twentieth-century medical practices in this wonderfully "oriental," almost
religious narrative of transformation. The passage is from *Conundrum*, the
story of Morris's "sex change" and the consequences for her life. Besides
the wink for luck, there is another obligatory ceremony known to male-
to-female transsexuals that is called "wringing the turkey's neck," although
it is not recorded whether Morris performed it as well. I will return to this
rite of passage later in more detail.

Making History

Imagine now a swift segue from the moiling alleyways of Casablanca to the
rolling green hills of Palo Alto. The Stanford Gender Dysphoria Program
occupies a small room near the campus in a quiet residential section of this
affluent community. The Program, which is a counterpart to Georges
Burou's clinic in Morocco, has been for many years the academic focus of
Western studies of gender dysphoria syndrome, also known as transsexualism. Here are determined etiology, diagnostic criteria, and treatment.

The Program was begun in 1968, and its staff of surgeons and psychologists first set out to collect as much history on the subject of transsexualism

as was available. Let me pause to provide a very brief capsule of their results. A transsexual is a person who identifies his or her gender identity with that of the "opposite" gender. Sex and gender are quite separate issues, but transsexuals commonly blur the distinction by confusing the performative character of gender with the physical "fact" of sex, referring to their perceptions of their situation as being in the "wrong body." Although the term transsexual is of recent origin, the phenomenon is not. The earliest mention of something that we can recognize ex post facto as transsexualism, in light of current diagnostic criteria, was of the Assyrian king Sardanapalus, who was reported to have dressed in women's clothing and spun with his wives.[2] Later instances of something very like transsexualism were reported by Philo of Judaea, during the Roman Empire. In the eighteenth century the Chevalier d'Eon, who lived for 39 years in the female role, was a rival of Madame Pompadour for the attention of Louis XV. The first colonial governor of New York, Lord Cornbury, came from England fully attired as a woman and remained so during his time in office.[3]

Transsexualism was not accorded the status of an "official disorder" until 1980, when it was first listed in the *American Psychiatric Association Diagnostic and Statistical Manual*. As Marie Mehl points out, this is something of a Pyrrhic victory.[4]

Prior to 1980, much work had already been done in an attempt to define criteria for differential diagnosis. An example from the 1970s is this one, from work carried out by Leslie Lothstein and reported in William A. W. Walters's and Michael W. Ross's *Transsexualism and Sex Reassignment*:

> Lothstein, in his study of ten ageing transsexuals [average age fifty-two], found that psychological testing helped to determine the extent of the patients' pathology [sic] . . . [he] concluded that [transsexuals as a class] were depressed, isolated, withdrawn, schizoid individuals with profound dependency conflicts. Furthermore, they were immature, narcissistic, egocentric and potentially explosive, while their attempts to obtain [professional assistance] were demanding, manipulative, controlling, coercive, and paranoid.[5]

Here is another example:

> In a study of 56 transsexuals the results on the schizophrenia and depression scales were outside the upper limit of the normal range. The authors see these profiles as reflecting the confused and bizarre life styles of the subjects.[6]

These were clinical studies, which represented a very limited class of subjects. However, the studies were considered sufficiently representative for them to be reprinted without comment in collections such as that of

Walters and Ross. Further on in each paper, though, we find that each investigator invalidates his results in a brief disclaimer that is reminiscent of the fine print in a cigarette ad: in the first, by adding, "It must be admitted that Lothstein's subjects could hardly be called a typical sample as nine of the ten studied had serious physical health problems" (this was a study conducted in a health clinic, not a gender clinic), and in the second, with the afterthought that "82 percent of [the subjects] were prostitutes and atypical of transsexuals in other parts of the world."[7] Such results might have been considered marginal, hedged about as they were with markers of questionable method or excessively limited samples. Yet they came to represent transsexuals in medicolegal/psychological literature, disclaimers and all, almost to the present day.

During the same period, feminist theoreticians were developing their own analyses. The issue quickly became, and remains, volatile and divisive. Let me quote an example.

> Rape . . . is a masculinist violation of bodily integrity. All transsexuals rape women's bodies by reducing the female form to an artifact, appropriating this body for themselves. . . . Rape, although it is usually done by force, can also be accomplished by deception.

This quotation is from Janice Raymond's 1979 book *The Transsexual Empire: The Making of the She-Male*, which occasioned the title of this paper. I read Raymond to be claiming that transsexuals are constructs of an evil phallocratic empire and were designed to invade women's spaces and appropriate women's power. Though *Empire* represented a specific moment in feminist analysis and prefigured the appropriation of liberal political language by a radical right, here in 1991, on the twelfth anniversary of its publication, it is still the definitive statement on transsexualism by a genetic female academic.[8] To clarify my stakes in this discourse let me quote another passage from *Empire*:

> Masculine behavior is notably obtrusive. It is significant that transsexually constructed lesbian-feminists have inserted themselves into the positions of importance and/or performance in the feminist community. Sandy Stone, the transsexual engineer with Olivia Records, an "all-women" recording company, illustrates this well. Stone is not only crucial to the Olivia enterprise but plays a very dominant role there. The . . . visibility he achieved in the aftermath of the Olivia controversy . . . only serves to enhance his previously dominant role and to divide women, as men frequently do, when they make their presence necessary and vital to women. As one woman wrote: "I feel raped when Olivia passes off Sandy . . . as a

real woman. After all his male privilege, is he going to cash in on lesbian feminist culture too?"[9]

This paper, "The *Empire* Strikes Back," is about morality tales and origin myths, about telling the "truth" of gender. Its informing principle is that "technical arts are always imagined to be subordinated by the ruling artistic idea, itself rooted authoritatively in nature's own life."[10] It is about the image and the real mutually defining each other through the inscriptions and reading practices of late capitalism. It is about postmodernism, postfeminism, and (dare I say it) posttranssexualism. Throughout, the paper owes a large debt to the work of Donna Haraway.

"All of Reality in Late Capitalist Culture Lusts To Become an Image for Its Own Security"[11]

Let's turn to accounts by the transsexuals themselves. During this period virtually all of the published accounts were written by male-to-females. I want to briefly consider four autobiographical accounts of male-to-female transsexuals, to see what we can learn about what they think they are doing. (I will consider female-to-male transsexuals in another paper.)

The earliest partially autobiographical account in existence is that of Lili Elbe in Niels Hoyer's book *Man into Woman* (1933).[12] The first fully autobiographical book was the paperback *I Changed My Sex!* (not exactly a quiet, contemplative title), written by the striptease artist Hedy Jo Star in the mid-1950s.[13] Christine Jorgensen, who underwent surgery in the early 1950s and is arguably the best known of the recent transsexuals, did not publish her autobiography until 1967; instead, Star's book rode the wave of publicity surrounding Jorgensen's surgery. In 1974 *Conundrum* was published, written by the popular English journalist Jan Morris. In 1977 there was *Canary*, by musician and performer Canary Conn.[14] In addition, many transsexuals keep something they call by the argot term "O.T.F.": The Obligatory Transsexual File. This usually contains newspaper articles and bits of forbidden diary entries about "inappropriate" gender behavior. Some transsexuals also collect autobiographical literature. According to the Stanford Gender Dysphoria Program, the medical clinics do not, because they consider autobiographical accounts thoroughly unreliable. Because of this, and since a fair percentage of the literature is invisible to many library systems, these personal collections are the only source for some of this information. I am fortunate to have a few of them at my disposal.

What sort of subject is constituted in these texts? Hoyer (representing Jacobson representing Elbe, who is representing Wegener who is representing Sparre),[15] writes:

> A single glance of this man had deprived her of all her strength. She felt as if her whole personality had been crushed by him. With a single glance he had extinguished it. Something in her rebelled. She felt like a schoolgirl who had received short shrift from an idolized teacher. She was conscious of a peculiar weakness in all her members . . . it was the first time her woman's heart had trembled before her lord and master, before the man who had constituted himself her protector, and she understood why she then submitted so utterly to him and his will.[16]

We can put to this fragment all of the usual questions: Not by whom but *for* whom was Lili Elbe constructed? Under whose gaze did her text fall? And consequently what stories appear and disappear in this kind of seduction? It may come as no surprise that all of the accounts I will relate here are similar in their description of "woman" as male fetish, as replicating a socially enforced role, or as constituted by performative gender. Lili Elbe faints at the sight of blood.[17] Jan Morris, a world-class journalist who has been around the block a few times, still describes her sense of herself in relation to makeup and dress, of being on display, and is pleased when men open doors for her:

> I feel small, and neat. I am not small in fact, and not terribly neat either, but femininity conspires to make me feel so. My blouse and skirt are light, bright, crisp. My shoes make my feet look more delicate than they are, besides giving me . . . a suggestion of vulnerability that I rather like. My red and white bangles give me a racy feel, my bag matches my shoes and makes me feel well organized. . . . When I walk out into the street I feel consciously ready for the world's appraisal, in a way that I never felt as a man.[18]

Hedy Jo Star, who was a professional stripper, says in *I Changed My Sex!*: "I wanted the sensual feel of lingerie against my skin, I wanted to brighten my face with cosmetics. I wanted a strong man to protect me." Here in 1991 I have also encountered a few men who are brave enough to echo this sentiment for themselves, but in 1955 it was a proprietary feminine position.

Besides the obvious complicity of these accounts in a Western white male definition of performative gender, the authors also reinforce a binary, oppositional mode of gender identification. They go from being unambiguous men, albeit unhappy men, to unambiguous women. There is no territory between.[19] Further, each constructs a specific narrative moment when their personal sexual identification changes from male to female. This moment is the moment of neocolporraphy—that is, of gender reassignment or "sex change surgery."[20] Jan Morris, on the night preceding surgery, wrote: "I went to say good-bye to myself in the mirror. We would never meet again, and I wanted to give that other self a last wink for luck."[21]

Canary Conn writes: "I'm not a muchacho . . . I'm a muchacha now . . . a girl [*sic*]."[22]

Hedy Jo Star writes: "In the instant that I awoke from the anaesthetic, I realized that I had finally become a woman."[23]

Even Lili Elbe, whose text is secondhand, used the same terms: "Suddenly it occurred to him that he, Andreas Sparre, was probably undressing for the last time." Immediately on awakening from first-stage surgery (castration in Hoyer's account), Sparre writes a note. "He gazed at the card and failed to recognize the writing. It was a woman's script." Inger carries the note to the doctor: "What do you think of this, Doctor. No man could have written it?" "No," said the astonished doctor; "no, you are quite right"—an exchange that requires the reader to forget that orthography is an acquired skill. The same thing happens with Elbe's voice: "the strange thing was that your voice had completely changed. . . . You have a splendid soprano voice! Simply astounding."[24] Perhaps as astounding now as then but for different reasons, since in light of present knowledge of the effects (and more to the point, the noneffects) of castration and hormones, none of this could have happened. Neither has any effect on voice timbre. Hence, incidentally, the jaundiced eyes with which the clinics regard historical accounts.

If Hoyer mixes reality with fantasy and caricatures his subjects besides ("Simply astounding!"), what lessons are there in *Man into Woman*? Partly what emerges from the book is how Hoyer deploys the strategy of building barriers within a single subject, strategies that are still in gainful employment today. Lili displaces the irruptive masculine self, still dangerously present within her, onto the God-figure of her surgeon/therapist Werner Kreutz, whom she calls The Professor, or The Miracle Man. The Professor is He Who molds and Lili that which is molded:

> What the Professor is now doing with Lili is nothing less than an emotional moulding, which is preceding the physical moulding into a woman. Hitherto Lili has been like clay which others had prepared and to which the Professor has given form and life . . . by a single glance the Professor awoke her heart to life, a life with all the instincts of woman.[25]

The female is immanent, the female is bone-deep, the female is instinct. With Lili's eager complicity, The Professor drives a massive wedge between the masculine and the feminine within her. In this passage, reminiscent of the "oriental" quality of Morris's narrative, the male must be annihilated or at least denied, but the female is that which exists to be continually annihilated:

> It seemed to her as if she no longer had any responsibility for herself, for her fate. For Werner Kreutz had relieved her of it all. Nor had she any longer a will of her own . . . there could be no past for her. Everything in the past belonged to a person who . . . was dead. Now there was only a perfectly humble woman, who was ready to obey, who was happy to submit herself to the will of another . . . her master, her creator, her Professor. Between [Andreas] and her stood Werner Kreutz. She felt secure and salvaged.[26]

Hoyer has the same problems with purity and denial of mixture that recur in many transsexual autobiographical narratives. The characters in his narrative exist in a historical period of enormous sexual repression. How is one to maintain the divide between the "male" self, whose proper object of desire is Woman, and the "female" self, whose proper object of desire is Man?

> "As a man you have always seemed to me unquestionably healthy. I have, indeed, seen with my own eyes that you attract women, and that is the clearest proof that you are a genuine fellow." He paused, and then placed his hand on Andreas's shoulder. "You won't take it amiss if I ask you a frank question? . . . Have you at any time been interested in your own kind? You know what I mean."
>
> Andreas shook his head calmly. "My word on it, Niels; never in my life. And I can add that those kind of creatures have never shown any interest in me."
>
> "Good, Andreas! That's just what I thought."[27]

Hoyer must separate the subjectivity of "Andreas," who has never felt anything for men, and "Lili," who, in the course of the narrative, wants to marry one. This salvaging procedure makes the world safe for "Lili" by erecting and maintaining an impenetrable barrier between her and "Andreas," reinforced again and again in such ways as two different handwriting styles and two different voices. The force of an imperative—a natural state toward which all things tend—to deny the potentialities of mixture, acts to preserve "pure" gender identity: at the dawn of the Nazi-led love affair with purity, no "creatures" will tempt Andreas into transgressing boundaries with his "own kind." "I will honestly and plainly

confess to you, Niels, that I have always been attracted to women. And today as much as ever. A most banal confession!"[28]—banal only so long as
the person inside Andreas's body who voices it is Andreas, rather than Lili.
There is a lot of work being done in this passage, a microcosm of the work
it takes to maintain the same polar personae in society at large. Further,
each of these writers constructs his or her account as a narrative of
redemption. There is a strong element of drama, of the sense of struggle
against huge odds, of overcoming perilous obstacles, and of mounting awe
and mystery at the breathtaking approach and final apotheosis of the Forbidden Transformation. Oboy. "The first operation . . . has been successful beyond all expectations. Andreas has ceased to exist, they said. His
germ glands—oh, mystic words—have been removed."[29]

Oh, mystic words. The *mysterium tremendum* of deep identity hovers
about a physical locus; the entire complex of male engenderment, the
mysterious power of the Man-God, inhabits the "germ glands" in the way
that the soul was thought to inhabit the pineal. Maleness is in the you-
know-whats. For that matter, so is the ontology of the subject; and therefore Hoyer can demonstrate in the coarsest way that femaleness is lack:
"The operation which has been performed here [that is, castration]
enables me to enter the clinic for women [exclusively for women]."[30]

On the other hand, either Niels or Lili can be constituted by an act of
insinuation, what the New Testament calls *endeuein*, or the putting on of
the god, inserting the physical body within a shell of cultural signification:

Andreas Sparre . . . was probably undressing for the last time. . . . For a lifetime these coverings of coat and waistcoat and trousers had enclosed him.[31]

It is now Lili who is writing to you. I am sitting up in my bed in a silk night-
dress with lace trimming, curled, powdered, with bangles, necklace, and
rings.[32]

All these authors replicate the stereotypical male account of the constitution of woman: Dress, makeup, and delicate fainting at the sight of blood.
Each of these adventurers passes directly from one pole of sexual experience to the other. If there is any intervening space in the continuum of sexuality, it is invisible. And nobody *ever* mentions wringing the turkey's neck.

No wonder feminist theorists have been suspicious. Hell, *I'm* suspicious.

How do these accounts converse with the medical/psychological texts?
In a time in which more interactions occur through texts, computer conferences, and electronic media than by personal contact—the close of the
mechanical age and the inception of the virtual, in which multiplicity and

prosthetic social communication are common—and consequently when individual subjectivity can be constituted through inscription more often than through personal association, there are still moments of embodied "natural truth" that cannot be avoided. In the time period of most of these books the most critical of these moments was the intake interview at the gender dysphoria clinic, when the doctors, who were all males, decided whether the person was eligible for gender reassignment surgery. The origin of the gender dysphoria clinics is a microcosmic look at the construction of criteria for gender. The foundational idea for the gender dysphoria clinics was first, to study an interesting and potentially fundable human aberration; second, to provide help, as they understood the term, for a "correctable problem."

Some of the early nonacademic gender dysphoria clinics performed *surgery on demand*, that is to say regardless of any judgment on the part of the clinic staff regarding what came to be called appropriateness to the gender of choice. When the first academic gender dysphoria clinics were started on an experimental basis in the 1960s, the medical staff would not perform surgery on demand, because of the professional risks involved in performing experimental surgery on "sociopaths." At this time there were no official diagnostic criteria; "transsexuals" were, ipso facto, whoever signed up for assistance. Professionally this was a dicey situation. It was necessary to construct the category "transsexual" along customary and traditional lines, to construct plausible criteria for acceptance into a clinic. Professionally speaking, a test or a differential diagnosis was needed for transsexualism that did not depend on anything as simple and subjective as feeling that one was in the wrong body. The test needed to be objective, clinically appropriate, and repeatable. But even after considerable research, no simple and unambiguous test for gender dysphoria syndrome could be developed.[33]

The Stanford clinic was in the business of helping people, among its other agendas, as its members understood the term. Therefore the final decisions of eligibility for gender reassignment were made by the staff on the basis of an individual sense of the "appropriateness of the individual to their gender of choice." The clinic took on the additional role of "grooming clinic" or "charm school" because, according to the judgment of the staff, the men who presented as wanting to be women did not always "behave like" women. Stanford recognized that gender roles could be learned (to an extent). Their involvement with the grooming clinics was an effort to produce not simply anatomically legible females, but *women* . . . that is, *gendered* females. As Norman Fisk remarked, "I now admit very candidly that . . . in the early phases we were avowedly seeking candidates who would have the best chance for success."[34] In practice this meant that the candidates for surgery were evaluated on the basis of their *performance* in the gender of choice. The criteria constituted a fully acculturated, consensual definition of gender, and *at the site of their enactment we can locate an actual instance of the apparatus of production of gender.*

This raises several sticky questions, the chief two being: Who is telling the story for whom, and how do the storytellers differentiate between the story they tell and the story they hear?

One answer is that they differentiate with great difficulty. The criteria that the researchers developed and then applied were defined recursively through a series of interactions with the candidates. The scenario worked this way: Initially, the only textbook on the subject of transsexualism was Harry Benjamin's definitive work *The Transsexual Phenomenon* (1966).[35] (Note that Benjamin's book actually postdates *I Changed My Sex!* by about ten years.) When the first clinics were constituted, Benjamin's book was the researchers' standard reference. And when the first transsexuals were evaluated for their suitability for surgery, their behavior matched up gratifyingly with Benjamin's criteria. The researchers produced papers that reported on this, and that were used as bases for funding.

It took a surprisingly long time—several years—for the researchers to realize that the reason the candidates' behavioral profiles matched Benjamin's so well was that the candidates, too, had read Benjamin's book, which was passed from hand to hand within the transsexual communities, whose members were only too happy to provide the behavior that led to acceptance for surgery.[36] This sort of careful repositioning created interesting problems. Among them was the determination of the permissible range of expressions of physical sexuality. This was a large gray area in the candidates' self-presentations, because Benjamin's subjects did not talk about any erotic sense of their own bodies. Consequently nobody else who came to the clinics did either. By textual authority, physical men who lived as women and who identified themselves as transsexuals, as opposed to male transvestites for whom erotic penile sensation was permissible, could not experience penile pleasure. Into the 1980s there was not a single preoperative male-to-female transsexual for whom data was available who experienced genital sexual pleasure while living in the "gender of choice."[37] The prohibition continued postoperatively in interestingly transmuted form, and remained so absolute that no postoperative transsexual would admit to experiencing sexual pleasure through masturbation either. Full membership in the assigned gender was conferred by orgasm, real or faked, accomplished through heterosexual penetration.[38] "Wringing the turkey's neck," the ritual of penile masturbation just before surgery, was the most secret of secret traditions. To acknowledge so natural a desire would be to risk "crash landing"; that is, "role inappropriateness" leading to disqualification.[39]

It was necessary to retrench. The two groups, on one hand the researchers and on the other the transsexuals, were pursuing separate ends. The researchers wanted to know what this thing they called gender dysphoria syndrome was. They wanted a taxonomy of symptoms, criteria for differential diagnosis, procedures for evaluation, reliable courses of treatment, and thorough follow-up. The transsexuals wanted surgery. They had very clear agendas regarding their relation to the researchers, and considered the doctors' evaluation criteria merely another obstacle in their path—something to be overcome. In this they unambiguously expressed Benjamin's original criterion in its simplest form: the sense of being in the "wrong" body.[40] This seems a recipe for an uneasy adversarial relationship, and it was. It continues to be, although with the passage of time there has been considerable dialogue between the two camps. Partly this has been made possible by the realization among the medical and psychological community that the expected criteria for differential diagnosis did not emerge. Consider this excerpt from a paper by Marie Mehl, written in 1986:

> There is no mental nor psychological test which successfully differentiates the transsexual from the so-called normal population. There is no more psychopathology in the transsexual population than in the population at large, although societal response to the transsexual does pose some insurmountable problems. The psychodynamic histories of transsexuals do not yield any consistent differentiation characteristics from the rest of the population.[41]

These two accounts, Mehl's statement and that of Lothstein, in which he found transsexuals to be depressed, schizoid, manipulative, controlling, and paranoid, coexist within a span of less than ten years. With the achievement of a diagnostic category in 1980—one which, after years of research, did not involve much more than the original sense of "being in the wrong body"—and consequent acceptance by the body police, that is, the medical establishment, clinically "good" histories now exist of transsexuals in areas as widely dispersed as Australia, Sweden, Czechoslovakia, Vietnam, Singapore, China, Malaysia, India, Uganda, Sudan, Tahiti, Chile, Borneo, Madagascar, and the Aleutians (this is not a complete list).[42] It is a considerable stretch to fit them all into some plausible theory.

Were there undiscovered or untried diagnostic techniques that would have differentiated transsexuals from the normal population? Were the criteria wrong, limited, or shortsighted? Did the realization that criteria were not emerging just naturally appear as a result of "scientific progress," or were there other forces at work?

Such a banquet of data creates its own problems. Concomitant with the dubious achievement of a diagnostic category is the inevitable blurring of boundaries as a vast heteroglossic account of difference, heretofore invisible to the "legitimate" professions, suddenly achieves canonization and simultaneously becomes homogenized to satisfy the constraints of the category. Suddenly the old morality tale of the truth of gender, told by a kindly white patriarch in New York in 1966, becomes pancultural in the 1980s. Emergent polyvocalities of lived experience, never represented in the discourse but present at least in potential, disappear; the *berdache* and the stripper, the tweedy housewife and the *mujerado*, the *mah'u* and the rock star, are still the same story after all, if we only try hard enough.

Whose Story Is This, Anyway?

I wish to point out the broad similarities that this peculiar juxtaposition suggests to aspects of colonial discourse with which we may be familiar: the initial fascination with the exotic, extending to professional investigators; denial of subjectivity and lack of access to the dominant discourse; followed by a species of rehabilitation.

Raising these issues has complicated life in the clinics.

"Making" history, whether autobiographic, academic, or clinical, is partly a struggle to ground an account in some natural inevitability. Bodies are screens on which we see projected the momentary settlements that emerge from ongoing struggles over beliefs and practices within the academic and medical communities. These struggles play themselves out in arenas far removed from the body. Each is an attempt to gain a high ground that is profoundly moral in character, to make an authoritative and final explanation for the way things are and consequently for the way they must continue to be. In other words, each of these accounts is culture speaking with the voice of an individual. The people who have no voice in this theorizing are the transsexuals themselves. As with men theorizing about women from the beginning of time, theorists of gender have seen transsexuals as possessing something less than agency. As with genetic women, transsexuals are infantilized, considered too illogical or irresponsible to achieve true subjectivity, or clinically erased by diagnostic criteria; or else, as constructed by some radical feminist theorists, as robots of an insidious and menacing patriarchy, an alien army designed and constructed to infiltrate, pervert, and destroy "true" women. In this construction as well, the transsexuals have been resolutely complicit by failing to develop an effective counterdiscourse.

Here on the gender borders at the close of the twentieth century, with the faltering of phallocratic hegemony and the bumptious appearance of heteroglossic origin accounts, we find the epistemologies of white male medical practice, the rage of radical feminist theories, and the chaos of lived gendered experience meeting on the battlefield of the transsexual body: a hotly contested site of cultural inscription, a meaning machine for the production of ideal type. Representation at its most magical, the transsexual body is perfected memory, inscribed with the "true" story of Adam and Eve as the ontological account of irreducible difference, an essential biography that is part of nature. A story that culture tells itself, the transsexual body is a tactile politics of reproduction constituted through textual violence. The clinic is a technology of inscription.

Given this circumstance in which a minority discourse comes to ground in the physical, a counterdiscourse is critical. But it is difficult to generate a counterdiscourse if one is programmed to disappear. The highest purpose of the transsexual is to erase him/herself, to fade into the "normal" population as soon as possible. Part of this process is known as *constructing a plausible history*—learning to lie effectively about one's past. What is gained is acceptability in society. What is lost is the ability to authentically represent the complexities and ambiguities of lived experience, and thereby is lost that aspect of "nature" that Donna Haraway theorizes as Coyote—the Native American spirit animal who represents the power of continual transformation that is the heart of engaged life. Instead, authentic experience is replaced by a particular kind of story, one that supports the old constructed positions. This is expensive, and profoundly disempowering. Whether desiring to do so or not, transsexuals do not grow up in the same ways as "GGs," or genetic "naturals."[43] Transsexuals do not possess the same history as genetic "naturals," and do not share common oppression prior to gender reassignment. I am not suggesting a shared discourse. I am suggesting that in the transsexual's erased history we can find a story disruptive to the accepted discourses of gender, that originates from within the gender minority itself and that can make common cause with other oppositional discourses. But the transsexual currently occupies a position that is nowhere, that is outside the binary oppositions of gendered discourse. For a transsexual, *as a transsexual*, to generate a true, effective, and representational counterdiscourse is to speak from outside the boundaries of gender, beyond the constructed oppositional nodes that have been predefined as the only positions from which discourse is possible. How, then, can the transsexual speak? If the transsexual were to speak, what would s/he say?

A Posttranssexual Manifesto

To attempt to occupy a place as speaking subject within the traditional gender frame is to become complicit in the discourse that one wishes to deconstruct. Rather, we can seize upon the textual violence inscribed in the transsexual body and turn it into a reconstructive force. Let me suggest a more familiar example. Judith Butler points out that the lesbian categories of "butch" and "femme" are not simple assimilations of lesbianism back into the terms of heterosexuality. Rather, Butler introduces the concept of *cultural intelligibility*, and suggests that the contextualized and resignified "masculinity" of the butch, seen against a culturally intelligible "female" body, invokes a dissonance that both generates a sexual tension and constitutes the object of desire. She points out that this way of thinking about gendered objects of desire admits of much greater complexity than the example suggests. The lesbian butch or femme both recall the heterosexual scene but simultaneously displace it. The idea that butch and femme are "replicas" or "copies" of heterosexual exchange underestimates the erotic power of their internal dissonance.[44] In the case of the transsexual, the varieties of performative gender, seen against a culturally intelligible gendered body *which is itself a medically constituted textual violence*, generate new and unpredictable dissonances that implicate entire spectra of desire. In the transsexual as text we may find the potential to map the refigured body onto conventional gender discourse and thereby disrupt it, to take advantage of the dissonances created by such a juxtaposition to fragment and reconstitute the elements of gender in new and unexpected geometries. I suggest we start by taking Raymond's accusation that "transsexuals divide women" beyond itself, and turn it into a productive force to multiplicatively divide the old binary discourses of gender—as well as Raymond's own monistic discourse. To foreground the practices of inscription and reading that are part of this deliberate invocation of dissonance, I suggest constituting transsexuals not as a class or problematic "third gender," but rather as a *genre*—a set of embodied texts whose potential for *productive* disruption of structured sexualities and spectra of desire has yet to be explored.

In order to effect this, the genre of visible transsexuals must grow by recruiting members from the class of invisible ones, from those who have disappeared into their "plausible histories." The most critical thing a transsexual can do, the thing that constitutes success, is to "pass."[45] Passing means to live successfully in the gender of choice, to be accepted as a "natural" member of that gender. Passing means the denial of mixture. One and the same with passing is effacement of the prior gender role, or the construction of a plausible history. Considering that most transsexuals choose reassignment in their third or fourth decade, this means erasing a considerable portion of their personal experience. It is my contention that this process, in which both the transsexual and the medicolegal/psychological establishment are complicit, forecloses the possibility of a life grounded in the *intertextual* possibilities of the transsexual body.

To negotiate the troubling and productive multiple permeabilities of boundary and subject position that intertextuality implies, we must begin to rearticulate the foundational language by which both sexuality and transsexuality are described. For example, neither the investigators nor the transsexuals have taken the step of problematizing "wrong body" as an adequate descriptive category. In fact "wrong body" has come, virtually by default, to *define* the syndrome.[46] It is quite understandable, I think, that a phrase whose lexicality suggests the phallocentric, binary character of gender differentiation should be examined with deepest suspicion. So long as we, whether academics, clinicians, or transsexuals, ontologize both sexuality and transsexuality in this way, we have foreclosed the possibility of analyzing desire and motivational complexity in a manner that adequately describes the multiple contradictions of individual lived experience. We need a deeper analytical language for transsexual theory, one that allows for the sorts of ambiguities and polyvocalities that have already so productively informed and enriched feminist theory.

Judith Shapiro points out that "to those . . . who might be inclined to diagnose the transsexual's focus on the genitals as obsessive or fetishistic, the response is that they are, in fact, simply conforming to *their culture's* criteria for gender assignment" (emphasis mine). This statement points to deeper workings, to hidden discourses and experiential pluralities within the transsexual monolith. They are not yet clinically or academically visible, and with good reason. For example, in pursuit of differential diagnosis a question sometimes asked of a prospective transsexual is: "Suppose that you could be a man [or woman] in every way except for your genitals;

would you be content?" There are several possible answers, but only one is clinically correct.[47] Small wonder, then, that so much of these discourses revolves around the phrase "wrong body." Under the binary phallocratic founding myth by which Western bodies and subjects are authorized, only one body per gendered subject is "right." All other bodies are wrong.

As clinicians and transsexuals continue to face off across the diagnostic battlefield that this scenario suggests, the transsexuals for whom gender identity is something different from *and perhaps irrelevant* to physical genitalia are occulted by those for whom the power of the medical/psychological establishments, and their ability to act as gatekeepers for cultural norms, is the final authority for what counts as a culturally intelligible body. This is a treacherous area, and were the silenced groups to achieve voice we might well find, as feminist theorists have claimed, that the identities of individual, embodied subjects were far less implicated in physical norms, and far more diversely spread across a rich and complex structuration of identity and desire, than it is now possible to express.[48] And yet in even the best of the current debates, the standard mode is one of relentless totalization. Consider the most perspicuous example in this paper, Raymond's stunning "all transsexuals rape women's bodies" (what if she had said, for example, "all blacks rape women's bodies"): For all its egregious and inexcusable bigotry, the language of her book is only marginally less totalizing than, for example, Gary Kates's "transsexuals . . . take on an exaggerated and stereotypical female role," or Ann Bolin's "transsexuals try to forget their male history." Both Kates's and Bolin's studies are in most respects fine work, and were published in the same collection as an earlier version of this essay;[49] but still there are no subjects in these discourses, only homogenized, totalized objects—fractally replicating earlier histories of minority discourses in the large. So when I speak the forgotten word, it will perhaps wake memories of other debates. The word is *some*.

Transsexuals who pass seem able to ignore the fact that by creating totalized, monistic identities, forgoing physical and subjective intertextuality, they have foreclosed the possibility of authentic relationships. Under the principle of passing, denying the destabilizing power of being "read," relationships begin as lies—and passing, of course, is not an activity restricted to transsexuals. This is familiar to the person of color whose skin is light enough to pass as white, or to the closet gay or lesbian, or to anyone who has chosen invisibility as an imperfect solution to personal dissonance. Essentially I am rearticulating one of the arguments for solidarity that has been developed by gays, lesbians, and people of color. The comparison extends further. To deconstruct the necessity for passing implies that transsexuals must take responsibility for *all* of their history, to begin to rearticulate their lives not as a series of erasures in the service of a species of feminism conceived from within a traditional frame, but as a political action begun by reappropriating difference and reclaiming the power of the refigured and reinscribed body. The disruptions of the old patterns of desire that the multiple dissonances of the transsexual body imply produce not an irreducible alterity but a myriad of alterities, whose unanticipated juxtapositions hold what Donna Haraway has called the promises of monsters—physicalities of constantly shifting figure and ground that exceed the frame of any possible representation.[50]

The essence of transsexualism is the act of passing. A transsexual who passes is obeying the Derridean imperative: "Genres are not to be mixed. I will not mix genres."[51] I could not ask a transsexual for anything more inconceivable than to forgo passing, to be consciously "read," to read oneself aloud—and by this troubling and productive reading, to begin to *write oneself* into the discourses by which one has been written—in effect, then, to become a (look out—dare I say it again?) posttranssexual.[52] Still, transsexuals know that silence can be an extremely high price to pay for acceptance. I want to speak directly to the brothers and sisters who may read/"read" this and say: I ask all of us to use the strength that brought us through the effort of restructuring identity, and that has also helped us to live in silence and denial, for a re-visioning of our lives. I know you feel that most of the work is behind you and that the price of invisibility is not great. But, although *individual* change is the foundation of all things, it is not the end of all things. Perhaps it is time to begin laying the ground-work for the next transformation.

Afterword

In the brief time, or so it seems, since this essay was first written, the situation both on the street with regard to articulating a specifically transgendered positionality and within the academy vis-à-vis theory has deeply changed, and continues to evolve. Whether the original *"Empire"* paper had the privilege of being a fortunately timed bellwether or whether it successfully evoked the build-it-and-they-will-come principle is unknown, but the results are no less gratifying for lack of that knowledge. Transgender (or for that matter, posttransgender) theory would appear to be successfully engaging the nascent discourses of Queer Theory in a number of graceful and mutually productive respects, and this is reason for guarded celebration. Needless to say, however, beginnings are most delicate and critical periods in which, while the foundation stones are still exposed, it is necessary to pay exquisite attention to detail. For this author, it is a most promising and interesting time in which to be alive and writing.

Notes

Thanks to Gloria Anzaldúa, Laura Chernaik, Ramona Fernandez, Thyrza Good-eve, and John Hartigan for their valuable comments on earlier drafts of this paper; Judy Van Maasdam and Donald Laub of the Stanford Gender Dysphoria Program for their uneasy help; Wendy Chapkis; Nathalie Magnan; the Olivia Records Collective, for whose caring in difficult times I am deeply grateful; Janice Raymond, for playing Luke Skywalker to my Darth Vader; Graham Nash and David Crosby; and to Christy Staats and Brenda Warren for their steadfastness. Especially I thank Donna Haraway, whose insight and encouragement continue to inform and illuminate this work.

1. Jan Morris, *Conundrum* (1974; Rpt., New York: Henry Holt, 1986) 139.

2. *Transsexualism and Sex Reassignment*, ed. William A. W. Walters and Michael W. Ross (Oxford: Oxford UP, 1986) 2.

3. This capsule history is related in the introduction to Richard Docter's *Transvestites and Transsexuals: Toward a Theory of Cross-Gender Behavior* (New York: Plenum Press, 1988).

4. In Marie Mehl's introduction to *Gender Dysphoria Syndrome: Development, Research, Management*, ed. Betty Steiner (New York: Plenum Press, 1985).

5. Don Burnard and Michael W. Ross, "Psychosocial Aspects and Psychological Theory: What Can Psychological Testing Reveal?" in Walters and Ross 58.

6. Walters and Ross 58.

7. Walters and Ross 58.

8. Janice Raymond, *The Transsexual Empire: The Making of the She-Male* (Boston: Beacon Press, 1979). There is some hope to be taken that Judith Shapiro's work ["Transsexualism: Reflections of the Persistence of Gender and the Mutability of Sex," in *Body Guards: The Cultural Politics of Gender Ambiguity*, ed. Kristina Straub and Julia Epstein (New York: Routledge, 1991)] will supersede Raymond's as such a definitive statement. Shapiro's accounts seem excellently balanced, and she is aware that there are more accounts from transsexual scholars that have not yet entered the discourse.

9. Raymond 20.

10. This wonderful phrase is from Donna Haraway's "Teddy Bear Patriarchy: Taxidermy in the Garden of Eden, New York City, 1908–1936," *Social Text*, vol. 11 (Winter 1984–85): 20.

11. Haraway, "Teddy Bear Patriarchy." The anecdotal character of this section is supported by field notes that have not yet been organized and coded. A thoroughly definitive and perhaps ethnographic version of this paper, with appropriate citations of both professionals and their subjects, awaits research time and funding.

12. Lili Elbe, *Man into Woman: An Authentic Record of a Change of Sex. The True Story of the Miraculous Transformation of the Danish Painter, Einar Wegener (Andreas Sparre)*, ed. Niels Hoyer (Ernst Ludwig Harthern Jacobsen), trans. from the German by H. J. Stenning, intro. Norman Haire (New York: E. P. Dutton & Company, 1933). The British sexologist, Norman Haire, wrote the introduction, thus making Hoyer's book a semi-medical contribution.

13. Hedy Jo Star (Carl Rollins Hammonds), *I Changed My Sex!* (publisher unknown, 1955). Star's book has disappeared from history, and I have been unable to find reference to it in any library catalog. Having held a copy in my hand, I am sorry I did not hold tighter.

14. There was at least one other book published during this period, Renée Richards's *Second Serve*, which is not treated here.

15. Niels Hoyer was a pseudonym for Ernst Ludwig Harthern Jacobson; Lili Elbe was the female name chosen by the artist Eider Wegener, whose give name was Andreas Sparre. This lexical profusion has rich implications for studies of boundaries of self; see, for example, Allocheiria Racine Stone, "Virtual Systems," in *ZONE 6: Fragments for a History of the Human Body, INCORPORATIONS* (New York: Urzone [MIT Press], 1992).

16. Hoyer 163.

17. Hoyer 147.

18. Morris 174.

19. In *Conundrum*, Morris does describe a period in her journey from masculine to feminine (from a few years before surgery to immediately afterward) during which her gender was perceived, by herself and others, as ambiguous. She is quite unambiguous, though, about the moment of transition from *male* to *female*.

20. Gender reassignment is the correct disciplinary term. In current medical discourse, sex is taken as a natural fact and cannot be changed.

21. Morris 140. I was reminded of this account on the eve of my own surgery. Gee, I thought on that occasion, it would be interesting to magically become another person in that binary and final way. So I tried it myself—going to the mirror and saying goodbye to the person I saw there—and unfortunately it did not work. A few days later, when I could next get to the mirror, the person looking back at me was still me. I still don't understand what I did wrong.

22. Canary Conn, *Canary: The Story of a Transsexual* (New York: Bantam, 1977) 271. Conn had her surgery at the clinic of Jesus Maria Barbosa in Tijuana. In this excerpt she is speaking to a Mexican nurse; hence the Mexicano terms.

23. Star.

24. I admit to being every bit as astounded as the good Doctor, since except for Hoyer's account there are no other records of change in vocal pitch or timbre follow-

ing administration of hormones or gender reassignment surgery. But there are more sufficient problems with Lili Elbe's true story, not the least of which is the scene in which Elbe finally "becomes a woman" by virtue of her physician's *implanting into her abdominal cavity a set of ovaries.* The attention given by the media in the past decade to heart transplants and diseases of the immune system have made the lay public more aware of the workings of the human immune response, but even in 1936 Hoyer's account would have been recognized by the medical community as questionable. Tissue rejection and the dream of mitigating it were the subjects of speculation in fiction and science fiction as late as the 1940s; for example, the miracle drug "collodiansy" in H. Beam Piper's *One Leg Too Many* (1949).

25. Hoyer 165.

26. Hoyer 170. For an extended discussion of texts that transmute submission into personal fulfillment see Sandy Stone, "Sweet Surrender: Gender, Spirituality, and the Ecstasy of Subjection; Pseudotranssexual Fiction in the 1970s," forthcoming.

27. Hoyer 53.

28. Hoyer 53.

29. Hoyer 134.

30. Hoyer 139. Lili Elbe's sex change took place in 1930. In the United States today, the juridical view of successful male-to-female sex change is still based upon lack; for example, a man is a woman when "the male generative organs have been totally and irrevocably destroyed." (From a clinic letter authorizing a name change on a passport, 1980.)

31. Hoyer 125.

32. Hoyer 139. I call attention in both preceding passages to the Koine Greek verb *endeuein*, referring to the moment of baptism, when the one being baptized enters into and is entered by the Word; *endeuein* may be translated as "to enter into" but also "to put on, to insinuate oneself into, like a glove"; viz. "He [*sic*] who is baptized into Christ shall have put on Christ." In this intense homoerotic vein in which both genders are present but collapsed in the sacrifi[c]ed body see such examples as Fray Bernardino de Sahagun's description of rituals during which the officiating priest puts on the flayed skin of a young woman in Sir James George Frazer, *The Golden Bough: A Study in Magic and Religion* (London: Macmillan, 1911) 589–591.

33. The evolution and management of this problem deserves a paper in itself. It is discussed in capsule form in *Proceedings of the Second Interdisciplinary Symposium on Gender Dysphoria Syndrome*, ed. Donald R. Laub and Patrick Gandy (Stanford: Division of Reconstructive and Rehabilitation Surgery, Stanford Medical Center, 1973); and in Janice M. Irvine, *Disorders of Desire: Sex and Gender in Modern American Sexology* (Philadelphia: Temple UP, 1990).

34. Laub and Gandy 7. Fisk's full remarks provide an excellent description of the aims and procedures of the Stanford group during the early years, and the tensions of conflicting agendas and various attempts at resolution are implicit in his account. For additional accounts, see both Irvine and Shapiro.

35. Harry Benjamin, *The Transsexual Phenomenon* (New York: Julian Press, 1966). The paper that was the foundation for the book was published as "Transsexualism and Transvestism as Psycho-Somatic and Somato-Psychic Syndromes" in the *American Journal of Psychotherapy*, vol. 8 (1954): 219–230. A much earlier paper by D. O. Cauldwell, "Psychopathia transexualis," in *Sexology*, vol. 16 (1949): 274–280, does not appear to have had the same effect within the field, although sex researcher John Money still pays homage to it by retaining Cauldwell's single-*s* spelling of the term. In early documents by other workers one may sometimes trace the influence of Cauldwell or Benjamin by how the word is spelled.

36. Laub and Gandy 8, 9.

37. The problem here is with the ontology of the term "genital," in particular with regard to its definition for such activities as pre- and postoperative masturbation. Engenderment ontologizes the erotic economy of body surface; as Judith Butler points out, engenderment polices which parts of the body have their erotic components switched off or on. Conflicts arise when the *same* parts become multivalent; for example, when portions of the [physical male] urethra are used to construct portions of the [gendered female in the physical male] neoclitoris. I suggest that we use this vertiginous idea as an example of ways in which we can refigure multivalence as intervention into the constitution of binary gendered subject positions; in a binary erotic economy, "who" experiences erotic sensation associated with these areas? (Judith Shapiro raises a similar point in her essay, "Transsexualism: Reflections on the Persistence of Gender and the Mutability of Sex" in *Body Guards*. I have chosen a site geographically quite close to the one she describes, but hopefully more ambiguous, and therefore more dissonant in these discourses in which dissonance can be a powerful and productive intervention.)

38. This act in the borderlands of subject position suggests a category missing from Marjorie Garber's paper "Spare Parts: The Surgical Construction of Gender," in *Differences*, vol. 1 (1990): 137–159; it is an intervention into the dissymmetry between "making a man" and "making a woman" that Garber describes. To a certain extent it figures a collapse of those categories within the transsexual imaginary, although it seems reasonable to conclude that this version of the coming-of-age story is still largely male—the male doctors and patients telling each other stories of what Nature means for both Man and Woman. Generally female (female-to-male) patients tell the same stories from the other side.

39. The terms "wringing the turkey's neck" (male masturbation), "crash landing" (rejection by a clinical program), and "gaff" (an undergarment used to conceal male genitalia in preoperative m/f transsexuals), vary slightly in different geographical areas but are common enough to be recognized across sites.

40. Based upon Norman Fisk's remarks in Laub and Gandy 7, as well as my own notes. Part of the difficulty, as I discuss in this paper, is that the investigators (not to mention the transsexuals) have failed to problematize the phrase "wrong body" as an adequate descriptive category.

41. Walters and Ross.

42. I use the word "clinical" here and elsewhere while remaining mindful of the "Pyrrhic victory" of which Mehl spoke. Now that transsexualism has the uneasy legitimacy of a diagnostic category in the DSM, how do we begin the process of getting *out* of the book?

43. The actual meaning of "GG," a m/f transsexual slang term, is "genuine girl" [*sic*], also called "genny."

44. Judith Butler, *Gender Trouble: Feminism and the Subversion of Identity* (New York: Routledge, 1990).

45. The opposite of passing, being *read*, provocatively invokes the inscription practices to which I have referred.

46. I am suggesting a starting point, but it is necessary to go much further. We will have to question not only how *body* is defined in these discourses, but to more critically examine who gets to say *what "body" means*.

47. In case the reader is unsure, let me supply the clinically correct answer: "No."

48. It is useful as well as gratifying to note that since the first version of this essay appeared in 1991, several coalition groups, one of which is appropriately named *Transgendered Nation*, have begun actively working to bring the rich diversity within transgendered communities to public attention. Their action at the 1993 conference of the American Psychological Association, which was debating the appropriateness of continuing to include transsexuality in the next edition of the official diagnostic manual (*DSM*), appeared brave and timely. Of course, several arrests (of transgendered demonstrators, not psychologists) ensued.

49. These essays appeared in Straub and Epstein.

50. For an elaboration of this concept, see Donna Haraway, "The Promises of Monsters: A Regenerative Politics of Gender for Inappropriate/d Others," in *Cultural Studies*, ed. Lawrence Grossberg, Cary Nelson, and Paula Treichler (New York, Routledge, 1990).

51. Jacques Derrida, "La loi du genre/The Law of Genre," trans. Avital Ronell, in *Glyph*, vol. 7 (1980): 176 (French), 202 (English).

52. I also call attention to Gloria Anzaldúa's theory of the Mestiza, an illegible subject living in the borderlands between cultures, capable of partial speech in each but always only partially intelligible to each. Working against the grain of this position, Anzaldúa's "new mestiza" attempts to overcome illegibility partly by seizing control of speech and inscription and by writing herself into the discourse. The stunning "Borderlands" is a case in point; Gloria Anzaldúa, *Borderlands/La Frontera: The New Mestiza* (San Francisco: Spinsters/Aunt Lute, 1987).

Works Cited

Anzaldúa, Gloria. *Borderlands/La Frontera: The New Mestiza*. San Francisco: Spinsters/Aunt Lute, 1987.

Benjamin, Harry. *The Transsexual Phenomenon*. New York: JulianPress, 1966.

Bolin, Ann. *In Search of Eve: Transsexual Rites of Passage*. Amherst, Massachusetts: Bergin and Garvey, 1988.

Bornstein, Kate. *Dear Sir or Madam: Confessions of a Gender Outlaw*. New York, Routledge, 1994.

Butler, Judith. *Gender Trouble: Feminism and the Subversion ofIdentity*. New York: Routledge, 1990.

Conn, Canary. *Canary: The Story of a Transsexual*. New York: Bantam, 1977.

Derrida, Jacques. "La loi du genre/The Law of Genre." Trans. Avital Ronell. In *Glyph*, vol. 7 (1980): 176 (French), 202 (English).

Docter, Richard F. *Transvestites and Transsexuals: Toward a Theory of Cross-Gender Behavior*. New York: Plenum Press, 1988.

Elbe, Lili. *Man into Woman: An Authentic Record of a Change of Sex. The True Story of the Miraculous Transformation of the Danish Painter, Einar Wegener (Andreas Sparre)*. Ed. Niels Hoyer (pseudonym for Ernst Ludwig Harthern Jacobsen), trans. from the German by H. J. Stenning, intro. Norman Haire. New York: E. P. Dutton & Company, 1933.

Faith, Karlene. *If It Weren't for The Music: A History of Olivia Records* [mss]. Forthcoming.

Foucault, Michel. *Herculine Barbin: Being the Recently Discovered Memoirs of a Nineteenth-century Hermaphrodite*. New York: Pantheon, 1980.

Frazer, Sir James George. *The Golden Bough: A Study in Magic and Religion*. London: Macmillan, 1911.

Gatens, Moira. *Feminism and Philosophy: Perspectives on Difference and Equality*. Cambridge: Cambridge UP, 1991.

Grahn, Judy. *Another Mother Tongue: Gay Words, Gay Worlds*. Boston: Beacon Press, 1984.

Greany, Markisha. "The Native American Berdache and the 'Non-Operative Transsexual': Towards a Case for the 'Non-Biological Sex Change.' " Unpublished paper.

Green, Richard, and John Money, eds. *Transsexualism and Sex Reassignment*. Baltimore: Johns Hopkins Press, 1969.

Grosz, Elizabeth. "Freaks." A paper delivered at the University of California, Santa Cruz Conference on Women and Philosophy, 1988.

Haraway, Donna J. "The Promises Of Monsters: A Regenerative Politics of Gender for Inappropriate/d Others." In *Cultural Studies*, Lawrence Grossberg, Cary Nelson, and Paula Treichler, eds. New York: Routledge, 1990.

———. "A Manifesto for Cyborgs: Science, Technology and Socialist Feminism in the 1980s." *Socialist Review*, vol. 80 (1985): 65–107.

———. "Teddy Bear Patriarchy: Taxidermy in the Garden of Eden, New York City, 1908–1936." *Social Text*, vol. 11 (Winter 1984–85): 20.

Hoyer, Niels. *Man into Woman*. (See Elbe, Lili.)

Irvine, Janice M. *Disorders Of Desire: Sex and Gender in Modern American Sexology*. Philadelphia: Temple UP, 1990.

Kates, Gary. "D'Eon Returns to France: Gender and Power and 1777." In *Body Guards: The Cultural Politics of Gender Ambiguity*, Kristina Straub and Julia Epstein, eds. New York: Routledge, 1991.

Laub, Donald R., and Patrick Gandy, eds. *Proceedings of the Second Interdisciplinary Symposium on Gender Dysphoria Syndrome*. Stanford: Division of Reconstructive and Rehabilitation Surgery, Stanford Medical Center, 1973.

Lothstein, Leslie Martin. *Female-to-Male Transsexualism: Historical, Clinical, and Theoretical Issues*. Boston: Routledge and Kegan Paul, 1983.

Morris, Jan. *Conundrum*. 1974. Rpt. New York: Henry Holt, 1986.

Nettick, Geri, and Beth Elliot. "The Transsexual Vampire." In *Lonely and a Long Way from Home: The Life and Strange Adventures of a Lesbian Transsexual* [mss]. Forthcoming.

Raymond, Janice. *The Transsexual Empire: The Making of the She-Male*. Boston: Beacon Press, 1979.

Riddell, Carol. *Divided Sisterhood: A Critical Review of Janice Raymond's The Transsexual Empire*. Liverpool: News From Nowhere, 1980.

Shapiro, Judith. "Transsexualism: Reflections of the Persistence of Gender and the Mutability of Sex." In *Body Guards: The Cultural Politics of Gender Ambiguity*, Kristina Straub and Julia Epstein, eds. New York: Routledge, 1991.

Spivak, Gayatri Chakravorty. *In Other Worlds: Essays in Cultural Politics*. New York: Routledge, 1988.

Star, Hedy Jo (Carl Rollins Hammonds). *I Changed My Sex!* Publisher unknown, 1955.

Steiner, Betty, ed. *Gender Dysphoria Syndrome: Development, Research, Management*. New York: Plenum Press, 1985.

Stoller, Robert J. *Presentations of Gender*. New Haven: Yale UP, 1985.

Stone, Allocheiria Racine. "Virtual Systems." In *ZONE 6: Fragments for a History of the Human Body, INCORPORATIONS*. New York: Urzone (MIT Press, 1992).

———. "Will the Real Body Please Stand Up?: Boundary Stories About Virtual Cultures." In *Cyberspace: First Steps*, M. Benedikt, ed. New York: MIT Press, 1991.

Stone, Sandy. "In the belly of the goddess: 'Women's Music,' Feminist Collectives, and the Cultural Arc of Lesbian Separatism, 1972–1979." Forthcoming.

———. "Sweet Surrender: Gender, Spirituality, and the Ecstasy of Subjection; Pseudotranssexual Fiction in the 1970s." Forthcoming.

Walters, William A. W., and Michael W. Ross, eds. *Transsexualism and Sex Reassignment*. Oxford: Oxford UP, 1986.

11

Beating the Meat/ Surviving the Text, or How to Get Out of This Century Alive

> This demise of feeling and emotion has paved the way for all our most real and tender pleasures—in the excitements of pain and mutilation; in sex as the perfect arena . . . for all the veronicas of our own perversions; in our moral freedom to pursue our own psychopathology as a game; and in our apparently limitless powers for conceptualization—what our children have to fear is not the cars on the highways of tomorrow but our own pleasure in calculating the most elegant parameters of their deaths.
>
> —J. G. Ballard, 1985[1]

Some time ago, in an issue of *Science-Fiction Studies*, I had occasion to rip into Jean Baudrillard's body—both his lived-body and his techno-body and the insurmountable, unthought, and thoughtless gap between them.[2] The journal had published an English translation of two of the French theorist-critic's short essays on science fiction and techno-culture,[3] one of them celebrating *Crash*, an extraordinary novel written by J. G. Ballard, first published in 1973 with an author's introduction added in 1974. My anger at Baudrillard arose from his willful misreading of a work whose pathological characters "get off" on the erotic collision between the human body and technology, and celebrate sex and death in wrecked automobiles and car crashes.

A moral tale written in the guise of a "pornographic" quasi-science fictional narrative, *Crash*'s cold and clinical prose robs the sex acts and the wounds the narrator describes of feeling and emotion and, I would assume in most cases, also of the ability to arouse the living flesh of the reader. Indeed, in his introduction, Ballard is explicit about his concerns and the novel's project. Viewing pornography as "the most political form of fiction, dealing with how we use and exploit each other in the most urgent and ruthless way," he describes *Crash* as "the first pornographic novel based on technology." It is, he says, "an extreme metaphor for an extreme situation, a kit of desperate measures only for use in an extreme crisis."[4] Excoriating the world around him in an explosive prose quite unlike that of the novel itself, Ballard's prescient introduction speaks of "voyeurism, self-disgust, the infantile basis of our dreams and longings" and suggests that, in a "communications landscape" of "sinister technologies," "mass merchandising," unlimited options, and "the dreams that money can buy," "these diseases of the psyche have now culminated in the most terrifying casualty of the century: the death of affect."[5] Feeling at a moral loss in the context of what is now—but was not then—called "postmodern" culture, Ballard is, nonetheless, moralistic. The "ultimate role of *Crash* is cautionary," he tells us. The novel "is a warning against the brutal, erotic and overlit realm that beckons more and more persuasively to us from the margins of the technological landscape."[6]

Baudrillard, however, refuses Ballard's warning while praising his work, and—as usual—succumbs to the brutal and erotic and techno-logical. Indeed, writing about *Crash*, the lived-body sitting at Baudrillard's desk must have forgotten itself to celebrate, instead, "a body with neither organs nor organ pleasures, entirely dominated by gash marks, cut-outs, and technical scars—all under the sign of a sexuality that is without referentiality and without limits."[7] Forgetting itself while invisibly grounding his fantasies of "a body commixed with technology's capacity for violation and violence," Baudrillard's lived-body is certainly disaffected, if not completely disavowed.[8] This is to say that Baudrillard's body is *thought* always as an object and never *lived* as a subject. And thought rather than lived, it can bear all sorts of symbolic abuse with indiscriminate and undifferentiated pleasure. This techno-body, however, is a porno-*graphic* fiction, objectified and written beyond belief and beyond the real—which is to say, it is always something "other" than the body Baudrillard lives as both "here" and "mine." Alienated from his own lived-body and its existence as the material premise for very real, rather than merely literal, pain, Baudrillard gets into the transcendent sexiness of the "brutal surgery" that

technology "continually performs in creating incisions, excisions, scar tissue, gaping body holes."[9] Rejecting Ballard's cautionary and moral gaze as
outmoded and inappropriate to the contemporary moment, he luxuriates
in the novel's wounds, "artificial orifices,"[10] and "artificial invaginations,"[11]
in the convergence of "chrome and mucous membranes," in "all the symbolic and sacrificial practices that a body can open itself up to—not via
nature, but via artifice, simulation, and accident."[12]

Where, in all this erotic technophilia, I asked at the time, was Baudrillard's
body? Both the one at the desk, the physical and intentional lived-body of the
man and the repressed or disavowed lived-body of the postmodernism for
which he and his disciples stand. At once decentered and completely extro-
verted, alienated in a phenomenological structure of *sensual thought* and
merely *psychic experience*, it was *re-signed* to being a *no-body*. The man's lived-
body (and, not coincidentally, the body of a man)—its material facticity, its
situatedness, finitude, and limitations—had been transubstantiated
through textualization into the infinite possibility and irresponsibility and
receptivity and legibility of the "pure" sign. Telling the "story" of this kind
of critical collapse of the materially real into "readable text," Fredric
Jameson points to how "finally the body itself proves to be a palimpsest
whose stabs of pain and symptoms, along with its deeper impulses and its
sensory apparatus, can be *read* fully as much as any other text."[13]

The sense of the body that Baudrillard privileges, then, is sense as it is
amputated from its origins in material existence. Baudrillard's body finds
its erotic pleasures located only in the *jouissance* of semiotic play, its pain
only in writer's block. And so—given that I first read Baudrillard on *Crash*
while I was recuperating from major cancer surgery on my left distal thigh
and knew all about gash marks, cut-outs, technical scars, and artificial orifices and invaginations—I wished the man a car crash or two, and a little
pain to bring him (back) to his senses.

Indeed, there is nothing like a little pain to bring us back to our senses,
nothing like a real (not imagined) mark or wound to counter the romanti-
cism and fantasies of techno-sexual transcendence that characterize so
much of the current discourse on the techno-body that is thought to occupy the cyberspaces of post-modernity. As Jameson reminds us: "History is
what hurts. It is what refuses desire and sets inexorable limits to individual
as well as collective praxis."[14] Thus, while it is true that, between operations, I could joke that my doctor "had gone where no man had gone
before," sitting there reading Baudrillard as I was living my artificial orifice and technical scars, I could attest to the *scandal* of metaphor and the
bad faith informing the "political economy of the sign." The "semiurgy of

contusions, scars, mutilations, and wounds" on *my* thigh were nothing like "new sexual organs opened in *the* body."[15] Even at its most objectified and technologically caressed, I lived this thigh—not abstractly on "the" body, but concretely as "my" body. Thus, sharp pain, dull aches, and numbness (which, after all, is not not-feeling, but the feeling of not-feeling), the cold touch of technology on my flesh, were distractions from my erotic possibilities, and not, as Baudrillard would have it, erotically distracting.

This critique, however, was leveled at Baudrillard some time ago— before I actually *became* a techno-body and experienced prosthetic pleasure. Fairly recently, my left leg was amputated above the knee and now I have a prosthetic replacement. Quickly done with pain (even the phantom sensations disappeared after five months), I went out and bought a whole new wardrobe of fancy underwear to don for my visits to the prosthetist—who is quite nice-looking, very absorbed in me, and generally positioned around crotch-level as he tinkers with my titanium knee. I love my prosthesis with its sculpted foam cosmetic cover—particularly the thigh which has no cellulite and is thinner than the thigh on my so-called "good" leg. With much effort, I have learned to walk again, the stump first thrust into the socket of a leg held on by a suspension belt and now into what is called a "suction" socket of a leg that—when it or I am working right—almost feels like "me." This new socket has also allowed me a kind of experience with "artificial orifices" that has none of the pain of surgery and all of the erotic play of technology. Every time I put the leg on, I literally "screw" a valve into a hole in my new thigh, depressing it to let the air out so that the prosthetic sucks my stump into the very depths of its fiberglass embrace.

I have also become a "lean, mean machine." After the amputation, I lost an extraordinary amount of weight—not from dieting in the mode of the self-loathing females of our culture, but from the intensive exercise of, first, merely getting from here to there on crutches and, now, from "pumping iron" to keep the rest of my body (the "meat" or "wetware" as we techno-bodies or cyborgs call it) up to the durability and strength of my prosthetic leg. Indeed—and here I admit to a certain confessional stance I don't usually condone in others—I gave up dieting years ago in anger at its built-in self-criticism and, hardly a glutton, worked on accepting myself "as I was." Now, however, all the clothes I never gave away fit me again. Quite frankly, I admit to feeling more positive about my loss of weight than negative about the loss of my leg. (This constitutes, I suppose, a "fair"—if hardly equitable—trade-off). The truth of the matter is that I feel more, not less, attractive than I used to. Hard body (however partial) that I am, I feel more erotically distracting and distracted than I have in years—although it is hard to find the time to do anything about it given all the hours I spend in physical therapy and at the gym. Indeed, over the year and a half since my amputation, I have come to learn that it's ridiculous (if not positively retrograde) to accept myself "as I am." I have found I can "make myself over," re-invent myself as a "harder" and, perhaps, even "younger" body. In fact, right now I am contemplating plastic surgery: getting my eyelids done, perhaps removing the crease that runs downward from the side of my mouth and makes me look less happy than I really am. This, then, is the power available to the "polymorphously perverse" cyborg woman—though hardly what Donna Haraway had in mind when she wrote her ironic manifesto.[16] If you've believed all of this, you probably think me less polymorphously perverse than extraordinarily self-deluded, bitter, or in some strange state of denial. Which, in fact, I'm not. Although a great deal of what I've revealed here is true, what is *not* true is that I've re-signed myself to being a cyborg, a techno-body. My prosthesis has not incorporated me. Rather, the whole aim of my physical existence over the last year and a half has been to incorporate it. Thus, my stance toward—and on—my prosthetic leg is quite a bit different from the one I've entertained here as a playful, yet ironic, response to the delights of the techno-body celebrated by Baudrillard and his followers. What many surgeries and my prosthetic experience has really taught me is that, if we are to survive into the next century, we must counter the millennial discourses that would de-contextualize our flesh into insensate sign or digitize it into cyberspace where, as one devotee put it, "it's like having had your everything amputated."[17] In the (inter)face of the new technological revolution and its transformation of every aspect of our culture (including our bodies), we have to recognize and make explicit the deep and dangerous ambivalence that informs the reversible relations we, as lived-bodies, have with our tools and their function of allowing us to transcend the limitations of our bodies.

Writing a number of years after her optimistic, if ironic, manifesto for cyborgs, Donna Haraway recognized the self-exterminating impulses of the discourses of disembodiment suggested by Baudrillard's porno-graphy of the body on the one hand and the *Mondo 2000/Wired*—let's download into the datascape and beat the meat—subculture on the other. In an interview she warns against the very "liberatory" cyborgism she once celebrated (however ironically) insofar as it jacks into (and off on) the "God trick," and denies mortality.[18] Our reversible relations with our technology, our confusion of consciousness with computation, of subjectively lived flesh with objective metal and hard-wiring, is—as Haraway points out—a "transcendentalist" move: "it produces death through the fear of it," disavowing as it does the fact that "we really do die, that we really do wound each other, that the earth really is finite, that there aren't any other planets out there that we know of that we can live on, that escape-velocity is a deadly fantasy."[19]

In *Technology and the Lifeworld*, philosopher Don Ihde discusses the ambivalent, or "doubled," desire that exists in our relations with any technology that extends our bodily sensorium and, thereby, our perceptions—be they eyeglasses or prosthetic legs, the motion picture camera or the computer. He tells us:

> On the one side is a wish for total transparency, total embodiment, for the technology to truly "become me." Were this possible, it would be equivalent to there being no technology, for total transparency would *be* my body and senses. . . . The other side is the desire to have the power, the *transformation* that the technology makes available. Only by using the technology is my bodily power enhanced and magnified by speed, through distance, or by any of the other ways in which technologies change my capacities. These capacities are always *different* from my naked capacities. The desire is, at best, contradictory. I want the transformation that the technology allows, but I want it in such a way that I am basically unaware of its presence. I want it in such a way that it becomes me. Such a desire both secretly *rejects* what technologies are and overlooks the transformational effects which are necessarily tied to human-technology relations. This illusory desire belongs equally to the pro- and anti-technology interpretations of technology.[20]

Obviously, transparency is what I wish—and strive—for in my relation to my prosthetic leg. I want to subjectively embody it. I do not want to regard it as an object or to think *about* it as I use it to walk. Indeed, in learning to use the prosthesis, I found that *looking objectively* at my leg in a mirror as an exteriorized thing to be thought about and manipulated did not help me improve my balance and gait so much as did *subjectively feeling* through all of my body the weight and rhythm of the leg in a *gestalt* of motor activity. Insofar as the leg remains an object external to me, a hermeneutic problem to be solved, a piece of technology to use, I cannot live it and be enabled by it to accomplish intentional projects that involve it but don't concern it. So, of course, I want it to become totally transparent. The desired transparency here, however, involves *my* incorporation of the prosthetic—and not the prosthetic's incorporation of me (although, seen by others to whom a prosthetic is strange, I may well seem its extension rather than the other way around). This is to say that although my new and enabling leg is made of titanium and fiberglass, I do not perceive myself as a hard body—even after a good workout at the gym, when my union with the weight machines (not the leg) momentarily reifies that metaphor. Nor do I think that because my leg may very well outlast me into the next millennium, it confers upon me invincibility or immortality. Prosthetically enabled, I am, nonetheless, not a cyborg. Unlike Baudrillard, I have not forgotten the limitations and finitude and naked capacities of my flesh—nor, more importantly, do I desire to escape them. They are, after all, what ground the concrete gravity and value of my life, and the very possibility of my partial transcendence of them through various perceptual technologies—be they my bi-focals, my leg, or my computer. That is, my lived-body—not my prosthetic leg which stands inert in a corner by the bed before I put it on in the morning—provides me the *material premises* and, therefore, the *logical grounds* for the intelligibility of those moral categories that emerge from a bodily sense of gravity and finitude.

I have been using the phenomenological term "lived-body" throughout to a purpose. Seeming redundant, it serves as a corrective to those prevalent objectifications that complacently regard the body, even one's own, as merely a conceptual or objective thing. One of the consequences of our high-tech millenarianism is that the moral material and significance of the lived-body is elided or disavowed, not only by the delusional liberatory rhetoric of technophiles who long to become either "pure" electronic information or self-repairing cyborgs like Schwarzenegger's Terminator, but also through the dangerous liberatory poetry of cultural formalists like Baudrillard who long to escape the lived-body and its limitations and write it off (quite literally) as just another sign of its times. This is to say, Baudrillard is of a piece with all those in our culture who revile the lived-body for its weaknesses and who wish to objectify its terrible mortality away—those, for example, who are obsessed with physical fitness (and through various and often perverse or pathological means attempt to transform themselves into hard bodies and lean machines), those who are turned on by images of the body being "blown away" and "riddled" by bullet holes (how clearly the vernacular speaks the substance of desire), those like Hans Moravec who want to "upload" into the datascape,[21] those who refer to their bodies contemptuously as "meat" and "wetware," and even those who, less overtly than Baudrillard, theorize and intellectually commodify "the body" as an *objective thing* that one can hold—dare I pun?—at arm's length, available to disinterested scrutiny. This alienated and highly fetishized fascination with the body-object (the body that we *have*) and the devaluation of the lived-body (the body that we *are*) is a consequence of a dangerous confusion between the agency that is our bodies/our selves and the power of our incredible new technologies of perception and expression.

In a recent article critiquing "technocriticism" and its underlying "rhetoric about age," Kathleen Woodward reads technological development in western culture as a "story about the human body":

> Over hundreds of thousand of years the body, with the aid of various tools and technologies, has multiplied its strength and increased its capacities to extend itself in space and overtime. According to this logic, the process culminates in the very immateriality of the body itself. In this view technology serves fundamentally as a prosthesis of the human body, one that ultimately displaces the material body, transmitting instead its image around the globe and preserving that image over time.[22]

As we increasingly objectify our thoughts and desires through modern technologies of perception and communication, our subjective awareness of our own bodies diminishes. As Woodward suggests, "there is a beguiling, almost mesmerizing relationship between the progressive vanishing of the body, as it were, and the hypervisuality of both the postmodern society of the spectacle . . . and the psychic world of cyberspace."[23] This disappearance (or increased "transparency") of the material, lived-body, its apparent displacement by technological prostheses that can enable and extend our perceptual and expressive powers, provokes in some the "heady" sensation of having "beat the meat." That is, the increasing transparency of one's lived-flesh enabled by new technologies as well as the ubiquitous visibility of new technologies leads to euphoria and a sense of the limitless extension of being beyond its materiality and mortality. This, however, is "false" consciousness—for it has "lost touch" with the very material and mortal body that grounds its imagination and imagery of transcendence. As Woodward emphasizes, "the possibility of an invulnerable and thus immortal body is our greatest technological illusion—that is to say, *delusion*."[24]

Thus, I have no desire, like Baudrillard or Moravec in their respective disembodying fantasies, to "beat the meat." Indeed, in light of Ihde's description of the doubled and contradictory structure of our relations with technology, this phrase resonates with contradictions that are tied to, but implicate more than, "sexual difference." Certainly, in American vernacular, it speaks of male masturbation. However, in today's world, it also speaks of a desire to get rid of bodily desire—perhaps once through orgasm, but now through technology. Simultaneously, then, the phrase expresses the contradictory wish, on the one hand, to get rid of the body and to overcome its material limitations and demands and, on the other, "to escape the newly extended body of technological engagement,"[25] and to *reclaim experience through the flesh.* Hence *Crash*, its narrator (an "other" Ballard) telling us, "The crash was the only real experience I had been through for years. For the first time I was in physical confrontation with my own body, an inexhaustible encyclopedia of pains and discharges."[26] Hence, the novel's conflation of wounds and orgasms and automobiles, its confusions of flesh and metal, its characters' imagination of "a sexual expertise that would be an exact analogue of the other skills created by the multiplying technologies of the twentieth century."[27] Hence, the dream "of other accidents that might enlarge [the] repertory of orifices, relating them to more elements of the automobile's engineering, to the ever-more complex technologies of the future." Hence Ballard's narrator asks, "What wounds would create the sexual possibilities of the invisible technologies of thermonuclear reaction chambers, white-tiled control rooms, the mysterious scenarios of computer circuitry?" and hence he visualizes "the extraordinary sexual acts celebrating the possibilities of unimagined technologies."[28] Throughout the discourses of cyborgism, there is extraordinary emphasis on the erotics of technology as flesh-based, on a transcribed and transubstantiated sexuality that is fatally confused as to the site of its experience.

Baudrillard, Moravec, the *Mondo 2000* and *Wired* folks, all want, as Ihde puts it, "what the technology gives but do not want the limits, the transformations that a technologically extended body implies."[29] Thus, the disavowal inherent in Baudrillard's celebratory description of the techno-body as "under the gleaming sign of a sexuality that is without referentiality and without limits." Wanting what "technology gives," but disavowing what it "limits," those who find the techno-body "sexy" forget that screwing the valve into place on my prosthetic thigh brings me no shudder of physical pleasure. This is a thigh that cannot make sense of the lacy lingerie that touches it, cannot feel the silk stockings that caress its artificial skin. In sum, my prosthetic leg has its limits and whatever it does to extend my being-in-the-world, whatever way it enhances and amplifies my perceptions and the significance of my existence, however much it seems to bring me in closer material contact with the technological world, I still had to give up my fleshy leg in trade, to lose something in the bargain. What is particularly dangerous about Baudrillard's erotics of technology—and utterly different from Ballard's pornography of technology in *Crash*—is that, despite its seeming heightened consciousness, it finally disavows the *technological status of technology.* Thus, unlike Ballard, Baudrillard's dizzying pro-technological rhetoric hides anti-technology desire and its self-deception promotes deadly, terminal confusions between meat and hardware.

At this millennial moment when high technology has given so many cultural critics and academics a technological "high," there might be some cachet in claiming for myself the "sexiness" of cyborg identity. Rather than—along with the century—being on my "last leg," I could describe myself as being on the "first leg" of some devoutly wished for transformation of my human frailty and mortality. This, however, is not the case. Living—rather than writing or thinking—my "newly extended body of technological engagement," I find the fragility of my flesh significantly precious. While I am deeply grateful for the motility my prosthetic affords me (however much in a transformation that is perceptually reduced as well as amplified), the new leg is dependent finally upon my last leg. Without my lived-body to live it, the prosthetic exists as part of a body without organs—a techno-body that has no sympathy for human suffering, cannot understand human pleasure, and, since it has no conception of death, cannot possibly value life.

And so, here as in *Science-Fiction Studies*, I wish Baudrillard a little pain—maybe a lot—to bring him to his senses. Pain would remind him that he doesn't just *have* a body, but that he *is* his body, and that it is in this material fact that "affect" and anything we might call a "moral stance" is grounded. Both significant affection and a moral stance (whether on prosthetic legs or not) are based on the lived sense and feeling of the human body not merely as a material object one possesses and analyzes among others, but as a material subject that experiences its own objectivity, that has the capacity to bleed and suffer and hurt for others because it can sense its own possibilities for suffering and pain. If we don't keep this subjective kind of bodily sense in mind as we negotiate our technoculture, we may very well objectify ourselves to death. It is only by embracing life in all its vulnerability and imperfection, by valuing the limitations as well as possibilities of our flesh, and by accepting mortality, that we will get out of this—or any—century alive.

Notes

1. J. G. Ballard, *Crash* (New York: Vintage Books, 1985) 1.

2. Vivian Sobchack, "Baudrillard's Obscenity," *Science-Fiction Studies* 18 (1991): 327–329.

3. Jean Baudrillard, "Jean Baudrillard: Two Essays," trans. Arthur B. Evans *Science-Fiction Studies* 18 (1991): 309–320.

4. Ballard 6.

5. Ballard 1.

6. Ballard 6.

7. Baudrillard 313.

8. Baudrillard 313.

9. Baudrillard 313.

10. Baudrillard 316.

11. Baudrillard 315.

12. Baudrillard 316.

13. Fredric Jameson, *Postmodernism, or The Cultural Logic of Late Capitalism* (Durham, NC: Duke UP, 1991) 186.

14. Jameson 102.

15. Baudrillard 314. Emphasis mine.

16. Donna Haraway, "A Manifesto for Cyborgs: Science, Technology and Socialist Feminism in the 1980s," *Socialist Review* 15 (1985): 65–107.

17. John Perry Barlow, "Being in Nothingness: Virtual Reality and the Pioneers of Cyberspace," *Mondo 2000* 2 (1990): 42. 18. Constance Penley and Andrew Ross, "Cyborgs at Large: Interview with Donna Haraway," *Social Text* 25/26 (1991): 18–23.

19. Penley and Ross 20.

20. Don Ihde, *Technology and the Lifeworld: From Garden to Earth* (Bloomington: Indiana UP, 1990) 75.

21. Hans P. Moravec, *Mind Children: The Future of Robot and Human Intelligence* (Cambridge, MA: Harvard UP, 1988).

22. Kathleen Woodward, "From Virtual Cyborgs to Biological Time Bombs: Technocriticism and the Material Body," in Gretchen Bender and Timothy Druckrey, eds., *Culture on the Brink: Ideologies of Technology* (Seattle: Bay Press, 1994) 50.

23. Woodward 50.

24. Woodward 51.

25. Ihde 75-76.

26. Ballard 39.

27. Ballard 100.

28. Ballard 179.

29. Idhe 76.

Ricahrd A. Cone and Emily Martin

12

Corporeal Flows

The Immune System, Global Economies of Food, and New Implications for Health

→ *Abstract*

Allergies and autoimmune disorders are increasing in incidence, especially among the urban poor. This paper,[1] which results from conversations and research that bring together knowledge and methods from anthropology and immunology,[2] considers the interrelated biological and social implications of the increasing incidence of immune dysfunctions, and the ways in which changes in food production, transport, and consumption, circulating through global markets, may be contributing to immune dysfunctions, especially through changes in "oral tolerance."

Is collaboration between a biologist and a cultural anthropologist possible today? Would bringing insights from biological science and cultural studies together produce a synergy that scholars on both sides would find enlightening? This paper could be seen as a test case for these questions. Richard Cone is a biophysicist who, for the first half of his career studied the fluid properties of membranes in the cell in order to further basic science. For the second half of his career he has been studying the physiological properties of sperm, the vagina, and the rectum, in order to develop a topical substance for the penis or vagina that would kill sperm and any pathogen found in human sexual orifices. Emily Martin is an anthropologist who, for the first half of her career studied cultural and social organization in the Taiwanese countryside. For the second half of her career, she has been studying the complex interplay among sciences like reproductive biology and immunology and concepts and practices that permeate the wider culture in the United States in order to understand, and influence, contemporary conceptions and practices related to health.

Reactions to drafts of this paper from our respective colleagues surprised us. We were both anxious that immunologists might be affronted by non-immunologists' suggesting new questions about the immune system. But we both felt confident that anthropologists and other students of culture would react with interest, the more so because the text is experimental in form and content. In spite of our worries, immunologists who read the paper were immensely encouraging, excitedly offering us related thoughts and references. One immunologist immediately made copies of the paper and assigned it to his students in an advanced immunology class, which he invited us to attend. Again confounding our expectations, colleagues in cultural studies were disapproving. Many felt that the paper conceded too much ground to science, and that it needed a stronger interpretive voice. No doubt future readers from the sciences will find many things to add or correct in this account, and we welcome that; but it would be dismaying if the paper were dismissed by students of culture because it speaks too much with the voice of science. In an effort to prevent this reaction, we would suggest that this account *is* an interpretation, of the body, of the globe, and of what it means to be healthy. It is an interpretation that dramatically rearranges in importance the parts of the body that biologists think have something to do with health, and it is an interpretation that postulates dramatic connections among things that ordinarily belong to separate disciplines: *the culture and economy of food production and consumption, the recent rise of autoimmune diseases,* and *the surfaces of our bodies that produce mucus.*

Prologue

This morning I awake with another stupifyingly painful headache, which I have been told is probably caused by an allergy to something in the air. Faced with the impossible choice of taking medicine that will make me unable to stay awake or trying to work in spite of the pain, I read the New York Times' Science Times *instead. I get absorbed in an article about a new form of treatment for autoimmune disorders, in which patients are fed orally the part of the body their immune systems are reacting to wrongly (i.e., since arthritis is caused by the immune system attacking and destroying collagen in the joints, arthritis sufferers are fed collagen from animal joints), and I am brought up short by the results: patients experience remission or significant relief from their symptoms.*

I am electrified by the implications of this. Isn't my immune system reacting to particles in the air that are harmless (pollen or mold), wrongly treating them as harmful substances that should be attacked, producing swelling and pain in my sinuses? Maybe I can simply eat *whatever is causing this reaction. . . .*

I call my husband, Richard, a biophysicist, in Baltimore and ask him how I can eat what is in the air, imagining pollinating flowers in soup, flowering grass on sandwiches, and spore forming molds on bread. (EM)

Eat what is in the air? [short pause] Well, you could eat local, unfiltered honey straight from the hive. The bees have done all the work of gathering up pollen of every kind along with all sorts of airborne particles. Whatever you are allergic to, it might be in there, and you would certainly be eating it. (RAC)

I immediately buy honey gathered from hives kept in a hamlet near Princeton (wondering why I never thought about how health food stores always seem to carry local, unfiltered honey) and after a few days of eating it, I experience profound relief from sinus pain. Ever since then, as long as I eat honey from the place I am in, my sinus problems have been dramatically reduced. Wanting to spread the news, Richard and I devise recipes so our friends who have allergies and autoimmune disorders can try oral tolerance, since the experiment might provide significant benefits at little risk or effort. One friend, whose immune system is attacking the melanin in her skin, tries eating melanin. Since melanin is found in high concentration in the eyes of any animal we suggest she can eat fish stock made out of fish heads. Same goes for another friend who has an autoimmune reaction to the vitreous fluid in her eyes. Still another friend, suffering from sinus congestion caused by allergy to molds, tries leaving her dishes out on the counter (where mold spores in the house will land on them) and then eating food from the dishes without rinsing them first. (EM)

Introduction

Immune disorders give rise to a diverse array of health problems, some of which, especially allergies and asthma, not only cause major suffering, but also are increasing in incidence. There are few effective therapies for immune disorders, and over the past few years immunologists have begun to investigate whether food ("oral exposure") might be used to help treat autoimmune diseases such as arthritis, multiple sclerosis, and diabetes. The results are promising. The recently demonstrated effects of oral exposures on immune functions also raise the possibility that major alterations in food production, transport, and diet may be playing a role in altering the incidence and severity of immune disorders. In this paper we describe some aspects of how food helps "instruct" the immune system to distinguish between what to attack, what to ignore, and what to protect. Occasionally the immune system can make false associations in this learning process and may start to attack something normal or innocuous as if it were a pathogen or toxin. In light of these recent immunological findings, we describe major changes in food transport, preparation, and consumption that might influence the incidence of immune disorders. Investigations of the connections between diet and immune function, "immuno-nutrition," may suggest ways to reduce the incidence or severity of immune disorders by changes in diet as well as changes in the global system of food production, processing, and transport.

Incidence of Allergy and Autoimmune Disease

What Is the Evidence the Incidence Is Rising?

The most thoroughly documented rise in incidence of these maladies is in asthma. The prevalence rate of asthma in the United States rose by 30 percent from 1980 to 1987 (Moslehi 1995). The National Institute of Allergy and Infectious Diseases reports that from 1990 to 1992 the number of people with self-reported asthma in the United States increased from 10.4 million to 12.4 million (Yunginger et al. 1992). Asthma has also been found to be more common by far (26 percent more prevalent) in African American children than in white children (Evans 1992).

In addition there is evidence that rates of death from asthma are increasing alarmingly despite recent advances in methods for treating asthma: while earlier treatments were based on the use of bronchodilators to relax the sphincter muscles that control the airways in the lungs, current therapies are based on the realization that asthma is an immune-dysfunction and hence include the use of anti-inflammatory drugs (such as cortico-steroids). Despite the resulting symptomatic improvements from this therapy, rates of death from asthma in the United States increased from 0.8 per 100,000 in 1977 to 2.0 in 1991 (Sly 1994). Another study showed that from 1980 to 1987 the rate of deaths from asthma increased by 30 percent (Moslehi 1995). Increases in death from asthma are also documented for Australia, Canada, Great Britain, and New Zealand, though Australia and New Zealand's rates have been falling recently (Sly 1994). As with the rates for asthma itself, the rates of death from asthma are highest in minorities in the United States. African Americans were three times as likely to die from asthma as whites in the period 1982–92 (CDC 1995). (See also Malveaux et al. 1993.)

Data on the incidence of allergies and autoimmune diseases are more difficult to come by. In the case of autoimmune disease, there is a pervasive impression among medical practitioners as well as the general public that they are dramatically increasing. But this impression is complicated because the number of maladies defined as autoimmune has itself been increasing, making it hard to prove an actual statistical increase in the number of cases.

Allergies are certainly pervasive. The National Institute of Allergy and Infectious Diseases says that, "while there are no solid statistics, estimates from a skin test survey suggest that allergies affect as many as 40 to 50 million people in the U.S." or one in five people (Gergen et al. 1987). Data are again scarce, but there are multiple indications that both allergies and autoimmune diseases affect women more than men (Schwartz and Datta 1989; CDC 1994). Not many statistics are available, but those we have indicate a rise in allergies in recent years. The number of children diagnosed with allergic dermatitis in the United States has increased from 3 percent in the l960s to 10 percent in the 1990s (Horan et al. 1992). In other countries, efforts have begun to document the widespread impression that the incidence of allergies is on the increase. Data from Sweden, Switzerland, Germany, Denmark, Japan, show a definite increase in allergic diseases (Kunz et al. 1991).

What Might Be Causing These Increases in Incidence?

Environmental toxins, both airborne and in food, might be implicated in the rise in allergies. Japanese investigators searching for causes of the dramatic increase in pollen allergies in Japan since the 1950s, have shown that exposure to diesel exhaust exacerbates allergic responses to pollens (Miyamoto et al. 1988; Kunz et al. 1991). French researchers found that severe food allergies in France from 1984 to 1992 were most commonly caused by foods that are "not of a primary nutritional importance: celery, crustaceans, fish, peanuts, mango, mustard" but that are often "hidden allergens in commercial foods" (Andre et al. 1994).

In addition, we have some evidence of the onset of autoimmune diseases in a community that has recently begun to eat transported and processed food for the first time. Narjan-Mar, a town of 20,000 on the Barents Sea in Russia, has been very isolated until recently. Because the surrounding area is so boggy, Narjan-Mar's access to the outside has been possible only by boat and within the last decade by plane and helicopter. Until a decade ago, virtually all the food they consumed was produced locally. But in the last 5 to 10 years, more and more of their food has been transported in from the outside. Concurrently, the medical staff of the local hospital has noticed an increasing number of allergies and "suppressed immune functioning." The medical staff thought the reason might be contact with outsiders or the poor quality of the food brought in from outside.[3] But the account we are about to give suggests quite a different explanation of why immune dysfunctions are increasing in places like Narjan-Mar and elsewhere, as well as how they may be linked in part to diet.

Immune Disorders

What Are the Main Types of Immune Disorders?

Allergies, such as hay fever and food allergies, occur when the immune system "overreacts" to airborne particles or components in food, treating benign or mildly toxic particles, such as ragweed pollen, as if they were highly toxic. The immune system expels these particles with such vigor that the immune reactions cause "bystander" damage to the lungs, gut, or other exposed tissue, and sometimes death by shock, dehydration, or suffocation. Autoimmune diseases occur when the immune system mistakenly attacks cells or tissues that are otherwise healthy "self"; in arthritis, the immune system attacks collagen or other tissues in the joints, in early-onset diabetes it attacks insulin-producing cells in the pancreas, and in multiple sclerosis it attacks nerve sheaths. Cancer can be considered a third type of immune disorder in that tumors grow only if the immune system fails to attack them, mistaking tumor cells for normal "self."

What Are the Roles of the Immune System?

The immune system consists of multiple arrays of continuously interact-ing cells, many of which move around throughout the body. This "mobile brain," as the immune system is sometimes called, constantly monitors or observes not only all the tissues of the body, but also all the things in the environment that impinge upon the surfaces of the lungs, intestines, and other mucosal surfaces as well as the skin. Mobile arrays of immune cells are continuously learning and memorizing, and sometimes forgetting, what to attack, what to leave alone, and what to protect. Immune system cells can distinguish what is "self" from what is "non-self" and they can "keep house" in the body, ridding it of unwanted debris.

How Does the Immune System Distinguish "Self" from "Non-self"?

For much of the past century, immunologists have focused on how the immune system learns to identify and attack pathogens, toxins, and other objects it recognizes as "foreign," such as parasites or tissue grafts, and how it learns to ignore cells it recognizes as "self." Interest in how the immune system distinguishes between "self and non-self" has led to major insights about how the immune system develops and matures. As each new immune cell begins to mature, if it reveals to its neighbors that it might later attack self, it is instructed to die before it matures (it is instructed to undergo "apoptosis," the dying process performed by normal cells at the end of their appropriate life-span); only if a maturing immune cell demon-strates no proclivity for attacking self is it permitted to continue maturing. However, this step in self/non-self discrimination is merely a single step in cell maturation, and many subsequent interactions continuously help reg-ulate all the activities of immune cells.

Who Does the Housework?

A major component of the immune system consists of phagocytic cells ("cell-eating" cells). In addition to attacking and eating invading pathogens, phagocytic cells of the immune system have another major role: macrophages ("big eaters") continuously explore around the body eating, digesting, and recycling the molecular subunits of dead cells and debris from the normal daily turnover of body tissues. Since the life-span of most cells in the body is a matter of days to weeks, phagocytosis of dead (apoptopic) cells is a major, though often ignored, activity of the immune system. Phagocytes spend *most* of their time eating, digesting, and recycling dead and dying "self"; encountering and eating a (foreign, "non-self") pathogen is a relatively *rare* event.

> *"Housekeeping" functions of the immune system have yet to become a major focus of interest in immunology—but I sometimes imagine what would happen if our phagocytes only chased after foreign invaders, but lost all interest in doing everyday housework, garbage removal, and recycling. We would literally clog up with our own garbage. (RAC)*

> *Like immunology, traditionally taught history highlighted the battles (men) fought, making maintenance activities (by women in the family and home) nearly invisible. Feminist accounts that attend to the importance of women's activities have revolutionized our understanding of history: it will be interesting to see whether a revolution in our understanding of the immune system could come about if the housekeeping activities of the lowly macrophage came to be regarded as more significant. (EM)*

What about the Food We Eat? Isn't It Foreign?

Despite nearly a half-century of research on how the immune system distinguishes "self" from "non-self," surprisingly little attention has been directed at problems posed by this self/non-self perspective: phagocytes eat dying cells that are in every way "self"; how do phagocytes know when to start eating this "self" debris? The food we eat presents an even more challenging problem if viewed from the self/non-self perspective: food is "non-self," packed with foreign cells and foreign surfaces. But the immune system does not react against most of the food we eat. This clearly demonstrates that the immune system is *not* dedicated to attacking all that is foreign or "non-self." The immune system is more sophisticated than the seductively profound "self/non-self" dichotomy implies. If it attacked food as "non-self," we wouldn't survive. This is clearly (and fortunately only occasionally) illustrated by the dire results of eating a small amount of food to which one is allergic: salivation, nausea, vomiting, diarrhea, headache, and sometimes death. How is it that most food, all of which is "foreign," is "tolerated" by the immune system? Amongst all the foreign surfaces and molecules the immune system encounters, how does it distinguish food from foe? Or, in the terms suggested by Matzinger (1994), how does it distinguish between what is dangerous and what is not dangerous?

The immune system in the gut, which forms a major part of what is called the *mucosal immune system*, learns to recognize and accept ("tolerate") food, allowing it to be absorbed into the blood and lymph. It also learns to recognize dangerous pathogens and toxins ingested along with food and helps prevent them from being absorbed, in part by secreting antibodies (especially a type called secretory IgA) that trap the pathogens and toxins in mucus. Once trapped, this part of the immune system helps attack, eat, and otherwise detoxify them. Similarly, in the lungs, the mucosal immune system learns to recognize innocuous particles of foreign materials, such as house dust, and to distinguish them from toxic pollutants that must be immediately expelled by coughing and increased mucus flow. This allows us to breathe with ease even in the presence of multitudes of nontoxic foreign particles of dust (as revealed by a beam of sunlight), while making us sneeze, gag, or otherwise stop inhaling air when it contains too many toxic particles. By their speed and severity, allergic responses help us to identify the allergen and to avoid further contacts with it (see Profet 1991). In this way, our "mobile" brain can instruct our neural brain to alter our behavior.

I find it intriguing that immunologists have devoted far more attention to the systemic immune system, the system that monitors the blood and lymph, than to the mucosal immune system, the system that monitors the mucus on the surfaces of the gut, lungs, eyes, and reproductive tracts. It is the mucosal system that must distinguish between foreign substances that are food from foreign substances that are foe. Mucosal immunology has emerged as a separate discipline only recently, in part because it is easier to study immune activities in the blood than in mucus. It seems that studying the blood is somehow more noble or "important" than studying mucus. The research in my laboratory is aimed at developing better methods for preventing sexually transmitted diseases and unwanted pregnancy and as a result students must work with semen, cervical mucus, and other unmentionable secretions. They joke, somewhat defensively, about being "masters of mucus." The lack of interest in immune functions in mucous secretions contributes to our current lack of understanding of allergic responses. Immunologists are still at a loss for understanding why we have IgE, the class of antibodies that mediate allergic reactions. They have even proposed that we might be better off without any IgE and have investigated methods for entirely eliminating this arm of mucosal immune function.[4] (RAC)

I can't believe it is an accident that mucosal immunology is relatively undeveloped. Much has been written by anthropologists like Mary Douglas and Victor Turner about the deep and complex cultural meanings that often become attached to bodily substances like blood or mucus and bodily orifices like the mouth or anus. Especially strong and troubled significance seems to be attached to substances that are "betwixt and between" (neither solid nor liquid, for example, but a sticky glop like mucus).[5] Such substances arouse horror, but not because of "lack of cleanliness or health," rather because they "disturb identity, system, order. [They are] what does not respect borders, positions, rules. The in-between, the ambiguous, the composite" (Kristeva 1982: 4). In Kristeva's phenomenological account, horror is aroused by these substances because they attest to the impossible task of maintaining a clear bodily boundary between the self and the world: "the fragile border . . . where identities (subject/object, etc.) do not exist or only barely so—double, fuzzy, heterogeneous, animal, metamorphosed, altered, abject" (p. 207).[6] Isn't it likely that scientists' disinclination to study mucus, and your lab members' joking about being "masters of mucus" would somehow be related to these cultural and phenomenological matters? Might not responses like Sartre's to "the viscous" come into play? "The slime is like a liquid seen in a nightmare, where all its properties are animated by a sort of life and turn back against me . . . the slimy offers a horrible image; it is horrible in itself for a consciousness to become slimy" (1981: 138, 140). (EM)

How Do the Mucosal and Systemic Immune System Interact with Each Other?

The mucosal immune system functions in partnership with the systemic immune system; each of the two systems performs markedly different functions, sometimes stimulating, sometimes opposing activities in the other system. Not only does the mucosal immune system learn to identify all the foreign substances in food as "food" (non-toxic, nonpathogenic), it also sends cellular messengers that can suppress systemic immune reactions against this food should it be encountered somewhere else in the body. This process is called *"oral tolerance,"* a somewhat cumbersome term used by immunologists to mean "orally induced inhibition of systemic (not oral) immune reactions." In plain words, if you eat a nontoxic substance, your mucosal system can inhibit your systemic immune system from reacting against that substance. Thus the mucosal system, in the process of monitoring the digestion and absorption of food, learns what is nontoxic and "teaches" the systemic system to "tolerate" it, even though the substance is foreign.

If a food substance is combined with what immunologists call an "adjuvant," such as a toxin, a pathogen, or components of a pathogen, both the mucosal and systemic immune systems react *against* the substance, abrogating oral tolerance to this substance. In short, if a toxin is attached to some food component, the mucosal immune system learns to treat that food component as dangerous and tells the systemic immune system to do the same. The details of how the presence of a toxin can switch oral tolerance (active immune suppression) to *"oral intolerance"* (active immune reaction) have yet to be clarified. Indeed, the potential abilities of toxins such as pesticides, pollutants, and food preservatives to switch oral tolerance to intolerance have yet to be investigated.

Oral tolerance was apparently discovered long ago: South American Indians are said to have fed their children poison ivy leaves to prevent the allergic skin reactions that otherwise occur if the skin contacts this plant prior to oral exposure (Dakin 1829). An early immunology experiment that demonstrated oral tolerance was reported in 1911 (Wells 1911): guinea pigs suffer a severe allergic response (sometimes fatal anaphylactic shock) if they are injected with chicken egg protein. However, guinea pigs can safely eat chicken egg protein, and if they are fed this protein for several weeks, they become tolerant to it. That is, they do not suffer a severe allergic response if it is injected into them. Oral exposure can thus produce systemic immune tolerance.

Can Autoimmune Disorders Be Treated by Oral Tolerance?

For much of the past century, oral tolerance has been viewed by most immunologists as merely a curiosity and given only passing mention in textbooks of immunology. Immunologic research has focused on systemic immune responses and on how to create vaccines that stimulate systemic immunity. Few immunologists have puzzled over how the immune system *learns* to tolerate that which is *not* dangerous, nor, until recently, have they focused on how it learns to distinguish between what is dangerous and what is not.[7] However, interest in autoimmune disorders has recently stimulated research on oral tolerance. Several clinical trials now in progress are testing whether oral tolerance can alleviate autoimmune diseases, such as arthritis and early-onset diabetes.

The question asked in these studies is remarkably simple: if you have arthritis, can you alleviate joint pain and swelling by eating collagen (the "antigen") to make your systemic immune system more "tolerant" of your

own collagen? In a recent clinical trial, people with arthritis who ate collagen supplements derived from chicken breast bones experienced significant reductions in joint swelling and pain, and in some cases complete
remission (Trentham et al. 1993). Similar trials are in progress in which
patients with multiple sclerosis are eating nerve protein (myelin basic protein) from cow brain, patients with uveitis, an autoimmune degeneration
of eye tissue that can lead to blindness, are eating a protein (S-antigen)
obtained from cow eyes; and trials are being planned for treating juvenile
and early-onset (type I) diabetes by eating human insulin (Weiner 1994).

Diet, Oral Tolerance, and Alternative Health Traditions

How Can Eating a Substance Cause Oral Tolerance? How Might Food Processing, Global Marketing of Food, and Diet Influence the Incidence of Allergies and Immune Dysfunctions?

Immunologists and anthropologists are only beginning to ask these questions, and before discussing what little they know we might learn more
by considering alternative or folk dietary practices that relate to these
questions.

Might Oral Tolerance Play a Role in Alternative Health Traditions?

Consider first the claims made for the healing properties of honey. From
the seventeenth century, honey has been described as a remedy for
coughs, labored breathing, and sore throats (Mintz n.d.: 6). A report from
Bulgaria claims to have found that more than half of over 17,000 patients
treated with honey for chronic bronchitis, asthmatic bronchitis, bronchial
asthma, chronic rhinitis, allergic rhinitis, and sinusitis achieved complete
remission of their symptoms (Brown 1993). Today honey is also widely
believed to have anti-bacterial effects (effects that have been demonstrated
in scientific studies [Subrahmanyam 1991; 1993]), anti-tumor effects as
well as beneficial effects on the heart and the digestive system (Crane
1975: 260, 263; Challem 1995).
   Popular contemporary sources that extoll the healing properties of consuming honey abound in public libraries and health food stores (Nasi 1978;
Jarvis 1960; Wade 1983). Jarvis, author of *Arthritis and Folk Medicine*,

exclaims, "Honey taken every day is the body cell's best friend" (p. 120). Testimonial letters written to a company that sells raw honey, the "Really Raw Honey Company" indicate the degree of passion felt by people who get relief from allergies in such a simple way.[8] Word of mouth recipes and directions for using honey to alleviate the symptoms of allergy to airborne pollens are widespread, and news groups on the Internet, such as alt.med.allergy frequently describe how people try using honey in various ways.

> *Here is a selection from an e-mail message written to me after I responded to a message this person posted on the news group. She regularly eats a piece of honeycomb from a hive in a neighborhood adjacent to hers. She explains:*

> > *The honeycomb grown locally contains much if not all of the very allergens I'm allergic to. Ingesting these in small amounts is just what I'm doing with the injections [from her allergist], to increase my body's tolerance of them. The theory is, in time, your body hardly reacts to them at all. Now, [my neighbor] told me that honey harvested . . . in one season will have different allergens than what's collected in another season. So at that point I get confused, so I'm just operating now like, it can't HURT me. Do you know about any of that? (EM)*

> > *Her allergist is injecting allergen to tolerize her immune system systemically; meanwhile, she is trying to help her mucosal immune system do its normal job of causing systemic tolerance by exposing it to the allergen orally. (RAC)*

The virtues of eating honey can be understood as providing the mucosal immune system a way to learn which airborne particulates are harmless: in the case of honey, the bees do the work of gathering up many of these particles (pollen, dust, and other particles in the air) and concentrating them in honey. When we eat honey and the airborne particles it contains, the particles contact the mucosa of the mouth and the gut. In the process the mucosal immune system can learn to tolerate them and instruct the systemic immune system not to react to them as toxic.

Consider second the health claims made for macrobiotics, a systematically devised program of diet and nutrition that stresses eating food that is local and seasonal. Macrobiotics was codified in its modern form in Japan by Sagen Ishizuka at the end of the nineteenth century (Kotzsch 1985: 28). Encouraged by his extensive study of traditional dietary practices around the world, as well as traditional Chinese and Japanese diet and medicine, Ishizuka also carried out systematic dietary experiments on himself and on patients he treated. One time he lived for a month on sweet potatoes alone to isolate their effect as a food. Since he was writing at a time of rising western influence in Japan, which some resented and resisted, it is important to note that Ishizuka in effect embraced a diet close to pre-western-influenced Japan, while at the same time proving its benefits through thoroughly western scientific experiments, theories, and record keeping. "He was above all a scientist in an age infatuated with science" (p. 27). In his two major books, Ishizuka sought to establish the "chemical and scientific" bases for his approach. One of Ishizuka's central tenets was that, for humans, health depends on a right relationship with their natural environment. This includes eating both whole, unmilled grain and food of the immediate locality. "It provides those foods which allow him to function healthily and happily in that particular place and climate. Man should eat, then, those foods which occur naturally and abundantly where he lives" (p. 29).

In Japan, later scholars continued to develop Ishizuka's ideas, with a continued emphasis on eating whole and local foods (p. 44). One of these, George Oshawa, developed the idea that local food is healthiest in connection with nationalist sentiments that were running high in Japan in the late 1930s. "Oshawa urges that the government should encourage the consumption of local foods and should discourage by high taxes imported and luxury items such as sugar . . . the government . . . should stop promoting Western medicine. It should instead develop preventive programs and therapies based on traditional diet, on acupuncture, herbalism, and massage" (p. 71). Although his purpose was nationalistic, Oshawa brought vividly to light the connections between the world trade in foodstuffs and the threat to a diet based on local food.

Without a direct historical connection to Japanese thinkers, western health food advocates often came up with similar principles. For example, The Rev. Sylvester Graham (immortalized by Graham flour and the Graham cracker) advocated whole grains, fresh, local fruits and vegetables (p. 268). Henry Thoreau was influenced by Graham, and Graham's influence can be heard in this lament in *Walden* over the decline of local food in New England:

> Every new Englander might easily raise all his own breadstuffs in this land of rye and Indian corn, and not depend on distant and fluctuating markets for them. Yet so far are we from simplicity and independence that, in Concord, fresh and sweet meal is rarely sold in the shops and hominy and corn in a still coarser form are hardly used by any. For the most part the farmer gives to his cattle and hogs the grain of his own producing, and buys flour,

which is at least no more wholesome, at a greater cost, at the store. (Thoreau 1930: 55; quoted in Kotzsch 1985: 268–269)

Thoreau, like Oshawa, draws a clear causal connection between distant food markets and the difficulty of obtaining local food, a connection we will explore in some detail later.

Graham also influenced the founders of the Seventh Day Adventists, whose ideas in turn were involved in the founding of the Battle Creek Sanitorium, the Kellogg diet, and the first Kellogg cereals, based on whole grains. "That the company they founded has become a giant manufacturer of products made with refined grains and white sugar is an ironic footnote" (Kotzsch 1985: 269). Regardless of the directions taken by the Kellogg company, contemporary advocates of the original principles of macrobiotics still explicitly stress eating whole and local foods. (For example, see Kushi and Esko 1985: 2–9) In the United States, among those who adopt what they consider healthy and natural, eating practices, advocating eating the "whole food" is exceedingly common even without explicit adherence to macrobiotics: as it is often said, "if you eat it, eat the whole thing."

Three major postulates repeatedly emerge from these alternative health traditions: (1) Eat whole food, not just refined, processed, or purified parts of animals or plants; (2) Eat seasonal and local food that is minimally processed, stored, and transported; and (3) Eating what you are allergic to can prevent the allergy (e.g., eat pollen in local honey to prevent hay fever).

The Global Food Industry, Dietary Changes, and the Immune System

Recent immunological findings and recent developments in our understanding of the political economy of food production bear on all three of these postulates. Since changes in the organization of the food industry involving multinational firms and a global market have led to far more highly processed food being produced and consumed, food that is generally not obtained locally, eating according to any of these three postulates becomes less and less a matter of course for most people in the world. Given the impact these changes in our diet may be having on health, understanding the interaction between the immune system and our diet has become extremely salient, and even urgent. We will discuss this interaction for each of the three postulates in turn.

1. Eat Whole Food, Not Just Refined, Processed, or Purified Parts of Animals or Plants

Why Might This Make Sense from the Point of View of the Immune System?

In addition to supplying vitamins and other diverse nutrients, eating whole, rather than refined or purified plant and animal foods, may broaden and enhance the efficacy of oral tolerance for suppressing autoimmune disorders. Recent research suggests there are at least two mechanisms by which food components can tolerize (suppress) systemic autoimmune responses (Weiner 1994). Mice can be experimentally induced to develop an autoimmune disorder that causes nerve degeneration. When such mice are fed low doses of a protein extracted from nerve tissue (myelin basic protein) they develop oral tolerance for this nerve protein, and suppress autoimmune activity against the entire surrounding nerve tissue (Miller et al. 1991), a form of "bystander protection." In addition, if such autoimmune mice are fed large doses of a protein (or "antigen"), they specifically suppress both antibody production and cellular immune responses against this protein. These and other experiments on autoimmune disorders in mice demonstrate that oral tolerance is best achieved by repeated feedings, and that a wide range of oral doses can induce oral tolerance. To date, immunologists have only tested the effects of feeding specific proteins, of "antigens," but the evidence now available suggests the broadest protection by oral tolerance might be obtained by feeding the entire tissue being attacked in an immune disorder, not just one of its molecular components.

Animal tests of oral tolerance for treating autoimmune diseases have also demonstrated that molecular components obtained from many different species can stimulate protective oral tolerance. Thus, although molecules obtained from the same species may produce the strongest oral tolerance, it is not necessary to eat food components obtained from the same species (i.e., cannibalism is not required) (Miller et al. 1992). This illustrates a general principle in biology, that molecular structures are conserved across many species, with some molecules being nearly identical in structure in plants, yeast, bacteria, and animals. Thus, regardless of the plant or animal species from which a molecule or food component is obtained, it may stimulate oral tolerance for similar molecules or components in the body. Broad-spectrum oral tolerance is thus most likely to be achieved by eating whole plant and animal tissues, not just purified or refined components.[9]

Restated Health Postulate: Eating a Wide Range of (Whole) Plant and Animal Food May Create Broad-spectrum Oral Tolerance for Reducing Autoimmunity and Allergies

- Both plant and animal food may be useful since there is remarkable conservation of molecular structures across species. Hence diverse foods may present the broadest range of antigens and thereby suppress the largest array of potentially allergic and autoimmune cells.
- Although current immunological research has focused on molecular antigens, the results to date suggest that eating complete joint tissue, not just collagen, might be more protective against arthritis; eating whole pancreas, not just insulin, more protective against diabetes; and whole nerve or brain tissue, not just myelin basic protein, more protective against multiple sclerosis. By eating the entire tissue, clonal energy and active tolerance (immune suppression) is more likely to be generated for all the antigens in the tissue, not just for a single molecule or its nearby ("bystander") neighbors.
- Processed foods, such as refined sugar and flour from which most parts of the plant tissue have been removed, and meat products derived exclusively from skeletal muscle from which all other bodily organs have been removed, may not provide broad-spectrum oral tolerance.
- There may be no need to eat large amounts of the relevant tissue; indeed small amounts might provide the best "bystander" protection; chicken soup, or other broths made from whole animal tissue contain diverse arrays of antigens that might produce broad-spectrum oral tolerance. (On the other hand, extensive cooking, baking, and other processing either at home or in industrial kitchens may well diminish or alter the antigen-array of the fresh, unprocessed food.)

How the Activities of the Global Food Industry Would Make Following This Postulate Difficult

The most obvious difficulty lies in the sheer growth in the proportion of processed food in contemporary diets, especially in developed countries. An obvious, but indirect measure of increased consumption of processed food is evidence by any number of different measures that the food processing industry has grown dramatically since the end of World War II (Connor 1988: 7–9). Processed food products, concentrated in a few countries, "account for nearly two-thirds of total world food and agricultural trade" (Henderson and Handy 1994: 167). From the perspective of consumption, it is estimated that as of the mid-1990s, 80 percent of the food consumed in the developed countries is processed by the food industries (Würsch 1994: 758S). In the developed countries, although food comes to represent a smaller proportion of total expenditures, purchases of processed food make up the bulk of what is spent on food, with estimates reaching as high as 70 percent (Goodman and Redclift 1991: 30). Some of this change is because

> in most of Europe [and the United States], married women now make up a significant proportion of the total labour force. Families with two adults at work have less time to prepare meals, but two incomes provide the household with the means to purchase the relatively expensive animal products, convenience and/or high quality foods as well as to buy take-away meals or to eat in restaurants. The growth of the convenience food market indicates that consumers are prepared to pay the extra costs in order to reduce the amount of time and effort associated with home preparation of meals (Frank and Wheelock 1988: 26).

Estimates of the dramatic growth in the amount of food eaten away from home, much of which would be processed, abound (Senauer et al. 1991: 32; Kinsey 1994: 47; Connor 1988: 15). In the United States "As incomes and the number of multiple-earner families rise, individuals eat out more often. The share of food expenditures away from home rose from 25 percent in 1954 to 46 percent in 1990. Most of this growth was in fast-food places" (Manchester 1991).

The amount of fresh fruit and vegetables in the American diet has been steadily decreasing in proportion to the amount of processed fruit and vegetables (Hadsell 1978: 137; Lebergott 1993: 83). Data from the U.S. Department of Agriculture shows the nature of change between 1960 and 1981: per capita consumption of fresh potatoes declined by half, while frozen potatoes increased nearly sevenfold. Per capita consumption of fresh vegetables stayed constant, while frozen vegetables nearly doubled. Consumption of fresh fruit declined somewhat, while consumption of canned fruit juices, frozen citrus juices, and chilled citrus juice significantly increased (Prescott 1982; *Food Consumption* 1968; 1977; *Food Consumption* Supplement 1968).

Changes in how much information the food processing industry discloses have made exact comparisons in some categories during the last few years difficult, but the rise in consumption of frozen potatoes, as well as processed fruits and vegetables continues through 1993 (Putnam 1994: 17, 43).

Not surprisingly, the impact of this increase in the amount of processed food consumed has had different effects on different ethnic and socio-economic groups.[10] Partly to express their ability to consume what is valued in the larger culture, low-income people do purchase processed foods: "finger foods, fun foods, snack foods, and fast and convenient foods" (Fitchen 1988: 323). But these foods have a different impact on the diets of the poor than on the affluent. An ethnographic study of poverty in the United States shows that the diets of low-income people nationwide "appear to be excessive in starches, fats, and sugars while being deficient in any or all of: meats and other proteins, vegetables and fruits, and milk products" (p. 318). "The well-to-do can afford both junk food and nutritious food; the poor can seldom afford both" (p. 324). In addition to the malnutrition that results from this diet, our argument suggests the preponderance of processed food eaten by low-income people might lead to a greater incidence of immune dysfunction.

What exactly does food processing do to food? In the following glowing contemporary description from a report commissioned by a professional organization of food technologists, we can hear echoes of the faith that science could transform food and eating into good, rational products and processes, a faith that had first been so enthusiastically embraced in industrializing America (Brumberg 1989; Levenstein 1988):

> Food processing requires the application of a wide variety of production inputs to transform lower-valued food materials into higher-valued food products. Labor, machinery, energy, and knowledge are combined on factory floors to convert raw animal, vegetable, and marine materials into intermediate food-stuffs or finished edibles. In establishments employing one worker or thousands, farm and fishery products are slaughtered and sliced, milled and mixed, blended and bottled, fried and frozen, or subjected to any of dozens of other processes. The result is that relatively bulky, perishable, and often inedible farm products are converted into more refined, concentrated, shelf-stable, and palatable foods (Connor 1988: 29).

Other analysts have different ways of describing what processing does to food. Richard Franke notes that transnational food firms, of which the 15 largest market most of the world's exported wheat, sugar, corn, pineapples, and bananas, "are in business to make a profit, and profits are maximized by two major factors: the cheapest possible land and labor and the maximum amount of processing" (1987: 463). For example, bananas, most of which are grown in Third World countries, return only 0.2 percent of the final price as gross margin to the producers. "The main profits go to packagers, insurance companies, shipping lines, and marketers, often owned by the same vertically integrated transnational" (pp. 463–464). Profits from pineapple, which is more processed than bananas, are increased by the processing itself, particularly when it occurs in the Third World. Profits from Dole pineapple in the Philippines are 17 times as high as in Hawaii (p. 463).

One result of increasing processing is what Magnus Pyke calls "the tendency towards *uniformity*." Many categories of processed foods are to be found in largely similar form over widening geographic areas. Breakfast cereals, for example, are consumed over much of Europe, North America, and Australasia (1972: 77–78).

> The style of 20th-century urban life, in which not only increasing numbers of people but also a steadily increasing proportion of the growing population are becoming involved, called for exactly the qualities that cornflakes provided: the cooking of maize in bulk in a factory rather than the domestic cooking of oatmeal in a thousand individual kitchens; service direct from the container rather than from a saucepan or serving bowl which would need subsequent cleaning; stability, allowing it to be put by in a cupboard without having to be covered or kept cool, thus allowing it to be taken out for a single individual living alone or eating alone separate from the rest of the household (pp. 77–78).

It seems paradoxical, but in addition to increased uniformity in its components, food processing now also involves increasing *product differentiation*: "the development of healthy foods for market 'niches,' often reflecting ethnic variety and traditions, but utilizing the full armoury of the food processing industry, and targeted to consumers willing to pay for high value-added products" (Goodman and Redclift 1991: 241; see also Kinsey 1994).[11] Some writers see the development of niche marketing of foods as an aspect of post-Fordist flexible accumulation which has supplanted homogeneous, industrially produced food (Goodman and Redclift 1991: 241). Others suggest a more complex phenomenon in which the same, uniform food components (soy powder, dried milk, wheat flour, sugar, flavorings, carageen, etc.) are combined and recombined in ever more sophisticated ways to create a diverse array of final products. The supermarket aisles appear to be filled with a cornucopia of different things, but underneath the packaging and flavoring, they are all made up of the same things: "Heightened differentiation—veal oreganata, francese, milanese, pizzaiola, limonata, etc.—is matched by the fact that any two packages of the same rare creation taste identical—and I mean *identical* (Mintz 1986: 17). Mintz's astute account of the cultural context of food differentiation ties it, among other things, to the belief, common in late capitalist societies, that "consumption is by definition morally good, so that more consumption is morally better" (p. 19). "Increasing individual opportunities to consume . . . can be perceived as increasing individual freedom of choice" (p. 19).

One feature of food processing that has been on the increase since World War II is *disassembly*.

> Chickens and turkeys were originally sold as whole birds (that is, not disassembled), but since the early 1960s, more and more birds have been cut up, and some are further processed by the manufacturer. More than half of all poultry is now cut up by the manufacturer. Milk is now routinely disassembled into the butterfat and skim portions, and the latter is often further disassembled into a variety of products. (Manchester 1992: 124–125)

One cannot doubt the appeal of fast food, restaurant food, or, for the well-off, luxury items such as skinless chicken breasts or broccoli tips to time-pressed working people, especially parents. The food industry is able to profit from highly processed food in part because the work people do to survive demands the time savings it allows. Our effort is to identify how the skin, joints, inner organs, roots, peel, and leaves that are now being removed from our food might be altering the incidence of immune disorders so that at the very least we might learn whether what we are missing is important. In addition, highly processed foods require increased use of preservatives, which brings us to the second postulate.

2. Eat Seasonal and Local Food That Is Minimally Processed, Stored, and Transported

Why Might This Make Sense from the Point of View of the Immune System?

Even though, to date, neither the food industry, nor immunologists, have addressed the effects of preservatives, food storage, and transport on immunological functions, we would like to suggest that some of the pesticides and fungicides ubiquitous in contemporary agriculture, as well as some of the preservatives required for prolonged storage and transport, may play some role in the increasing incidence of immune dysfunctions. Such molecules, though demonstrated to be of relatively low acute toxicity for humans, may still be capable of occasionally triggering the mucosal immune system to switch from oral tolerance to intolerance. In addition, food handled and consumed in the presence of high levels of toxic substances in urban environments such as heavy metals (lead), solvents (gasoline), cigarette smoke, and other automobile and industrial exhaust products, must necessarily become contaminated with these toxic substances. Thus the array of pesticides, preservatives, and urban airborne toxins consumed with food may contribute to allergies and autoimmune diseases. This conjecture is based on the following immunological findings.

It has long been known that the end products of digestion, small soluble molecules, rarely if ever can stimulate immune responses—they are not effective "antigens" that generate antibodies. Most of the food we eat is in fact digested into small molecules; proteins are digested into amino acids, starches and carbohydrates into simple sugars. But some of the food we eat is only partially digested before it is absorbed into the blood and lymph. Indeed, some of the food molecules nursing mothers eat, remain incompletely digested after being secreted into their milk and even after being absorbed into the infant's blood. Thus, every time we eat a meal, despite all the digestive actions of the gut, our systemic immune systems are exposed to a vast array of foreign proteins, carbohydrates, and other incompletely digested cellular debris that is absorbed into the blood and lymph.[12]

Even though foreign molecules, oil drops, and other substances absorbed by the gut have not been fully digested, they usually do not stimulate the immune system to generate antibodies against them. Indeed, although they are foreign and obviously "non-self," most proteins are not "immunogenic"; only certain subsets carry "markers" of foreign-ness, like the molecules on bacterial cell walls called lipopolysaccharides (Janeway 1989).

Antibodies are likely to be generated only when "adjuvants" tell immune cells to attack the antigen. Adjuvants are sometimes called, even by immunologists, their "dirty secret." To "immunize" an animal against some molecule (the antigen), immunologists have found they must deliver the antigen together with an "adjuvant," typically Freund's adjuvant. Adjuvants are a sort of witch's brew containing toxins, pathogens, bacterial fragments, or other irritants of bacterial origin combined in a dispersion of microscopic drops of oil or other particles coated with the antigen; the process of making this oil/water dispersion is somewhat like making a toxic mayonnaise. Only if antigens are delivered in such an adjuvant do they usually stimulate strong immune reactions. Thus the toxic or pathogenic components of the adjuvant appear to instruct the immune system to recognize the antigen as "dangerous" and to generate antibodies against it and/or a cellular responses that attack or expel it.

Adjuvants are such an important part of immunizing an animal against an antigen (and such a crude aspect of it) that immunologists have often forgotten to mention that they included an adjuvant in the process; they simply report that the animal was "immunized with the antigen" or "injected with the antigen," and fail to mention that the antigen was delivered in an adjuvant. This leads to difficulties in understanding since it obscures that the antigen generated immune reactions only when it was somehow labeled as dangerous. And just what labels an antigen as dangerous has yet to be investigated. (RAC)

Some recent experiments in which a protein antigen was delivered with, and without, an adjuvant are especially revealing (Sun et al. 1994; Weiner 1994). In mice, if nerve sheath protein (myelin basic protein) is used as the antigen, and this antigen is combined with an adjuvant, in this case, cholera toxin, the combination acts like a vaccine, a vaccine against nerve sheaths. Mice injected with this anti-nerve vaccine develop an autoimmune disease that attacks their nerves. However, as mentioned above, when these autoimmune mice are fed repeated doses of the nerve sheath antigen alone (no toxin or adjuvant) the antigen induces oral tolerance that alleviates or cures their symptoms. In contrast, if a toxin is attached to the antigen, an oral exposure to this "oral vaccine" can abolish (abrogate) oral tolerance previously obtained by feeding the antigen alone, and generates both mucosal and systemic immune reactions against the antigen. In short, when an antigen is eaten without an adjuvant it is likely to stimulate the immune system to tolerate the antigen and suppress autoimmune reactions against tissues that display this antigen, oral tolerance. In contrast, if the antigen is combined with an adjuvant, it is likely to stimulate immune reactions that attack the antigen, and nearby cells, anywhere in the body that the antigen occurs, resulting in oral "intolerance."

When we eat food, most of the time the molecules we eat arrive in the *absence* of toxins, pathogens, or other things that act as adjuvants. Hence most of the time the immune system treats the food we eat as a "friend" and develops active tolerance that suppresses immune reactions against this food, as well as suppressing immune reactions against all the components in the body, or "self," that are closely similar to this food. In contrast, if a component of food is labeled with or attached to a toxin or a pathogen, the immune system treats it as "dangerous" and develops active immune reactions against it.

It is the potential "adjuvant-like" character of pesticides, preservatives, and toxic pollutants that suggests that local seasonal food that requires minimal storage and transport and requires minimal use of preservatives and exposure to pollutants may be least likely to stimulate immune disorders.

To avoid possible misunderstanding: we are not advocating any kind of simple valorization of "the local." We are only too aware that idealizations of localized communities and their cultures can play a role in nationalistic or ethnic movements with disturbing desires to achieve purity by expelling anyone who does not share the right "blood" or have a long enough historical link to local territory.[13] Since we know so little about how immuno-nutrition works, we can only speculate, but it may be that optimum conditions for the immune system do not require an unchanging locale. At either end of the class hierarchy, perhaps both itinerant farm workers and jet-setting businessmen would have less allergies if they were able to eat local food wherever they were: even though their locations might frequently change, their immune systems could benefit if, in each place, their guts could teach their noses not to sneeze.

Restated Health Postulate: Eating Local Plant and Animal Food (and Honey) May Produce Most Effective Oral Tolerance Against Local Airborne Allergens

- Local plant and animal food, if produced and processed in ways that reduce the presence of pesticides, pollutants, and pathogens (to reduce adjuvant effects) may promote oral tolerance against airborne antigens from these same local plants and animals, and may help counteract the adjuvant effects of urban pollution. (See Profet 1991.)

How the Activities of the Global Food Industry Would Make Following This Postulate Difficult

First of all we should note that the difficulty is recent. Only a little more than 100 years ago, most perishable food in Europe and America was bought at local markets. Dairy products, poultry, eggs, fruit, vegetables, meat, and fish were mainly produced locally and sold at nearby markets (Pyke 1972: 25). From almost all food passing through local markets 100 years ago, we have arrived at a situation today where almost none of it does (p. 25). Since the factors that contributed to this dramatic change are so many and complex, we can only briefly mention some of them here. They include the needs and demands of expanding industrial society to feed more workers more cheaply (Tannahill 1988: 306); the innovations of the Henry Ford of food supply, Thomas Lipton, who devised means of mass production in food processing, centralized production, and advertising for food; technological developments in transportation and preservation of food (railways, canning, and refrigeration to mention only a few) (Tannahill 1988: 306–313); and scientific innovations in hybrid seeds and fertilizer (Kloppenburg 1984: 303).

Emblematic of these changes is the situation of rural farm workers, who in a study done in Suffolk, England, in the early 1970s, "only rarely and infrequently consume[d] the food she or he produce[d]—and even then it [was] mainly in a fashion familiar to most suburban gardeners" (Newby 1983: 31). Using their deep freezer, ubiquitous among farm workers in this area, families could manage with infrequent trips to shops, located inconveniently far away. This purchased, non-local food, together with produce from their vegetable garden and gleanings from the fields after they had been harvested for Bird's Eye, made up their larder. "A deep freeze was a necessity, forced on such workers by changes in retailing and, more indirectly, by the specialization of most farm production itself" (Goodman and Redclift 1991: 30). The people whose labor most directly produced food now purchased most of what they ate in the form of products that had gone through many stages of wholesaling, processing, packaging, retailing before it reached their hands (Newby 1983: 36).

To understand the increase in the amount of transported (not local) food consumed, we must first turn to the organization of the agricultural industry. Like many others, this industry has been marked by increasing concentration and internationalization. Indeed, in the United States, "average concentration is much higher in the food industry than in American manufacturing industry as a whole" (Leopold 1985: 320). Concentration into ever fewer and larger firms has characterized both the retail branch and the manufacturing branch of the food industry (Manchester 1991: 3). For example, until recently food wholesaling was "typically a local business" (Manchester 1992: 41) because grocery wholesalers usually did not handle perishables. But in the 1950s and 1960s U.S. wholesalers began to handle produce, frozen foods, and meat, and as they grew in size through mergers and acquisitions, distribution to retail outlets became more and more centralized. The retail source of food also became increasingly centralized with fewer stores (supermarkets) serving larger areas rather than more stores serving smaller local areas (Newby 1983: 42).

Data on the transportation of processed foods bears out the increasingly small role of consuming locally produced foods. In the United States some products are still marketed locally or regionally because of their perishability or high transportation costs: cottage cheese, fluid milk, ice cream, bread, soft drinks, and ice. But these are the *only* "industries where 80% of the value of shipments was delivered within 200 miles of manufacturing points" (Marion 1986: 210).[14] All other food industries are essentially "national in geographic scope: meat packing, most canned goods, dried and frozen fruits and vegetables, and beverages" (Marion 1986: 210). In other words, plants are located close to sources of major raw materials, and the finished products are distributed from there around the whole country.

Rapid acceleration of the rate of internationalization of U.S. food production may also bear on the decline of consumption of local foods. This internationalization is not just a matter of trade in food produced abroad, which would perforce not be local, it is a matter of firms themselves becoming multi-national.

> When measured in terms of the value of sales, foreign operations of firms that have direct investment abroad are larger than direct trade in food and related goods by an order of several magnitudes. As a result of foreign investment and overseas operations, many firms have lost their national identities. For example, many Europeans are surprised to learn that the Kellogg Company is a U.S. firm, and many Americans are equally surprised to learn that Pillsbury is a British firm (Henderson and Handy 1994: 166–167)

To achieve economies of scale across huge international markets, these firms are turning to such processes as "global ingredient procurement." For example, the New Zealand Milk Products company is owned by the multi-national firm, New Zealand Dairy Board. All NZMP's raw material comes from New Zealand, and most of its dairy products are produced at its Hawera plant in New Zealand.

> "You have to look at the economics of scale. It's better to supply global customers from one source," notes Patricia Boone, NZMP's vice president of sales and marketing. For instance, the Hawera plant can produce a milk protein for Kraft's specifications here in the U.S. and with its 10 ton/hour spray dry capacity, can just as easily produce that same protein for Kraft's global operations. (Mancini 1993: 101)

These firms also seek beneficial economic conditions within a global market. A spokesperson for Sysco, the giant distributor that supplies the "away-from-home-eating-market" in North America, explains how "economics" have led to importing from abroad many crops and products that could be obtained in the United States: seedless red bunch grapes from Chile, tomato paste from Hungary, and apricots from Spain. In some cases, to take advantage of low wage rates, California packing plants for quick frozen vegetables were "disassembled, put on barges, shipped down to the West Pacific Coast ports of Mexico and Central America, trucked into the interior and set up" (Woodhouse 1993: 208).[15]

The increase in the proportion of food that is now being stored and transported great distances suggests that the amount of preservatives consumed with this food is also increasing. Until careful research is performed to determine whether, or which, preservatives have adjuvant-like effects, the impact of increasing global food transport on immune disorders will remain unanswered.

3. Eating What You Are Allergic to Can Prevent the Allergy

Does This Make Sense from the Point of View
of the Immune System?

When people eat food produced in the place they usually live, the substances they ingest pass through, and are intimately monitored by, the mucosal immune system of the gut, giving it a chance to "learn" whether these substances are benign parts of the environment. When people eat food shipped across great distances, the substances eaten can be disjunct with local, airborne substances. In other words, if you eat local food (including particulate matter from the local air), your immune system may learn whether the pollen, dust, and other airborne particles you breathe are harmless. In urban environments with heavy burdens of airborne toxins, your immune system may also be more capable of distinguishing airborne toxins from benign airborne particulates.

As we discussed above, Wells demonstrated oral tolerance in 1911 by repeatedly feeding hen's egg protein to a guinea pig and thereby suppressing an otherwise fatal allergic response to an injection of this protein. More recently, an analogous process has been demonstrated in the laboratory: if mice are repeatedly fed extracts of ragweed pollen they suppress allergic reactions (production of IgE) against this allergen (Aramaki et al. 1994; see also Cooke and Wraith 1993; Hoyne et al. 1993; Metzler and Wraith 1993). These experiments in mice parallel, and help corroborate, the traditional use of honey to prevent hay fever, sinus headaches, and other human allergies.

Restated Health Postulate: Eat the Antigen (without an Adjuvant) to Prevent the Allergy

How the Global Political Economy of Food
Makes This Difficult

The proliferation of highly processed food in tandem with growth in the food processing industry means that food has become more and more alike. The food we buy has less and less of the local physical environment in which it was grown attached to it. Compare carrots bought from a local Farmer's Market with their roots and leaves intact and still dusty from the field to washed, frozen, diced, and peeled carrots processed by Bird's Eye in a plant far away. Food has become less and less likely to be eaten near its place of production, in tandem with the internationalization of the food industry and the growth of a global food market. All these factors mean that what we eat is often disjunct with local, airborne substances. Our immune systems are learning about one set of substances through the food we eat and another quite different set through the air we breathe. The mucosal immune system is given little chance to learn which local pollen, mold, and dust can be eaten without harm, and hence can also be breathed without harm.

Conclusions and Future Directions in Immuno-Nutrition

Immunological research now makes clear that if an antigen, such as an airborne particle or a food component, is delivered to a mucosal surface in the absence of a toxin or other adjuvant, the mucosal immune system is likely to learn to treat the antigen as a benign "friend" and actively suppress systemic immune reactions against this antigen, oral tolerance. To obtain oral tolerance, the antigens in food need not be identical to "self" antigens, they can be obtained from other species. Repeated feeding of antigens similar to a self-antigen in a tissue undergoing autoimmune attack may thus induce oral tolerance that can help alleviate or prevent autoimmune disease in that tissue. Similarly, oral doses of airborne antigens, delivered in the absence of toxins, pollutants, or other adjuvants, might alleviate allergies.

In contrast, if an antigen is combined with a toxin or other adjuvant and delivered to a mucosal surface, the mucosal immune system is likely to learn to treat the antigen as "dangerous," and stimulate both mucosal and systemic immune reactions against it. If the antigen is a self-antigen and it is delivered with an adjuvant, it can induce an autoimmune disease that attacks all cells displaying the self-antigen, and this autoimmune attack can spread to bystander cells as well, just as in allergic reactions.

Adjuvants, such as toxins and pollutants, can switch mucosal immune actions from tolerance to intolerance, or attack. Mucosal adjuvants have yet to be carefully studied or identified, but at present they are known to include toxins, such as choler toxin, pathogenic bacteria including fragments of such bacteria, and probably smoke, solvents, and other industrial pollutants. It follows that reducing adjuvant loads, toxic air pollutants and toxins, pathogens, and other adjuvants in food may minimize the incidence of allergies and autoimmunity. Minimizing airborne toxins, such as diesel exhaust, gasoline and other solvents, lead and other heavy metals, may reduce the incidence of asthma and respiratory allergies (Profet 1991). Similarly, in food, reducing toxins, pathogens, and pesticides and preservatives with adjuvant-like activity, may minimize the likelihood of inducing food allergies and autoimmune reactions.

Pesticides play a major role in modern agriculture and food preservatives play a major role in reducing food spoilage and disease, but the potential role of pesticides and preservatives as adjuvants that might increase the incidence of immune disorders has yet to be investigated.

To achieve protective oral tolerance, optimum dose and frequency are important, yet virtually unexplored. As with vitamins and other nutrients, to develop and maintain oral tolerance, antigens need to be eaten repeatedly and in appropriate doses since the mucosal immune system is continuously learning, and forgetting, over time-spans of weeks to months. Optimal doses and frequencies for obtaining oral tolerance are still unknown.

The most protective antigens, and the most injurious adjuvants, have yet to be investigated or identified. For example, do vegetarian diets increase, or decrease, the risk of autoimmune diseases? Vegetarian diets might increase this risk by reducing oral tolerance toward self-antigens (all of which are of animal origin). On the other hand, a vegetarian diet might decrease the incidence of autoimmune disease by reducing the likelihood that animal antigens will be present in the gut whenever it becomes infected or irritated by toxins or other adjuvants.[16]

Conclusions and Future Questions in the Political Economy of Food

Our argument links processes at very different levels: how the mucosal immune system operates, how the rate of allergy and autoimmunity is rising globally, and how both of these may be influenced by changes in the kinds of foods people have available to eat. Many elements in our argument are not demonstrable at the present time for lack of evidence. But unless the argument is set forth, surely no one will bother to look! Our primary motivation in writing this paper is to stimulate studies that would investigate these links.

The ideal way to end the paper would be to discuss what is happening in a number of mediating sites, which would illustrate concretely whether and how the connections we describe are operating. The case of Narjan Mar mentioned above, could, with the appropriate particulars, reveal how recent changes in diet, together with a high level of environmental toxins, have affected the rates of autoimmune problems. Or, if we had more information, we could discuss the extremely high rates of asthma in the south Bronx (hospitalization rates are 8 times the national average): "asthma is so common that the pockets of men on street corners bulge with small breathing pumps the way they might bulge with cigars elsewhere" (Nossiter 1995: A1). These rates are already being investigated in relation to both indoor and outdoor pollution, but not in relation to recent increases in the proportion of processed and transported food (Nossiter 1995).[17]

In another place, Nogales, Arizona, rates of autoimmune diseases like lupus are extremely high (Walsh et al. 1993). For lupus alone, and considering only medically confirmed or probable cases, the rate is the highest ever found (Cone 1996: A15).

> "To tell you the truth, it scares the hell out of me," said Anna Acuna, one of many longtime Nogales residents afflicted with lupus. "It frightens me when I see young people diagnosed, it frightens me when I see mothers incapacitated. I think of us as being on the cutting edge of something that is happening all over the world." (Cone 1996: A14).

Scientists are now using new techniques to decide whether these high rates are connected to Nogales's high level of toxic contamination (mostly from industrial runoff produced by U.S.-owned maquiladoras on the Mexican side of the town), but so far no one is looking at the additional role diet might play (pp. A14–15).

The reach and scope of the global forces now bearing on the food processing and transporting industries makes it plain there is no easy way to implement the lessons that can be learned about optimal health from immuno-nutrition. Unless the food industry's domination of food production and transport for the purpose of maximizing returns could be reduced or reversed (an unlikely prospect), diets made up of foods maximally processed and minimally local will continue to provide the path of least resistance for most, and, for the poor, the only possible path. Our hope might be overly optimistic, but one of our purposes in writing this paper is to encourage directions in scientific research that, communicating clearly and effectively to the general population, would, through consumer pressure, make some impact on food production and marketing. The food industry has responded many times—often led or forced by federal public health agencies—to new scientific discoveries about healthful diets and to consumer pressure to modify food accordingly. The stories of how vitamins, bran, calcium, or whole grains came to be added to foods would provide many examples.

It is quite possible that the outcome of such pressure might be a technological fix: remedy the faults of highly processed and transported food by further processing, such as close monitoring of the use of certain preservatives, or adding a "globally representative" cocktail of airborne particles. This would require careful evaluation! It is also possible that some consumers (if they were able) would react by withdrawing from the market, giving up their skinless chicken breasts or broccoli tips for homemade chicken stew or vegetable soup. Beyond these possibilities, there are many small ways people could at low risk experiment with variations in their diet without waiting for either the food industry or scientific research to catch up.

Revealing the operations of the powerful forces that bear on health in the interface between the body, diet, and the environment carries both encouraging benefits as well as frightening risks and we will end on this disquieting note. On the one hand, if the mucosal immune system could be harnessed to educate the body about what is and is not toxic, the incidence of autoimmune illness might be reduced. On the other hand, who will be in a position to say what the content of that education should be? For example, who will bear the costs if our bodies can be taught to "tolerate" higher levels of industrial pollution?

Notes

1. We would like to thank readers of earlier drafts of this paper for their insights and suggestions: Albert Bendelac, Lauren Berlant, Norma Field, Lorna Rhodes, Sharon Stephens, Adria Trowbridge, Rick Trowbridge, Martin Weigert, and Donna Haraway. We will answer for any faults that remain.

2. The conventions of biophysics about multiple authors generally place the senior author and head of the lab in the place of honor, last. The conventions of anthropology generally order multiple authors alphabetically. We are following the latter convention.

3. Thanks to Sharon Stephens for reporting this case to us after her trip to Narjan-Mar with a group from the University of Trondheim, Norway.

4. Janeway and Travers 1994.

5. See Mary Douglas (1980) and Victor Turner (1967) for the classic accounts in anthropology.

6. Grosz 1994: 192ff cogently discusses Kristeva, Douglas, and Sartre on the in-between and the viscous.

7. For an insightful discussion of this question, see Matzinger 1994.

8. Thanks to Mimi Roha at "Really Raw Honey Company" for showing me some of these letters and allowing me to use their extensive library of books and articles on honey.

9. Of considerable practical interest for treating autoimmune disorders, if certain non-toxic subunits of bacterial origin are coupled to the food component (e.g., lipopolysaccharide, subunit B of cholera toxin), they *enhance* oral tolerance, as if their bacterial origin acts as a recognition enhancer that, in the absence of a toxin, increases the vigor with which the mucosal immune system instructs the systemic immune system to tolerate the food component (Khoury et al. 1992; Sun et al. 1994).

10. Space limitations prevent us from dealing adequately with the enormously important cultural meanings attached to food and all aspects of its preparation. Exemplary works on this subject include Mintz 1985; Douglas 1984; Goody 1982; Levenstein 1988; Feeley-Harnik 1994.

11. Jerome notes the dramatic increase in the variety of foods carried in supermarkets in the United States from the 1920s to the 1970s (1975: 93).

12. One of the most striking examples of how undigested food enters the blood and lymph is the way undigested droplets of oils and fat ("chylomicrons"), along with any other food components adhering to their surfaces, are transported directly from the lumen of the gut to the lymph. Milk, like mayonnaise, is white in color because it is a suspension of fat droplets. After eating milk, or any meal high in fat content, the lymph vessels in the gut (the "lacteals") turn white as they collect all these transported drops of oil and fat.

13. See Balibar 1991: 21 on culture, territory, and racism in Europe. See Holston and Appadurai 1996: 191 on exclusionary local movements across the globe.

14. For lack of space we do not discuss it here, but the enormous growth in marketing and consumption of specialty water, "spring" water often shipped far from its place of origin, would be an interesting additional case to consider in comparison to foodstuffs.

15. Gretel and Pertti Pelto have coined the term "delocalization" to refer to processes in which "food varieties, production methods, and consumption patterns

are disseminated throughout the world in an ever-increasing and intensifying network of socio-economic and political interdependency" (1983: 309). They argue that
delocalization has improved the nutrition of people in industrialized nations through
an increase in diversity of the diet, while it has deteriorated food diversity in less
industrialized nations. Our argument would question whether there might be deleterious health effects from delocalization even when it leads to increased food diversity.

16. In all types of animals including insects, reduced food intake may contribute to increasing life-span. The mechanism by which reduced food intake has
this virtually universal effect is not known, but it has been suggested that reduced
food intake, especially reduced fat intake, may reduce the incidence of autoimmune diseases. Since fat and molecules associated with it are absorbed relatively
undigested into the lymph and blood in the form of droplets (chylomicrons), and
since many toxins are oil soluble, foods high in fats may be more likely to increase
the incidence of immune disorders, especially in the presence of high burdens of
toxins and pollutants.

17. Other studies that are investigating the impact of chemical toxins on the
immune system include Germolec 1994 and Frolov et al. 1993.

References

Andre, F., C. Andre, L. Cacarace F. Colin, and S. Cavagna. 1994. "Role of new
     allergens and of allergens consumption in the increased incidence of food sensi-
     tizations in France." *Toxicology* 93(1): 77–83.
Aramaki, Y., Y. Fujii, H. Suda, I. Suzuki, T. Yadomae, and S. Tsuchiya. 1994.
     "Induction of oral tolerance after feeding of ragweed pollen extract in mice."
     Immunology Letters 40(1): 21–25.
Brown, Royden. 1993. *Royden Brown's Bee Hive Product Bible*. Garden City Park,
     NY: Avery Publishing Group.
Brumberg, Joan Jacobs. 1989. "Beyond meat and potatoes: A review essay." *Food
     and Foodways* 3(3): 271–281.
Centers for Disease Control (CDC). 1995. "Asthma-United States." *Mortality and
     Morbidity Weekly Report* 43(51–52): 952–955.
Centers for Disease Control and Prevention (CDC). 1994. *Vital and Health Statis-
     tics, National Ambulatory Medical Care Survey 1991 Summary*. DHHS Publica-
     tion (No. PHS 94-1777). Washington, DC: U.S. Department of Health and
     Human Services; Public Health Service; National Center for Health Statistics.
Challem, Jack. 1995. "Medical journals document value of bee propolis, honey,
     and royal jelly." *Natural Foods Merchandiser.*
Connor, John M. 1988. *Food Processing: An Industrial Powerhouse in Transition*. Lex-
     ington Books.
Cooke, A., and D. C. Wraith. 1993. "Immunotherapy of autoimmune disease."
     Current Opinion in Immunology 5(6): 925–933.

Crane, Eva. 1975. *Honey: A Comprehensive Survey*. London: Heinemann.

Dakin, R. 1829. "Remarks on a cutaneous affection produced by certain poisonous vegetables." *American Journal of Medical Science* 4: 98–100.

Douglas, Date, and Cathryn Prince. 1995. "Eating away at disease?" *New Scientist* 145: 36–40.

Douglas, Mary, Ed. 1984. *Food in the Social Order: Studies of Food and Festivities in Three American Communities*. New York: Russell Sage Foundation.

Evans, R. 1992. "Asthma among minority children: A growing problem." *Chest* 101(6): 368s–371s.

Farb, Peter, and George Armelagos. 1980. *Consuming Passions: The Anthropology of Eating*. Boston: Houghton Mifflin.

Feeley-Harnik, Gillian. 1994. *The Lord's Table: The Meaning of Food in Early Judaism and Christianity*. Washington: Smithsonian Institution Press.

Fitchen, Janet M. 1988. "Hunger, malnutrition, and poverty in the contemporary United States: Some observations on their social and cultural context." *Food and Foodways* 2: 309–333.

Food Consumption, Prices, and Expenditures. 1977. Agricultural Economic Report (no. 138, 1977 Supplement). Washington, DC: U.S. Department of Agriculture; Economics, Statistics and Cooperatives Service.

Food Consumption, Prices, Expenditures. 1968. Agricultural Economic Report (no. 138). Washington, DC: U.S. Department of Agriculture, Economic Research Service.

Food Consumption, Prices, Expenditures Supplement for 1968. 1968. Supplement to Agricultural Economic Report (no. 138). Washington, DC: U.S. Department of Agriculture, Economic Research Service.

Frank, Judith, and Verner Wheelock. 1988. "International trends in food consumption." *British Food Journal* 90(1): 22–29.

Franke, Richard W. 1987. "The effects of colonialism and neocolonialism on the gastronomic patterns of the Third World." Pp. 455–79 in *Food and Evolution: Toward a Theory of Human Food Habits*, ed. M. Harris and E. B. Ross. Philadelphia, PA: Temple University Press.

Gergen, P. J., P. C. Turkeltaub, and M. G. Kaovar. 1987. "The prevalence of allergic skin reactivity to eight common allergies in the US population: Results from the second National Health and Nutrition Examination Survey." *Journal of Allergy and Clinical Immunology* 800: 669–679.

Gofton, Leslie. 1989. "Sociology and food consumption." *British Food Journal* 91(1): 25–31.

Goodman, David, and Michael Redclift. 1991. *Refashioning Nature: Food, Ecology, and Culture*. London: Routledge.

Goody, Jack. 1982. *Cooking, Cuisine, and Class: A Study of Comparative Sociology*. New York: Cambridge University Press.

Hadsell, Robert M. 1978. "Food processing: Search for growth." Pp. 131–140 in *The Feeding Web*, ed. J. Dye. Palo Alto, CA: Bull Publishing.

Henderson, Dennis R., and Charles R. Handy. 1994. "International dimensions of the food marketing system." Pp. 166–95 in *Food and Agricultural Markets: The Quiet Revolution*, ed. L. P. Schertz and L. M. Daft. Washington, DC: National Planning Association.

Horan, R. F., L. C. Schneider, and A. L. Scheffer. 1992. "Allergic skin disorders and mastocytosis." *Journal of the American Medical Association* 268(20): 2858–2868.

Hoyne, G. F., R. E. O'Hehir, D. C. Wraith, W. R. Thomas, and J. R. Lamb. 1993. "Inhibition of T cell and antibody responses to house dust mite allergen by inhalation of the dominant T cell epitope in naive and sensitized mice." *Journal of Experimental Medicine* 178(5): 1783–1788.

Janeway, C. A. 1989. "Approaching the asymptote? Evolution and revolution in immunology." *Cold Spring Harbor Symposium in Quantitative Biology* 54: 1–13.

Janeway, Charles, and Paul Travers, 1994. *Immunobiology: The Immune System in Health and Disease*. New York: Garland Publishing.

Jarvis, D. C. 1960. *Arthritis and Folk Medicine*. New York: Fawcett Crest.

Jerome, Norge W. 1975. "On determining food patterns of urban dwellers in contemporary United States society." Pp. 91–110 in *Gastronomy: The Anthropology of Food Habits*, ed. M. L. Arnott. The Hague: Mouton.

Khoury, S. J., W. W. Hancock, and H. L. Weiner. 1992. "Oral tolerance to myelin basic protein and natural recovery from experimental autoimmune encephalomyelitis are associated with downregulation of inflammatory cytokines and differential upregulation of transforming growth factor beta, interleukin 4, and prostaglandin E expression in the brain." *Journal of Experimental Medicine*. 176(5) 1355–1364.

Kinsey, Jean. 1994. "Changes in food consumption from mass market to niche markets." Pp. 44–57 in *Food and Agricultural Markets: The Quiet Revolution*, ed. L. P. Schertz and L. M. Daft. Washington, DC: National Planning Association, Report no. 270.

Kloppenburg, J., Jr. 1984. "The social impacts of biogenetic technology in agriculture: Past and Future." In *The Social Consequences and Challenges of New Agricultural Technologies*, ed. G. M. Berardi and C. C. Geisler. Boulder, CO: Westview Press.

Kotzsch, Ronald E. 1985. *Macrobiotics Yesterday and Today*. Tokyo: Japan Publications.

Kunz, B., J. Ring, and O. Braun-Falco. 1991. "Are allergies really increasing?" *Fortschritte der Medizin* 109(17): 353–356.

Kushi, Aveline and Wendy Esko. 1985. *The Changing Seasons Macrobiotic Cookbook*. Wayne, NJ: Avery Publishing Group.

Lebergott, Stanley. 1993. *Pursuing Happiness: American Consumers in the Twentieth Century*. Princeton, NJ: Princeton University Press.

Leopold, Marion. 1985. "The transnational food companies and their global strategies." *International Social Science Journal* 37(3): 315–320.

Levenstein, Harvey. 1988. *Revolution at the Table: The Transformation of the American Diet*. New York: Oxford University Press.

Malveaux, F. J., D. Houlihan, and E. L. Diamond. 1993. "Characteristics of asthma mortality and morbidity in African-Americans." *Journal of Asthma* 30(6): 431–437.

Manchester, Alden C. 1991. "The food marketing revolution, 1950–90." *Agriculture Information Bulletin, Economic Research Service* (627): 1–8.

———. 1992. *Rearranging the Economic Landscape: The Food Marketing Revolution, 1950–1991*. Agricultural Economic Report (660). Washington, DC: Economic Research Service, U.S. Department of Agriculture.

Mancini, Leticia. 1993. "The global ingredients supermarket." *Chilton's Food Engineering* 65: 95–101.

Marion, Bruce W. 1986. *The Organization and Performance of the U.S. Food System*. Lexington, MA: Lexington Books.

Matzinger, P. 1994. "Tolerance, danger, and the extended family." *Annual Review of Immunology* 12: 991–1045.

Metzler, B., and D. C. Wraith. 1993. "Inhibition of experimental autoimmune encephalomyelitis by inhalation but not oral administration of the encephalitogenic peptide: Influence of MHC binding affinity." *International Immunology* 5(9): 1159–1165.

Miller, A., O. Lider, A. al-Sabbagh, and H. L. Weiner. 1992. "Suppression of experimental autoimmune encephalomyelitis by oral administration of myelin basic protein from different species." *Journal of Neuroimmunology* 39(3): 243–250.

Miller, A., O. Lider, and H. L. Weiner. 1991. "Antigen-driven bystander suppression following oral administration of antigens." *Journal of Experimental Medicine* 174: 791–798.

Mintz, Sidney W. 1986. "American eating habits and food choices: A preliminary essay." *Journal of Gastronomy* 2(3): 15–22.

———. N.d. "The conquest of honey by sucrose: A psychotechnical achievement." *Sugar: Essays to Mark the 125th Anniversary of F.O. Licht*, ed. G. Hagelberg.

———. 1985. *Sweetness and Power*. New York: Viking.

Miyamoto, T., S. Takafuji, S. Suzuki, K. Tadokoro, and M. Muranaka. 1988. "Environmental factors in the development of allergic reactions." Pp. 553–64 in *Toxicological and Immunological Aspects of Drug Metabolism and Environmental Chemicals*, ed. R. W. Estabrook. New York: F.K. Schattauer Verlag.

Moslehi, Javid. 1995. "Asthma gene localized by Hopkins researchers." *Johns Hopkins Newsletter* (Baltimore, MD), A (Part 1): B1–11.

Nasi, Andrea. 1978. *The Honey Handbook*. New York: Everest House.

National Institute of Allergy and Infectious Diseases. 1995. *Asthma and Allergy Statistics*. Washington, DC: National Institutes of Health, Public Health Service.

Newby, Howard. 1983. "Living from hand to mouth: The farmworker, food and agribusiness." Pp. 31–44 in *The Sociology of Food and Eating*, ed. A. Murcott. Hants, England: Gower.

Paul, William E., ed. 1989. *Fundamental Immunology*. 2nd ed. New York: Raven Press.

Pelto, Gretel H., and Pertti J. Pelto. 1983. "Diet and delocalization: Dietary changes since 1750." Pp. 308–29 in *Hunger and History: The Impact of Changing Food Production and Consumption Patterns on Society*, ed. R. I. Rotberg and T. K. Rabb. Cambridge: Cambridge University Press.

Prescott, Richard, Compiler. 1982. *Food Consumption, Prices, and Expenditures, 1960–81*. Statistical Bulletin (694). Washington, DC: Economic Research Service, U.S. Department of Agriculture.

Profet, Margie. 1991. "The function of allergy: Immunological defense against toxins." *Quarterly Review of Biology* 66(1): 23–26.

Putnam, Judith Jones. 1994. "Food consumption, prices, and expenditures, 1970–93." *Statistical Bulletin* (915). Washington, DC: Economic Research Service, U.S. Department of Agriculture.

Pyke, Magnus. 1972. *Technological Eating*. London: John Murray.

Randolph, Theron G., and Ralph W. Moss. 1989. *An Alternative Approach to Allergies*. New York: Harper and Row.

Schertz, Lynn P., and Lynn M. Daft, Eds. 1994. *Food and Agricultural Markets: The Quiet Revolution*. Washington, DC: National Planning Association, Report no. 270.

Schwartz, Robert S., and Syamal K. Datta. 1989. "Autoimmunity and autoimmune diseases." Pp. 819–66 in *Fundamental Immunology*, 2nd ed., ed. W. E. Paul. New York: Raven Press.

Senauer, Ben, Elaine Asp, and Jean Kinsey. 1991. *Food Trends and the Changing Consumer*. St. Paul, MN: Eagan Press.

Sharman, Anne. 1991. "From generation to generation: Resources, experience, and orientation in the dietary patterns of selected urban American households." Pp. 174–203 in *Diet and Domestic Life in Society*, ed. A. Sharman. Philadelphia, PA: Temple University Press.

Sly, R. M. 1994. "Changing asthma mortality." *Annals of Allergy* 73(3): 259–268.

Subrahmanyam, M. 1993. "Honey impregnated gauze versus polyurethane film (OpSiter) in the treatment of burns—a prospective randomised study." *British Journal of Plastic Surgery* 46: 322–323.

———. 1991. "Topical application of honey in treatment of burns." *British Journal of Surgery* 78: 497–498.

Sun, J.-B., J. Holmgren, and C. Czerkinshy. 1994. "Cholera toxin B subunit: An efficient transmucosal carrier-delivery system for induction of peripheral immunological tolerance." *Proceedings of the National Academy of Sciences USA* 91: 10795–10799.

Tannahill, Reay. 1988. *Food in History*. New York: Crown Publishers.

Taylor, W. R., and P. W. Newacheck. 1992. "Impact of childhood asthma on health." *Pediatrics* 90(5): 657–662.

Thoreau, Henry David. 1930. *Walden*. London: J.M. Dent and Sons.

Trentham, D. E., R. A. Dynesius-Trentham, E. J. Orav, D. Combitchi, C. Lorenzo, K. L. Sewell, D. A. Hafler, and H. L. Weiner. 1993. "Effects of oral administration of collagen on rheumatoid arthritis." *Science* 261: 1727–1730.

Würsch, Pierre. 1994. "Carbohydrate foods with specific nutritional properties— a challenge to the food industry." *American Journal of Clinical Nutrition* 59(suppl.): 758s–762s.

Wade, Carlson. 1983. *Propolis: Nature's Energizer: Miracle Healer from the Beehive.* New Canaan, CT: Keats Publishing.

Weiner, Howard L. 1994. "Oral tolerance." *Proceedings of the National Academy of Sciences USA* 91: 10762–10765.

Wells, H. 1911. "Studies on the chemistry of anaphylaxis. III. Experiments with isolated proteins, especially those of hen's egg." *Journal of Infectious Destases* 9: 147–151.

Woodhouse, John A. 1993. "Sourcing fruits and vegetables in a global food system." Pp. 207–9 in *The Emerging Global Food System: Public and Private Sector Issues*, ed. G. E. Gaull and R. A. Goldberg. New York: John Wiley and Sons.

Yunginger, U. S., D. E. Reed, E. J. O'Connell, L. J. Melton, W. M. O'Fallon, and M. D. Silverstein. 1992. "A community-based study of the epidemiology of asthma: Incidence rates, 1964–1983." *American Review of Respiratory Disease* 146(4): 888–894.

Additional Reference List

Balibar, E. 1991. "Is There a 'Neo-Racism'?" Pp. 17–28 in *Race, Nation, Class: Ambiguous Identities*, eds. E. Balibar, and I. Wallerstein. London: Verso.

Cone, M. 1996. "Human immune systems may be pollution victims." *Los Angeles Times*, May, pp. 1, A14–15.

Douglas, M. 1980. *Purity and Danger: An Analysis of the Concepts of Pollution and Taboo.* London: Routledge and Kegan Paul.

Frolov, V. M., N. A. Peresadin, V. Ya. Vitrishchak, and A. M. Petrunya. 1993. "Assessment of immune status in employees of large chemical plants in Don- bass." *Immunologiya* (5): 57–59.

Germolec, D. R. 1994. "Immune alterations resulting from exposure to chemical mixtures." In *Toxicology of Chemical Mixtures: Case Studies, Mechanisms and Novel Approaches*, ed. R. S. H. Yang. San Diego, CA: Academic Press.

Grosz, E. 1994. *Volatile Bodies: Toward a Corporeal Feminism.* Bloomington: Indiana University Press.

Holston, J., and A. Appadurai. 1996. "Cities and citizenship." *Public Culture* 8(2): 187–203.

Kristeva, J. 1982. *Powers of Horror: An Essay on Abjection.* New York: Columbia University Press.

Nossiter, A. 1995. "Asthma common and on rise in the crowded South Bronx."
    New York Times, September 5, pp. A1, B2 col. 3.
Sartre, J.-P. 1981. *Existential Psychoanalysis*. New York: Philosophical Library.
Turner, V. 1967. *The Forest of Symbols*. Ithaca, NY: Cornell University Press.
Walsh, B. T., M. Reed, J. Emerson, E. P. Gall, L. Clark, and Living For Everyone
    Community Group (USA). 1993. "A large cluster of systemic lupus erythe-
    matosus individuals in a Mexican-American border town in Arizona." *Arthritis
    and Rheumatism* 36(9 suppl.): S145.

13

Tales from the Crypt

Contamination and Quarantine in Todd Haynes's *[Safe]*

In a scene about a third of the way into Todd Haynes's film *[Safe]* (1993), ten-year-old Rory White, the stepson of Carol and the son of Greg White, reads his school project on the rise of Los Angeles gangs to his parents at the dinner table. Rory describes in lurid detail the alleged crimes of the gangs, "rapes, riots, shooting innocent people, slashing throats, arms and legs being dissected . . .," and concludes, "today Black and Chicano gangs are coming into the valleys and mostly white areas more and more. That's why gangs in L.A. are a big American issue." It is this paranoid image of a violent and threatening "Other" that upper-middle class families like the aptly named Whites increasingly define themselves against and ostensibly strive to be "safe" from in southern California. Life in the suburbs far from dangers of the city has become the contemporary dream for many southern Californians, and its appeal is furthered by the promotion of such a lifestyle in the popular media. On television and in magazines the suburban lifestyle of the upper middle class is often portrayed as *the* desirable lifestyle against which everything else is measured.

As the title of Haynes's movie suggests, members of the upper middle class distinguish and display their difference in status from lower classes by the level of security they have achieved, not only financial security and security of legitimate social roles, but also security of person and property. To a large extent, issues of privacy and personal safety govern the daily lives of those who can afford to isolate themselves from the street. Control, for them, is defined by the degree to which they are able to shut themselves off from the outside world.[1] The media's sensationalist coverage of crime reinforces the paranoia of the upper middle class, who believe that they are constantly under threat from an underclass of undesirable types. As Mike Davis says in his critical social history of Los Angeles, *City of Quartz*, "Middle class imagination, absent from any first-hand knowledge of inner-city conditions, magnifies the perceived threat through a demonological lens."[2] It is through such exaggerated fears about personal security that the upper middle class justifies their movement within an enclosed social sphere with minimal contact with those outside their class. However, as Haynes makes clear in *[Safe]*, the discourse around personal safety also serves to hold in place conservative assumptions about social roles and gender that reinforce the traditional patriarchal structure of the nuclear family.

Despite their attempts to quarantine themselves from bad influences, the Whites' security does become threatened. Yet it is not from a realization of the "perceived threat" of the violent "Other," so vividly described by Rory, rather the danger lurks within their immediate environment, emanating, it seems, from the very trappings of their achievement of a successful upper-middle-class lifestyle. The member of the household directly affected by this interior intrusion is also the one most contained physically and psychologically by her social sphere—the "homemaker," Carol White—and the damage is done to an important site of control for the bourgeoisie, the body—the homemaker is made sick by her own environment.

Carol suffers from allergic reactions seemingly brought on by the pollution and chemical fumes she encounters as she listlessly carries out her daily tasks. As these reactions increase in severity, the decline of her health begins to interfere with her ability to maintain the gendered social role expected of her. Not wanting to rock the boat, she initially blames these mysterious reactions on stress and general poor health, continually apologizing to her husband for being unable to carry out her marital duties satisfactorily. However, after attending a support group of (mostly) women with similar symptoms to her own, she finds out that she has an immune system disorder that is known by various names, including "environmental illness," "multiple chemical sensitivity," "chemical AIDS," and "twentieth-century disease," which means the body can no longer tolerate the low-level toxins and forms of pollution that are part of modern life.

Although its symptoms have been reported by an increasing number of sufferers since the early eighties, environmental illness is not yet recognized as a discrete condition by the medical profession.[3] There has been more research carried out in recent years to determine why people are affected by this disorder, but in 1987, the year in which *[Safe]* is set, much less was known about it. Subsequently, Carol's doctor refuses to accept her explanation that her illness is a reaction to chemicals because, as he says, "from a medical standpoint there is just no proof that this thing is an immune system breakdown much less one based on environmental factors." While recuperating in the hospital after a violent allergic reaction to pesticide, Carol sees a television infomercial on a chemical-free retreat in New Mexico called Wrenwood that describes itself as a "communal settlement dedicated to the healing individual" and a "safe haven for troubled times." In the absence of recognition or support from other sources, she decides to give it a try, leaving behind the safety of her home, her family, and her homemaker role.

In keeping with the tradition of the "disease-of-the-week" movie to which Haynes refers in *[Safe]*, the audience is led to believe that Carol's departure from the claustrophobic atmosphere of her domestic life in the San Fernando Valley, which seemed to be as much the cause of her malaise as the toxins in the air, can only result in a positive outcome. Yet Haynes refuses to provide the audience with any such reassuring resolution. Instead of finding a place where, as we would like to hope, she can not only get well but develop a more solid sense of identity, Carol merely moves from one oppressive environment to another. At Wrenwood she falls under the sway of New Age guru Peter Dunning, who urges his followers to stop blaming the external environment and instead to look inward for a cure by learning to love themselves. However, his teachings fail to arrest the continuing decline in Carol's state of health.

The current rhetoric about preventative health and well-being, with its leanings toward a holistic philosophy, has perhaps lulled us into believing that alternative therapies can fix what traditional medicine is unable to. Yet Haynes's depiction of the various systems of belief that Carol (mal)functions in relation to, reveals the limitations of any one paradigm to explain in full the causes of illness, or to offer complete remedies. He

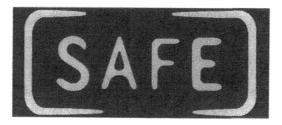

Figure 13.1   Title, Todd Haynes's *[Safe]*.

further subverts the "disease-of-the-week" genre of films by negating the possibility that Carol can still overcome the limitations of the various systems she encounters and fight her way back to good health through sheer determination and strength of character. Instead, she is a character who has a weak sense of identity and is easily cowed into submission by figures of authority that have the backing of more powerful belief systems than her own.

By posing Carol as an already vulnerable character made even more so by her illness, and by refusing to provide any access to her inner psychological state, Haynes never allows the audience to be completely on her side. At times her passivity and lack of self-awareness become so infuriating that we believe along with her husband, her doctor, and her guru that Carol is really the one to blame for her illness and that it is "all in her head." Her weak position in relation to the patriarchal figures of authority she is up against, and her desperate need to be accepted by the systems they represent, raises issues about the ways that we negotiate our sense of identity in relation to external influences and pressures in society and about how our need to feel valued and secure ties into this identity formation.

The brackets that enclose the word "safe" in the film's title point to the way Carol seeks to secure a sense of identity by conforming to the roles expected of her within such closed systems as patriarchy, medicine, and alternative therapies—discourses that seemingly offer orderly, rational, and complete answers. Yet *[Safe]* leaves the viewer far from reassured that any reductive system, even an alternative one, can fully satisfy our individual needs and desires or represent the totality of our identity. Although Carol readily plays by the rules of these systems, she pays an enormous personal price for doing so. It is the limitations and dangers of such systems, which aim for closure through self-serving discourses, and the way they affect the identity of the individual in relation to illness, particularly illness that is coded feminine, that Haynes addresses in *[Safe]*. The film investigates the extent to which we depend on distinctions between inside and outside and between self and other, both as a society and as individuals, in creating a sense of order and control and in maintaining coherent belief systems. While Haynes shows us how such distinctions are sustained, he is perhaps even more interested in situations and circumstances where these rule-of-thumb distinctions become muddied or can no longer be applied.

[Safe] presents a number of "sites of confusion" where exteriority and interiority can no longer be clearly circumscribed. There is Carol's shaky sense of identity, which means her boundaries that separate self and other are far from solid, making it difficult for her to discriminate between what is useful for her to absorb from her external environment and what she would be better off resisting. There is the disruptive effect of illness generally, which can throw our body boundaries into chaos, and there is the particular nature of environmental illness, which weakens the immune system's ability to function as a barrier between damaging elements of the external environment and the internal functioning of the body. And finally there is the holistic rhetoric that Carol absorbs at Wrenwood, which suggests that boundaries between inside and outside do not really exist. This third aspect is particularly complex as it poses a rhetoric that breaks down distinctions between inside and outside within a system that is the most closed of all the discourses presented in the film. Haynes has said that it is in illness and the chaos it causes that hope can be found in *[Safe]*,[4] and it is our need to resolve this confusion and reinstate the boundaries between inner space and outer space with which the film deals.

The first half of the film traces Carol's quotidian routine as an upper-middle-class homemaker in Los Angeles suburbia and the gradual disruption of this routine by her illness. She lives with Greg and Rory in an expensively furnished and spotlessly clean, color-coordinated mansion in a housing development on the edges of the San Fernando valley, and she spends most of her days within the enclosed spaces of her home, her car, friends' houses, the gym, or shopping malls. On the few occasions she is seen outside, it is within the fenced perimeters of the Whites' property, tending her stunted roses and, later, during nocturnal wanderings in the garden. Haynes has described L.A. as a "transitional carpeted hum zone" where "you never breathe real air; you're never in any real place."[5] Through the use of long shots, he captures the sterility and claustrophobic feel of the airless interiors that Carol moves through, transforming domestic spaces into impersonal, pastel-toned dollhouse settings. Carol is positioned as an awkward Barbie-like figure within these spaces, where

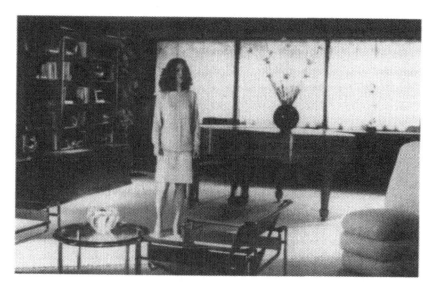

Figure 13.2   Still from Todd Haynes's *[Safe]*.

the incessant drone of vacuum cleaner, talk radio, and television and the buzz of fluorescent lights is heard more often than conversation.

While Carol's existence within this bell-jar environment supposedly stems from concerns over personal safety, it also serves as an indicator of class privilege. Within the upper-middle-class society portrayed in *[Safe]*, the high level of income achieved by the breadwinner husbands means that there is no need for the wives to work, even at home. Thus in their roles as homemakers Carol and her friends become conspicuous markers of their husbands earning power. Affluence is displayed not only through material consumption but also by the consumption of services such as home help, which "free" upper-middle-class wives from mundane tasks. Haynes makes a wry reference to the degree to which Carol and her friends are emancipated from the smallest task in the baby shower scene when Carol admires the wrapping on a gift and asks her friend if she wrapped it herself. Her friend replies, "Are you kidding? I wish I were that creative." Creativity is reduced to the ability of these women to make over their homes and themselves in an image that appropriately complements their husbands' social standing and level of income. In *[Safe]* a woman's place is as firmly in the home as it was in the fifties, yet by the eighties her position reflects class status more than a gendered division of labor.

The image of upper-middle-class women that Haynes presents in *[Safe]* is something of an anachronism, harking back not only to the fifties housewife and, as a number of critics have noted, the Stepford wives,[6] but also the ideal of the middle- and upper-class Victorian wife. Barbara Ehrenreich and Deirdre English recount descriptions of the affluent wife contemporary to the late nineteenth and early twentieth century that could be just as easily applied to Carol and her peers:

> She did not work: that is, there was no serious, productive work to do in the home, and the tasks which were left—keeping house, cooking and minding the children—she left as much as possible to the domestic help. She was, biologically speaking, specialized for one function and one alone—sex.[7]

> [Her other role] was to do precisely nothing, that is nothing of any economic or social consequence. A successful man could have no better social ornament than an idle wife. Her delicacy, her culture, her childlike ignorance of the male world gave a man the "class" which money alone could not buy.[8]

Like their Victorian predecessors, the upper-middle-class "ladies" of the late eighties portrayed in *[Safe]* have marriages based on what Charlotte Perkins Gilman called a "sexuo-economic relation," where in exchange for financial security provided by the husband, they perform sexual, reproductive, and home management duties.[9] They live their lives in a historical and political vacuum unaffected by almost a century of social change. Although part of Haynes's critique of the upper middle class in 1987 focuses on their "political amnesia, social isolationism and cultural myopia,"[10] characteristics of the Reagan era, it is difficult to conceive that one of the most profound social interventions of the second half of the twentieth century—feminism—could have completely passed these women by. It is often claimed that the second wave of feminism primarily influenced and benefited white-middle class women, and if this is so, it seems surprising that Carol and her peers would readily accept such limiting social roles as the entirety of their personality. Yet apparently this kind of life guarantees a certain kind of protection, comfort, and social status, albeit on patriarchal terms, which makes redundant the need or desire for any expression of independence.

Haynes does not set out to condemn Carol's choice of vocation but rather to critique the greater patriarchal system in which she is enmeshed. Yet in the process of showing just how retrograde and conservative such a system is, he also portrays the women within in it as hapless victims who by their passive acceptance of the status quo become complicit in maintaining it. In the absence of a feminist consciousness that could possibly grant them some sense of agency or power, Carol and her friends remain enclosed within the traditional patriarchal structure of the family where their prescribed social roles becomes the sum total of their identity. With no other avenue of self-expression available, interior decorating takes on an exaggerated significance becoming "not only the limit of the characters' interest in reality, but also a displaced arena for exercising control, a therapy that helps make up for helplessness in the face of chaos."[11]

For Carol, who is entirely a product of this environment, the concept of an existence or an identity outside of her entrenched lifestyle is unimaginable. Nothing else is real for her. Faced with the horrifying possibility that the only life she knows and understands cannot deliver what it promised, it is no wonder that her discontent can only manifest itself in (equally horrifying) physical symptoms. Unable to consciously acknowledge that her "perfect" lifestyle may have something to do with her lack of energy and her extreme reactions to environmental toxins (after all, she has no "reason" to get sick), Carol repeats the stock phrase that passes as an acceptable explanation for all ills these days, which is that "she has been under a lot of stress and a little run down lately." Yet the thing that probably causes the most stress in her life is her struggle to repress the feeling that her social role is ultimately dissatisfying. While her mind refuses to accept that her lifestyle is suffocating her, her body clearly states the truth of the matter. She is literally unable to breathe in the claustrophobic environment that she inhabits and begins escaping her house at night to wander like a sleepwalker around her garden.

The baby shower scene make clear the extent to which Carol must struggle to keep up the appearances that ensure her inclusion in this social milieu. While she follows social convention by conforming in dress and behavior to her peers' expectations, she is obviously troubled by the sense of dislocation between her need to be affirmed socially and her realization on some level that this kind of life is ultimately shallow and empty. When she escapes the stilted, lifeless conversation of the party to go to the bathroom, she lingers there, gazing uncomprehendingly at herself in the mirror. As she opens the sliding door to leave, her image, reflected on the door's mirrored inside surface, is abruptly erased. In her desire for social acceptance, Carol has cultivated her homemaker persona so well that it has obliterated any other aspects of her identity. Beyond this "selfless" image that she seems no longer able to recognize, she has no solid existence. It is little wonder then that, in the absence of any other models of self-definition, Carol is unable to consciously confront her rejection of this particular lifestyle. Yet she can no longer conceal her abhorrence of the expectations placed upon her.

When Carol returns to the party, she compliments the daughter of the hostess on her drawing of a princess and is informed by the girl that this "princess" is, in fact, Carol. As the "big present" (a stroller) is being opened, Carol invites the girl to sit on her lap but almost immediately starts to experience a reaction, which turns into a serious, asthmalike attack. Throughout this distressing incident, Carol's first priority is to maintain her ladylike demeanor, and she sits poised and smiling as if nothing out of the ordinary is taking place. Although her attack could be attributed to the ice-cream cake she had just been eating, it seems equally as likely that it is a reaction against assumptions about childbearing as it is informed by consumerism. Her body literally rejects this aspect of her prescribed role by refusing to carry the weight of the child she "bears" on her lap. Despite her best efforts, Carol can no longer outwardly maintain her image as a domestic princess.

[Safe] demands that we read environmental illness, and Carol's susceptibility to it, in a number of contradictory ways simultaneously. In the broadest sense, it can be read in the first half of the film as a metaphor, personified in Carol, for the sense of disease and alienation that lies beneath the glossy exterior of contemporary upper-middle-class life. More specifically, as the last two paragraphs suggest, within the context of Carol's unbearably restrictive social role, we cannot avoid reading it psychologically as a classic hysterical reaction. Yet the film clearly shows that Carol's reactions directly correspond to her contact with chemicals, pollutants, and some foods, so we must also recognize Carol's suffering as a concrete response to physical substances. Finally, we can regard her illness, as does the leader of Wrenwood in the second half of the film, as simply an "attitude problem" bought about by faulty thinking. Despite a bias towards the physical explanation, Haynes makes it impossible to settle definitively on one reading over another because of the complicating factors of Carol's fragile sense of identity, which enters into both her and our response to her illness, and the absence of concrete knowledge about environmental illness. *[Safe]* sets up these possible readings, only to throw their validity into doubt, so that our understanding of what and who is to blame for Carol's illness constantly fluctuates.

Although the word "hysterical" is never used in *[Safe]*, it is clearly implied in the way Carol is treated both by her doctor and her husband after she falls ill. This diagnosis is also strongly suggested by the similarity of Carol's circumscribed social position to that of the classic victims of hysteria—the Victorian wives described above. As Elaine Showalter recounts, hysteria—"the quintessential female malady"—had its "golden age" between 1870 and World War I and emerged forcefully during this time largely as a response to the particular constraints on intellectual and sexual freedom endured by bourgeois women.[12] Nervous disorders such as hysteria, "expressed the insoluble conflict between their desires to act as individuals and the internalized obligations to submit to the needs of the family, and to conform to the model of self-sacrificing "womanly" behavior."[13] The symptoms of hysteria were many and varied and included fainting, vomiting, sobbing, impaired hearing and vision, loss of voice, and heart palpitations, but two of its defining characteristics were the seizure and the sensation of choking or suffocation.[14] In addition to malaise, Carol repeatedly experiences sensations of suffocation, and this is perhaps the clearest suggestion that the cause of her illness, like that of her Victorian sisters, lies in her immediate familial environment.

We must conclude then that within the context of Carol's particular situation, it seems her illness is at least in part a hysterical reaction to an intolerable situation. But if we accept this diagnosis, how are we to take seriously the existence of environmental illness as a real physical condition rather than writing it off as a psychiatric problem, as many in the medical profession have done? And how are we to continue to sympathize with Carol when she is mistreated by practitioners that interpret her illness to suit their own agenda? I think it is possible to see Carol's reactions as both symptoms of hysteria *and* of environmental illness if we take hysteria to be a form of environmental illness, instead of regarding environmental illness as a form of hysteria. After all, in both cases Carol's sickness can be traced back to her environment and in both cases the symptoms manifest themselves through the body. In the case of hysteria, it is an aspect of her *social* environment that makes her sick, namely the suffocating constraints of patriarchy, while in the case of environmental illness, her sickness is caused by chemicals and toxins in her *physical* environment. Both the social and the physical environments are integral aspects of the sphere in which Carol exists.

The way that hysteria was regarded by the medical profession at the turn of the century also bears comparison with the contemporary medical establishment's attitude towards environmental illness. As well as primarily affecting women, hysteria was also seen as having distinctively "feminine" traits because of its particular "nature." Showalter points out a number of links that were made between hysteria and the notion of an essential femininity: "Its vast, unstable repertoire of emotional and physical symptoms and the rapid passage from one to another suggested the lability and capriciousness traditionally associated with the feminine nature. . . . Like other aspects of the feminine, it seemed elusive and enigmatic, resistant to the powers of masculine rationality."[15] The difficulty in reaching a clear diagnosis prompted one doctor, as Showalter notes, to suggest that it would be more appropriate to name the illness "mysteria."[16]

Like hysteria, as well as disorders such as chronic fatigue syndrome, the symptoms of environmental illness were initially reported primarily in white, upper-middle-class women and it, too, has been treated as something of a "female malady."[17] While physicians today do not, understandably, go so far as to place a gender on the manifestations of environmental illness, the disease shares with hysteria many of the elusive "feminine" traits that confound attempts to medically diagnose it. One article concludes that such conditions as multiple chemical sensitivity (MCS) do not exist, but rather represent "junk science" not based on "rational thought"; unlike such diseases as diabetes, with clearly definable external markers, MCS displays a range of symptoms that "is virtually endless; the onset can be abrupt or gradual and may or may not be linked to any specific exposure or causative factor; and symptoms may vary in intensity, may come and go and typically do not correlate with objective physical findings and laboratory results."[18]

The difficulty in providing a medical definition for environmental illness has led researchers within the medical establishment to conclude that people who believe they have the illness are, in fact, suffering from forms of "psychologic distress," such as depression, anxiety reactions, and somatization, and to recommend psychiatric treatment.[19] However its sufferers and those who support the existence of the illness argue that the psychological problems stem from distressing physical symptoms and not the reverse. They point out that sick building syndrome, a similar chemical-related illness, was initially dismissed as a "psychogenic illness"[20] but is now recognized as a real physical reaction. The disbelief and the negative attitudes of the medical profession and the greater society may also contribute to sufferers' feelings of distress and alienation. Carol responds to such skepticism from her doctor and her husband by taking on the blame for her sickness herself, apologizing repeatedly to Greg for not being "normal." Within the context of a culture she has fully internalized, there can be no other explanation. In the same way that hysteria and other women's "illnesses" and bodily functions have traditionally been pathologized by the medical profession, so too has environmental illness. As Roy Grundmann points out, "If a woman's illness cannot be determined scientifically, society puts the onus on her."[21]

Unable to formulate a satisfactory clinical diagnosis within the paradigm of traditional medicine, the medical profession has no alternative but to cite psychological causes for environmental illness if it is to retain a stake in its treatment. As one psychiatrist put it, "psychiatric syndromes offer a simpler explanation for these symptoms."[22] Yet simplification seems to be counterproductive in addressing so complex and puzzling a disorder. Haynes is clearly skeptical that psychiatry can help Carol and treats it as another means by which the medical network of male "professionals" dictate the terms of her "female malady." He points to the conservative old boy paternalism of the medical profession by having the doctor present Greg rather than Carol with the psychiatrist's card.

Her visit to the psychiatrist is, predictably, a flop. Rather than offering a nonthreatening atmosphere in which she could perhaps begin to understand the factors contributing to her illness, both the psychiatrist and his office are cold and intimidating. Carol faces him over the expanse of his enormous desk as if she were a disobedient student in the principal's office. The expectation that she is to accept and understand her illness in terms that are fully contained by the internal logic of the psychiatric paradigm is underlined by the "interior" decor of the office. The most dominant feature of this decor is the lacquered wall panels of stylized landscapes that negate the need for any reference to the unseen external environment outside the curtained windows. As usual Carol struggles to express herself verbally, and her level of discomfort is increased by her inability to grasp the rules of this particular social situation and her role within it. When the psychiatrist points out that she is the one who is expected to do the talking she is rendered speechless. Again, in her desire to please and to gain acceptance from authoritative systems, Carol readily subjects herself to a discourse that will not adapt to her individual needs.

Carol's strong desire for affirmation from the society in which she lives, which perhaps stems in part from the frightening possibility that she really does not belong, makes it essential for her to understand and play by the rules of whatever system she finds herself in. She willingly defers to the male authority figures around her, always privileging their language over her own tentative voice. Consequently, like the sufferers of hysteria, she loses the ability to speak for herself and has difficulty articulating even the most simple sentences. When she does attempt to convey her feelings, she is often demeaned or silenced. She is frequently interrupted or leaves sentences hanging, and she never contradicts the assumptions that people make about what she is feeling. When she begins to explore the possibility that her illness may have some connection to the environment, she makes herself particularly vulnerable to Greg's "father-knows-best" disapproving attitude. As she starts to tell him about the first meeting she attended of people with environmental illness, he demands, "Who told you to go to this?" and belittles her further explanations by implying that it is absurd for Carol to believe that she is sick because of "bug spray." In the face of Greg's disdain at her attempt to act on her own behalf without his prior approval, she quickly clams up, saying, "I don't know why (I got sick)." When she is not functioning within the safe bounds of a social role that is guaranteed by a circumscribed discourse, Carol has little certainty of voice, and at a later meeting that she attends with Greg, she looks to him to speak for her about why they came.

However Carol's confidence does grow as she finds out more about her illness and realizes that many other people suffer the same feelings of disorientation. During this brief period in the middle of [Safe] when Carol learns the language of environmental illness, she speaks with more clarity and confidence than at any other time. Finding out that her illness does in fact exist outside her head and is suffered by others alleviates temporarily her terrible confusion and sense of alienation. As she takes steps to improve her health she develops a point of focus that she previously lacked. Her discovery that she has a genuine physical illness revives her lagging energies, and she seizes on the concrete reality of environmental illness as an explanation for the chaotic state of her life. She readily abandons her increasingly problematic social role of homemaker to embrace her new, more purposeful role as a sufferer of environmental illness. Carol demonstrates her grasp of the language of her new role when she eagerly relates her newly acquired knowledge about her disorder to her friend over lunch. She claims that finding out about chemicals and their effects has made her more "aware" than she used to be. Forced by illness to step outside her closed-off world and look at her life from a different perspective, Carol shows her potential for achieving greater self-awareness, (although the film repeatedly undercuts this possibility).

It is during this time that Carol visits a clinical ecologist, who performs allergy tests to ascertain what substances most affect her. Clinical ecology, which is not recognized as a medical specialty, is a fringe area of medicine connected to allergy-immunology[23] to which many sufferers of environmental illness eventually turn. Its practitioners believe that many illnesses are caused by low-level exposures to chemicals, and they recommend diet and lifestyle changes based on an avoidance of substances that cause reactions.[24] In what has been described as "the closest thing the medical profession has to a streetfight,"[25] the traditional medical community strongly disputes the theories and methods of clinical ecology, dismissing them as unprovable and "pseudoscientific." They accuse clinical ecologists of recommending lifestyle alterations that are restrictive and isolating for patients, without necessarily offering any relief.[26] Yet their efforts to discredit clinical ecologists and to disprove the existence of environmental illness point to greater concerns than simply a regard for the welfare of patients. In the same way that the upper middle class has sealed itself off from external "threats," so too has the medical profession attempted to close its ranks against "alternative" practices that challenge its supremacy. Haynes is less critical of clinical ecology than he is of the medical profession and of the alternative treatment Carol receives at Wrenwood, perhaps because it engages in a debate with the medical status quo rather than wholly rejecting it as Wrenwood does. But like the other self-contained worlds that the filmmaker critiques, he presents it as yet another system in which a man in a position of authority dictates the terms of Carol's illness.

As part of her treatment by the clinical ecologist, Carol begins a "clearing" process designed to decrease her "total body load" of pollutants so that she can "start from scratch." "Unloading" involves reducing her exposure to toxins as much as possible, which in turn means stripping away the most conspicuous markers of her lifestyle, such as furniture (her new couch is "totally toxic"), fashionable clothing, makeup, food, and even—when she moves into her own "safe" room—her husband. This "getting clear" can also be read metaphorically in the context of the film as a stripping away of one identity to make way for a new one, and indeed, Carol switches easily from one externally defined role to another, clinging to the safety of a social role as the primary expression of her identity rather than confronting the deeper issues that contribute to her illness.

Before we or Carol are given the chance to find out if her new regime of healthy living has any effect, she suffers a seizure—bought on, ironically, by the very bug spray Greg dismissed—and lands in the hospital. Despite continued skepticism from Greg and her doctor, Carol insists that it is "the chemicals" that are making her sick and comes to probably the bravest and most ambitious decision of her life—to move to the chemical-free retreat of Wrenwood in New Mexico. The upbeat music that accompanies the shots of her journey there conveys a sense of escape and adventure, but the greeting she initially receives on her arrival at Wrenwood does not bode so well. When the taxi drives through an unmarked gate into the retreat, a woman emerges from a cabin screaming and gesticulating at Carol and the driver to stop and go back because the car is contaminating the whole area. As Carol stumbles across the rocky ground with her luggage the woman

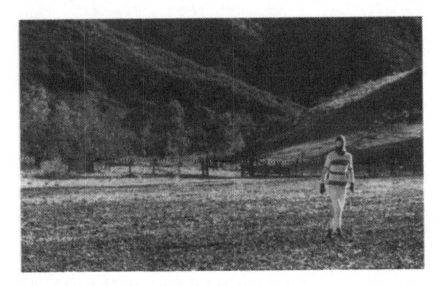

Figure 13.3   Still from Todd Haynes's *[Safe]*.

continues to stare at her saying in a sinister voice, "I see you." Carol's sense
of disorientation is echoed stylistically in this scene and throughout *[Safe]*
by withholding or delaying establishing shots. Once Carol is well inside the
compound, we do get a shot of the main building, but it is difficult to grasp
a sense of the overall layout of Wrenwood.

    This creepy incident is one of several in *[Safe]* that invokes a trope of
the horror film genre, and the absence of any clearly delineated entrance
into Wrenwood is the first suggestion that Carol is entering a place even
more insulated from, and hostile to, the outside world than the one she
came from. The subsequent warm welcome that Carol receives from the
facilitators at the retreat, the appearance for the first time of an African
American person in the film, the revelation that the center's leader Peter
Dunning has AIDS and the implication that he is gay are all factors that
encourage the presumably progressive audience to have a favorable opinion of Wrenwood and to dismiss the doubts raised by earlier events. But
our temporary good vibrations about the place are almost immediately
thrown into question. From the haranguing tone of Peter's "sermon" at
the group meeting she attends that evening, it becomes apparent that
Carol has once more placed herself in an environment where she must
submit to the language of an authoritative male. It is no wonder, then, that
on returning to her cabin later that night, she displays unrepressed emotion for the first time in the film and bursts into tears.

Although we see some of the practical steps taken at the spartan retreat to quarantine its inhabitants from the chemical-laden world outside, such as the installation of light boxes and "safe" televisions, the focus quickly shifts to the psychological approach of Peter. Contrary to what we might expect from a chemical-free retreat "dedicated to the healing individual," the Wrenwood community comes across as a quasi-religious New Age cult, presided over by Peter as evangelistic cult leader, where "love" replaces "God" or "Christ" as the object of worship and the key to redemption. Its rules include silent meals with separate seating for men and women, moderation in dress, and restraint in sexual interaction. The group meetings have a painfully familiar revivalist tone about them: the "congregation" shouts in approval as Peter lists the positive things he sees happening in the world such as "a decline in drugs and promiscuity," there are sing-alongs accompanied by guitar (the first line of the song "Give Yourself to Love" is, "Love has made a circle that holds us all inside"), and the group holds hands as they intone their motto, "We are one with the power that created us, we are safe, and all is well with the world."

While this portrayal of Wrenwood borders on satire, I do not believe that Haynes wishes to completely dismiss the ideology of the New Age movement. Rather, he wants to show how a familiar rhetoric can be employed not as a progressive alternative to conservative beliefs about the individual and her relationship to the world, as we might imagine, but as a retrograde reinforcement of such beliefs. Rosalind Coward describes the alternative movement's philosophy of health and the body as "profoundly religious," with its roots specifically in Christian Puritanism.[27] This puritan impulse, which has produced the "entangling of health and morality and the implication of personal responsibility for well being,"[28] is what Haynes criticizes in his depiction of Wrenwood. It is useful here to discuss in more depth the way that a New Age philosophy of health and well-being has come to pervade popular thought and to examine the critique of this approach made by both Haynes (in [Safe]) and Coward.

Andrew Ross says that "while most New Age practices today are still restricted to a minority culture, the influence of their ethical principles is quite mainstream and quite middle-class, permeating suburban life and corporate philosophy alike."[29] While such principles have taken hold in corporate thinking fairly recently, they earlier entered public consciousness in relation to health and medicine and emphasized preventative rather than curative approaches to illness. Although preventative medicine may take the form of broad public health measures (environmental and occupational safety regulations, for example), its New Age incarnation tends to be individualistic, with the responsibility for maintaining good health placed squarely on the individual.[30] During the eighties, this ethos of personal responsibility was articulated to economic deregulation and other antigovernment positions.

This "look-after-yourself"[31] approach to maintaining good health, with its focus on diet and fitness, became immensely popular throughout the middle class during the eighties, as witnessed by the explosion of interest in sports such as aerobics and jogging. The success of public awareness campaigns focusing on eating habits and the introduction of foods onto supermarket shelves that were marketed specifically for their health benefits also indicate the influence of the preventative approach to health on mainstream culture. Whereas previously a reasonably good state of health—indicated primarily by an absence of illness and disease—was the necessary backdrop for an active life, since the early eighties good health has taken center stage, expressing personal control and a successful lifestyle. "Total" health is the ultimate if unattainable goal, to be sought constantly, the true indicator of an "optimal state of well being."[32]

This continuing preoccupation with health paved the way for a more mainstream acceptance of alternative medicine and therapies, and the philosophies on which they were based, and carried the concept of personal involvement in sustaining a sense of well-being beyond physical health to encompass all aspects of the individual's being—mind, body, and spirit. The pervasive reach of this holistic approach into suburban life is invoked in [Safe] when Carol's friends chat in the locker room after their aerobics class about a self-help book that encompasses issues of "exercise, diet, healthy food, emotional maintenance and stress management." Coward, too, notes the degree to which this notion of the fully integrated individual that she calls the "fantasy of the whole person" has influenced the way that we as a society talk and think about health. She believes that our "national obsession" with good health has made us especially receptive to the holistic philosophy expounded by the alternative health movement, a philosophy that she claims opens the way for a "potentially highly moralistic approach to health."[33] She states,

> By relating the state of the body, the level of stress and so on to a deep meaning expressed by this kernel of the whole person, everything is made comprehensible by reference to this inner core. In the idea of the whole person, the possibility that an individual has control over health and the possibility that an individual is to be blamed for the disease often shade into one another. And there are numerous ways in which a holistic approach to health gets tipped towards this more guilt-provoking idea of illness.[34]

Peter Dunning's moralistic teachings and their effect on Carol and the other "inmates" of Wrenwood could be viewed as a worst-case scenario of this tendency to merge personal responsibility with personal blame. In an especially torturous scene where Peter is conducting a group therapy session, he asks each member why they got sick and prompts them to provide the "correct" answer, which is that they made themselves sick because of negative attitudes. One women, Nell, whose husband has just died from a chemical-related illness that Peter claims was caused by his inability to "give up the rage," refuses to toe the line and take the blame; when she expresses anger at the world for making her sick, he angrily concludes, "The only person who can make you get sick is you. If our immune system is damaged, it's because we have allowed it to be through anger . . . does anyone have a problem with that?"

In this paradigm, the state of our physical health is completely dictated by the state of our emotions, which are invested with the ability to cause or cure physical illness. The individual is accorded unlimited power to transform her own fate and that of the world through love. Conversely, negative feelings must be avoided at all costs, even if it means limiting one's experience of the world. Although Wrenwood ostensibly offers a safe haven from chemicals and toxins—a claim that is debatable given its proximity to built-up areas, roads, and flight paths—its insularity really works to control incoming information. In one of his speeches during a group meeting, Peter says that he has stopped reading the newspapers and watching the news on television because he has heard the "media doom and gloom" and the "fatalistic negative attitudes" the media promotes. He refuses to subject himself to such negativity because if he does, "my immune system will believe what I believe." Yet by dismissing the media outright, Peter not only overlooks the positive empowering effect that the information it disseminates can have on individuals' lives but also betrays his belief that he is powerless to affect positive change in the outside world. He seems to forget as well that the "positive" effects of the Wrenwood community are advertised through the very media that he so roundly condemns.

Without a free flow of "contaminating" information into Wrenwood, its inhabitants cannot place their illness within a social context, they thus have no basis from which to engage politically with the environmentally based issues that have directly affected them. In the absence of external sources of knowledge, the residents have little choice but to fall back on Peter's wholly internal explanation of the cause and cure of their disease. While the purpose of quarantine is usually to isolate a small group of people with a contagious illness in order to control the spread of disease in the greater population, Wrenwood functions as a kind of reverse quarantine station where its inhabitants are protected from the spread of "unhealthy" information that permeates the larger "diseased" society, information that may be frightening and confusing, thus threatening to their illusion of control.

The appealingly simple and manageable internal approach to attaining well-being proffered by New Age gurus like Peter may give the individual some sense of agency in negotiating an illness or disease that confounds attempts by medical science to locate a cause or cure. But it also constitutes an extremely vicious circle in which illness becomes an ongoing expression of one's failure to love oneself enough, which in turn leads to negative feelings of guilt and blame, which in turn feed the illness. Although Carol's sickness manages to disrupt some of the assumptions and practices of the earlier systems of traditional patriarchy and medicine in which she was enclosed, Peter's rhetoric of personal culpability feeds on and completely contains the sickness by locating both its cause and cure within the perimeters of her self. Despite the fact that Wrenwood is an "alternative" to these other systems, it represents the most perfectly closed and thus the most damaging example of a reductive discourse in the entire film. Yet Carol, in her overriding need to find a "safe" environment, accepts another limiting, controlling discourse at face value, believing that she can adjust to and benefit from the Wrenwood environment simply, as she puts it, by "learning the words."

Haynes has said that his harsh criticism in *[Safe]* of this particular manifestation of New Age philosophies was in response to Louise Hay's book, *The AIDS Book: Creating a Positive Approach*, popular in the eighties among people with AIDS.[35] This book advocates, along with her earlier, immensely successful book, *You Can Heal Your Life*, a very similar philosophy to that put forward by Peter in *[Safe]*. Perhaps the most telling indication of Hay's attitude toward illness is her inserting a hyphen into the word "disease" in her books so that it stands for the general disease or malaise of the jaded citizens of the late twentieth century. Like Peter, Hay believes the answer to this "dis-ease" is a "positive approach." What bothers and interests Haynes about the appeal of this approach for people with incurable illnesses is that they would willingly accept "culpability over chaos" in order to maintain some sense of control, however illusory, over their situation.[36] Its attraction is that it possesses an internal circular logic that offers a neat and easily understandable explanation for diseases that often do not make much sense within any other paradigm. Within the personal sphere, sufferers are able to completely dictate and control the meanings of their illnesses even if they cannot cure them. Complicated external factors, both social and physical, become irrelevant because they exist outside this logic. While internalizing illness in this way may greatly simplify the links between cause and cure, it also means deliberately choosing ignorance over information by turning away from the messy outside world.

It is sometimes argued that sufferers of AIDS and environmental illness who have turned to such a philosophy—through sheer desperation and frustration at being unable to find help elsewhere—have at least managed to take their health out of the hands of a medical establishment that has been more of a hindrance than a help to them. But Haynes utterly rejects the kind of alternative offered by Wrenwood, not only because it places individuals suffering from perplexing illnesses in a no-win situation but more crucially because it completely ignores the social and structural factors that produce ill health and thus negates collective political engagement as a form of struggle. Social action is at odds with the personal responsibility rhetoric of the New Age movement because it shifts the focus away from the self and onto society as the most desirable site for change. As a result, in Coward's words, "[w]hat could be a political critique of conventional medicine is instead a critique based on a *philosophical* opposition to orthodox medicine and attitudes towards health."[37]

It is not difficult to see similarities between the alternative philosophy of personal responsibility exemplified by Wrenwood in *[Safe]* and the populist notion of individualism that characterized the politics of the Reagan era and the lifestyle of the 'Whites and that continues today. Indeed shifts in thinking about health in the last two decades are indicative of more "general changes in ideas about the individual's role in society."[38] As Ross has pointed out, "In the eighties, conservative forms of populism were quite successful in collapsing the perception that individuals *count* into the laissez-faire principle of self-reliance as the foundation of social good,"[39] and the pervasiveness of New Age language has no doubt contributed to the acceptance of this conservative understanding of social responsibility.

While Haynes criticizes the lack of social consciousness of the highly individualistic upper middle class in the eighties, personified by the Whites, he is perhaps even more sharply critical of individualism as he believes it has played out in the politics of the left through the New Age movement. In a recent interview, he cites the "implosion" of ideas that developed out of the counterculture of the sixties as an example of the failure of the left to sustain an effective voice in political and cultural spheres.[40] Yet both Ross and Grundmann dispute this "narrative of decline" of the left that "recounts the falling off of radicalism, and the absorption, recuperation, commodification, or yuppification of counter-cultural politics" because it does not acknowledge leftist political activism centered around issues such as feminism, racism, sexual preference, anti-nationalism, AIDS, and ecology.[41] Grundmann has argued that *[Safe]* lacks a critical perspective because "not only does the film ignore the most viable left-wing agendas, it also fails to account for their absence."[42]

I believe Haynes's intentionally excludes overt political references so as to seal the audience firmly inside the claustrophobic environment of both the Whites' upper-middle-class lifestyle and the equally conservative Wrenwood community. He wants us to experience these environments from within and get caught up in the rhetoric they espouse rather than placing us at a safer, if more politically informed, distance from them. Haynes does briefly suggest the possibility of political activism in the middle part of the film when Carol encounters the support group for sufferers of environmental illness, but after this short-lived breath of fresh air, which holds the potential for change, we are quickly plunged back into another oppressive environment that has withdrawn from the outside world.

The absence of a political context in *[Safe]* is in keeping with the film's refusal to provide any viable solutions to Carol's predicament, so that at the end of the film "we leave (her) almost where we found her at the beginning . . . —suffering in a repressive system that is supposed to have been the answer to everything."[43] The cures offered to Carol are far more damaging than the effects of her illness, and although it may be true, as Grundmann says, "It is [her] lack of critical consciousness that keeps her from empowering herself, her utter political apathy that makes her such a pathetic character,"[44] Haynes ultimately reserves his condemnation for the ideological systems that envelop her. Because of her need for confirmation from external sources, Carol is particularly vulnerable to being subsumed into the "natural" logic of the discourses of patriarchy, medicine, and the New Age movement she encounters. All of these discourses take it upon themselves to speak for Carol and position her according to their require-ments, rather than providing an environment where she can begin to rec-ognize and articulate an identity that is not wholly governed by the expectations of others.

Carol's containment by the inward-looking rhetoric espoused at Wren-wood becomes total when she readily moves into a porcelain-lined igloo that Claire reassures her is "perfectly safe as long as on one else sets foot inside." Carol does not question if this "room of her own" may have a less-than-therapeutic effect on her declining health. Although this is the same space that Nell's husband occupied shortly before his death, she accepts Claire's claim that Nell's husband "actually improved" during his stay there. The price that Carol willingly accepts for the safety that she achieves through her isolation in this chilly space is the complete surrender of autonomous speech and action. Yet this outcome is preferable to her than risking the possibility that her attempts to speak for herself may lead to rejection and condemnation.

When Carol is called upon to make a speech for her birthday in the penultimate scene, the vulnerable position from which she speaks is made apparent. Unable to put together an intelligible sentence of her own, she stumbles over and mangles snatches of rhetoric from the various systems she has passed through, turning them into an almost incoherent jumble. But it is less her inability to speak clearly than what she does manage to convey that threatens her acceptance into the Wrenwood family. When, drawing on the language of the environmental illness support group she was briefly involved with, she claims that awareness of external factors is important because the problem is "out there," she exposes to the others just how little she has really assimilated the Wrenwood philosophy. While her failure to "get it" indicates that Carol has retained some resistance to the rhetoric of personal responsibility, any hope that this could lead her to reject this approach to healing is dashed when later that night she returns to her igloo and begins to "learn the words" that will guarantee her acceptance into the community. As she did in earlier roles, Carol has once again chosen to dedicate her energies to memorizing and faultlessly performing her part in a scenario that she had no part in writing, rather than questioning the appropriateness of her assigned role. Playing the "dutiful daughter" has granted Carol the protection of a paternalistic culture, but the fatal cost of this protection is the permanent burial of her own voice.

A parallel between Carol's circumstances and those of the classic hysteric can once again be seen in the marked similarity between the New Age "cure" prescribed by Peter at Wrenwood and the rest cure that was commonly employed to treat the female sufferers of neurasthenia and hysteria during the Victorian era. Haynes makes an obscure reference to the rest cure in a group therapy scene where Carol mentions, when participants are asked to recall a room from their childhood, that hers had a yellow wallpaper. This seemingly irrelevant detail alludes to the celebrated short story by Charlotte Perkins Gilman about the destructive effects that the rest cure had on the mental health of women who were subject to it. First published in 1892, "The Yellow Wallpaper"[45] draws on Gilman's experience with the famous American nerve specialist, Dr. S. Weir

Mitchell, whom she consulted when she was unable to overcome severe postpartum depression after the birth of her only child. The rest cure that Mitchell invented and prescribed involved isolating the patient, confining her to her bed, forbidding any kind of intellectual stimulus, and giving her copious amounts of soft, bland food. It reduced women to an infantile state and aimed to ensure their complete submission to the expertise of the doctor and eventual return to their "proper" roles of wife and mother. Mitchell recommended to Gilman that she live as domestic a life as possible, keep her child close to her, and never touch "pen, brush or pencil" as long as she lived. As a result of this advice, Gilman said that she almost lost her mind. She wrote "The Yellow Wallpaper" in the hope that doctors such as Mitchell would reconsider their treatment for sufferers of nervous disorders.[46]

In the story a women describes her gradual descent into madness after being prescribed the rest cure by her husband-doctor. Just as Peter insists that his patients surrender fully to his interpretation of their illness, and in the same way that Dr. Mitchell demanded "complete obedience" of Gilman, so too does the women's husband in the story insist on her total submission to his authority. He ridicules any suggestions that she makes toward improving the terms of her cure, treating her as if she were nothing more than a petulant child, and dismisses her increasing obsession with the wallpaper in the room to which she is confined as simply another example of her overactive imagination. In the face of such confident assertions of his superior knowledge, the woman, like Carol, "drops back into the posture of helplessness which her culture has helped her view as more acceptable than argumentation."[47] As she says, "If a physician of high standing, and one's own husband, assures friends and relatives that there is really nothing the matter with one but temporary nervous depression—a slight hysterical tendency—what is one to do?"[48] Indeed Carol's eventual submission to the language of Wrenwood suggests that exactly the same question has passed through her mind. Even though she managed to reject her doctor's diagnosis of her illness and to escape her homemaker role, she, too, eventually comes to the conclusion that she has little option but to accept the assertions of another authoritative male if she wants to retain some modicum of social immunity.

Although the husband-physician in "The Yellow Wallpaper" and Carol's husband, her doctor, and Peter in [Safe] may be genuinely concerned about the well-being of the women who turn to them for care, they are unable or unwilling to allow the specificities of the women's respective illnesses to interfere with the construction and maintenance of their masculine discourses. Tied as they are to the rationalism that justifies their privileged position in the world, these men simply cannot interpret the obvious symptoms of deterioration in the women they treat and so they bury the experiential language of the female patients under the weight of their own seemingly more sensible pronouncements. At one point in *[Safe]*, when Carol tells Peter that she is "still learning the words," he says that "words are just a way to get at what is true." Yet the words Peter uses to expound his point of view only conceal the truth that is spoken by Carol's body. In *[Safe]* and "The Yellow Wallpaper," the women's verbal speech is effectively silenced. As Hélène Cixous has said of hysterical women, "their tongues are cut off and what talks isn't heard because it's the body that talks and man doesn't hear the body."[49]

The woman in "The Yellow Wallpaper" finally gets her husband to pay attention to her mental instability by tearing the maddening wallpaper off the walls of the room. Yet, as Linda Wagner-Martin points out, even though she finally expresses her anger at her husband's incomprehension of her mental state by physically rebelling against her situation, she remains the "good girl" throughout her madness. Rather than leaving the house or taking an even more extreme action such as suicide that she understands would be "improper," she vents her rage in a "tentative and hidden way": "Her escape into madness may have won her continuing argument with John . . . but it is only a Pyrrhic victory because her present life is valueless to anyone, particularly to herself.[50] Carol's more pronounced concern with being "good girl" does not even allow her to claim this kind of sad victory. She herself seems unable to understand that her body is screaming out against the cure prescribed for her. Like the rest cure, it isolates her, deprives her of external stimulus and information, and subjects her to a rigid set of inappropriate beliefs. By accepting the terms of her cure Carol ensures her validity to the Wrenwood community, but she does so at an enormous personal cost. Not only does she give up any likelihood of developing the resources that would enable her to exercise personal and political agency, and thus establish an identity more appropriate to her particular needs, she practically sacrifices her life for the sake of social acceptance.

Yet while Carol is particularly susceptible to being martyred by the external structures that govern the terms of her identity, there are at Wrenwood a few sparks of resistance to Peter's insidious totalizing philosophy. In a scene I mentioned earlier, Peter goes around the group and makes each person confess culpability for their own illness, but Nell, angrily grieving the loss of her husband, refuses to submit to his logic.

When Nell says, "I wanted to get a gun and blow the heads off everyone who got me like this," Peter tells her to "put the gun away" and to "learn to love Nell and her disease." Still she refuses to deny or internalize her anger and stares stubbornly out toward the horizon. The force of Nell's outwardly turned rage, drawing attention to the part that external forces beyond her control have played in her and her husband's illness, contains more positive energy and potential for personal empowerment than the rest of the group's resolution to learn to love themselves more. Her resistance also destabilizes Peter's rhetoric about turning away from negative emotions and embracing love, and he is unable to conceal his anger at this challenge to his despotic control.

While Nell's path of resistance gives us hope that she may yet escape the Wrenwood community, another character who has slipped out of Peter's grasp has taken a direction similar to that of the woman in "The Yellow Wallpaper," who was finally reduced to creeping about her room. Lester, who Peter describes as "very, very afraid, afraid to eat, afraid to breath," is an eerie figure who is always seen alone and from a distance stumbling about the open spaces of Wrenwood like a victim of a nuclear holocaust. His uncanny appearances and his lack of incorporation into the community reveal that, contrary to its motto, all is not well in the Wrenwood world. Both Nell and Lester are reminders that while ideological systems work to both contain and confine individuals by offering protection in exchange for conformity within a prescribed space, there will always be openings where the logic of such systems can and will be contested and disrupted. Haynes illustrates this point by using brackets around the film's title rather than fully enclosing the word "safe" within a box. The gaping space between each bracket signifies the parameters of the systems within which Carol seeks to protect herself, suggesting that no amount of ideological work can guarantee any system full immunity from the "corrupting" influence of the external environment, nor can the reactions of individuals functioning in relation to such dogmatic discourses be fully determined. Although Carol's readiness to submit to the dictates of repressive systems make her a perfect example of Foucault's notion of the "docile body," it is this very body that disrupts the smooth running of patriarchy by collapsing into chaos.

Carol's fate is literally sealed at the end of the film as she locks herself in her igloo and intones the words of self-love that destroy the final remnants of her individuality. Haynes's refusal to allow the audience to imagine that there is even a glimmer of a chance of redemption for Carol is extremely difficult to bear, and we are left trying to imagine different circumstances that could have saved her from such a tragic end. Yet in our desire to redeem Carol, we take it upon ourselves to come up with a means by which she can solve her dilemma, thus aligning ourselves with the structures in the film that also believe they know what is best for her. By highlighting our desire for a more satisfactory sense of closure in this way, Haynes reveals how difficult it is for us as humans to resist the appeal of discourses that purport to provide surefire answers. Yet *[Safe]* suggests that retreating to places that seemingly resolve the chaos that can arise around illness and identity can be more dangerous to the individual and to society than engaging fully with the messy contradictions of the late twentieth century.

Notes

1. Roy Grundmann, "How Clean Was My Valley: Todd Haynes's *Safe*," *Cineaste* 21.4 (1995): 22.
2. Mike Davis, *City of Quartz* (New York: Vintage Books, 1990) 224.
3. For reasons as to why this is the case, see Michael Castleman, "This Place Makes Me Sick," *Sierra* (September/October 1993): 105–116; Thomas Orne and Paul Benedetti, *Multiple Chemical Sensitivity*, ed. Stephen Barrett (American Council on Science and Health, 1991): see also on the internet, http://www.primenet.com/'nchaf/acsh/mcsdoc.html
4. In Amy Taubin, "Nowhere to Hide," *Sight and Sound* 6.5 (May 1996): 33.
5. In Collier Schorr, "Diary of a Sad Housewife," *Artforum International* 33.10 (Summer 1995): 87.
6. This expression comes from the film *The Stepford Wives* (1975), directed by Bryan Forbes, in which a group of men replace their wives with identical robots who are perfect homemakers. For a recent article on the film, see *Film Review* (August 1996): 44–47.
7. Barbara Ehrenreich and Deirdre English, *For Her Own Good: 150 Years of Expert Advice to Women* (New York: Anchor Books, 1978) 105.
8. Ehrenreich and English 106.
9. Ehrenreich and English 105.
10. Grundmann 22.
11. Grundmann 22.
12. Elaine Showalter, *The Female Malady: Women, Madness and English Culture, 1830–1980* (New York, Toronto: Pantheon Books, 1985) 129–132.
13. Showalter 144.
14. Showalter 129
15. Showalter 129.
16. Showalter 130.

17. It is estimated that 70 to 80 percent of people who have reported suffering from symptoms of environmental illness are women. See Castleman 109; William J. Rea, *Chemical Sensitivity: Vol.* 1 (Boca Raton, Fla.: Lewis Publishers, 1992); *Archives of Environmental Health* 48.1 (January/February 1993): 6–12.

18. Orne and Benedetti 4.

19. Gregory Simon et al., "Immunologic, Psychological, and Neurophysiological Factors in Multiple Chemical Sensitivity: A Controlled Study," *Annals of Internal Medicine* 19.2 (15 July 1993): 97–103.

20. Eric Nelson, "The MCS Debate: A Medical Streetfight," *Washington Free Press* (February/March 1994); see also on the internet, http://www.speakeasy.org/wfp/08/Boing4.html

21. Grundmann 23.

22. Donald W. Black in Castleman 110.

23. Castleman 108.

24. Orne and Benedetti 7–8.

25. Nelson 1.

26. Castleman 110.

27. Rosiland Coward, *The Whole Truth: The Myth of Alternative Health* (London: Faber and Faber, 1989) 87

28. Coward 87.

29. Andrew Ross, "New Age Technoculture," *Cultural Studies*, ed. Lawrence Grossberg, Cary Nelson, and Paula A. Treichler (New York: Routledge, 1992) 533.

30. Coward 2–3.

31. I have taken this term from Anne Karpf's book, *Doctoring the Media* (London: Routledge 1988). It is one of four frameworks (the others being the medical approach, the consumer approach, and the environmental approach) identified by Karpf that the media commonly employ in discussing health and medical issues.

32. Coward 2.

33. Coward 13, 69.

34. Coward 69.

35. Louise Hay, *The Aids Book: Creating a Positive Approach* (Santa Monica, Calif.: Hay House, 1988).

36. In "Gentlemen Prefer Haynes: Of Dolls, Dioramas and Disease: Todd Haynes's *Safe* Passage," *Film Comment* 31.4 (July/August 1995): 81.

37. Coward 11.

38. Coward 6.

39. Ross 541.

40. In Taubin 33.

41. Ross 544; Grundmann 24.

42. Grundmann 24.

43. In Schorr 88.

44. Grundmann 24.

45. Charlotte Perkins Gilman, "The Yellow Wallpaper," *"The Yellow Wallpaper" and Selected Stories of Charlotte Perkins Gilman*, ed. Denise D. Knight (Newark: U of Delaware P, 1994) 39–53.

46. Showalter 138–144; Ehrenreich and English 101–102, 131–133.

47. Linda Wagner-Martin, "Gilman's 'The Yellow Wallpaper': A Centenary," *Charlotte Perkins Gilman: The Woman and her Work*, ed. Sheryl L. Meyering (Ann Arbor, Mich.: U.M.I. Research Press, 1989) 55.

48. Gilman 39.

49. In Showalter 161.

50. Wagner-Martin 60.

Contributors

MICHAEL BÉRUBÉ teaches at the University of Illinois at Urbana-Champaign. Bérubé is the author of several books, most recently *Life As We Know It* (1996).

LISA CARTWRIGHT is Associate Professor of English and Visual and Cultural Studies at the University of Rochester. She is the author of *Screening the Body: Tracing Medicine's Visual Culture* (1995) and numerous articles on gender, media, and health care.

STACIE A. COLWELL is an M.D. and Ph.D candidate in history at the University of Illinois at Urbana-Champaign as part of the Medical Scholars Program. She is writing her dissertation on the history of East African women's health development and family planning programs.

RICHARD A. CONE is Professor of Biophysics and Biology at Johns Hopkins University. His research on photoreceptors and vision led to the discovery of the fluid nature of cell membranes for which he, together with Michael Edidin, received the Cole Award from the Biophysical Society. For the past 15 years, he has pursued research to develop improved barrier methods for preventing unwanted pregnancy and sexually transmitted diseases. Recently, he cofounded ReProtect, LLC, to develop consumer products that protect reproductive health.

ANNE K. ECKMAN is a post-doctoral fellow in the Department of Epidemiology at the University of North Carolina at Chapel Hill and a member of the Women's Health Communities Project at the Institute for Southern Studies in Durham, NC. Her research has focused on the impact of the women's health movement and community activism on medicine and community health organizations.

VALERIE HARTOUNI is Associate Professor of Communication and Women's Studies at the University of California, San Diego. Her book, *Cultural Conceptions: On Reproductive Technologies and the Remaking of Life* (1997), considers as a problem of discourse and culture the controversies surrounding the development and use of the new technologies of human genetics and reproduction.

JANET LYON teaches at the University of Illinois at Urbana-Champaign. She is completing a book entitled *Revamping the Revolution: Feminist Polemics and the Manifesto's "Hostile Hand."*

EMILY MARTIN is Professor of Anthropology at Princeton University. Her work on ideology and power in Chinese society was published in *The Cult of the Dead in a Chinese Village* (1972), *Chinese Ritual and Politics* (1981) and, with Hill Gates, *The Anthropology of Taiwanese Society* (1981). Beginning with *The Woman in the Body: A Cultural Analysis of Reproduction* (1987), which won the Eileen Basker Memorial Prize of the Society for Medical Anthropology, she has been working on the anthropology of science and reproduction in the United States. Focused on the interplay between scientific and popular conceptions of the immune system, her latest book is *Flexible Bodies: Tracking Immunity in American from the Days of Polio to the Age of AIDS* (1994).

GAYE NAISMITH is currently in the honors program in Visual Arts and English at Monash University in Melbourne, Australia. As part of this program, she has recently completed a year of study and research at the

University of California, Santa Barbara. Her studies encompass film, popular culture, and women's issues.

CONSTANCE PENLEY is Professor of Film Studies and Women's Studies at the University of California, Santa Barbara. A founding editor of *Camera Obscura*, she is the author of *The Future of an Illusion: Film, Feminism, and Psychoanalysis* and *NASA/TREK: Popular Science and Sex in America*. Her edited books include *Feminism and Film Theory*, *Technoculture* (with Andrew Ross), and *Male Trouble* (with Sharon Willis).

MARK ROSE is Professor of English at the University of California, Santa Barbara, and the author, most recently, of *Authors and Owners: The Invention of Copyright* (1993), which was nominated for a National Book Critics Circle Award. He is currently preparing The Norton Shakespeare Workshop, an electronic publication to be issued in connection with the forthcoming Norton Shakespeare.

ELLA SHOHAT is Associate Professor of Women's Studies and Cultural Studies at the City University of New York-Graduate Center, and the coordinator of the Cinema Studies Program at CUNY-Staten Island. She is the author of *Israeli Cinema: East/West and the Politics of Representation* (1989) and co-author (with Robert Stam) of *Unthinking Eurocentrism: MultiCultural Studies in the Media Age* (1994).

VIVIAN SOBCHACK is Associate Dean and Professor of Film and Television Studies at the UCLA School of Theater, Film, and Television. Her books include *Screening Space: The American Science Fiction Film* (1987) and *The Address of the Eye: A Phenomenology of Film Experience* (1992), and she has edited a recent anthology, *The Persistence of History: Cinema, Television, and the Modern Event* (1996). Currently, she is completing a volume of her own essays called *Carnal Thoughts: Bodies, Texts, Scenes, and Screens*.

CAROL STABILE is Associate Professor of Communication at the University of Pittsburgh. She is the author of *Feminism and the Technological Fix* (1994).

ALLUCQUÈRE ROSANNE (SANDY) STONE is an assistant professor in the Department of Radio-TV-Film at the University of Texas at Austin. She is the director of the Advanced Communication Technologies Laboratory and the author of *The War of Desire and Technology at the Close of the Mechanical Age* (1995).

PAULA A. TREICHLER teaches at the University of Illinois at Urbana-Champaign in the College of Medicine, the Institute of Communications Research, and the Women's Studies Program. Her books include *A Feminist Dictionary* (with Cheris Kramarae, 1986), *Language, Gender, and Professional Writing* (with Francine Frank, 1989), and *Cultural Studies* (with Lawrence Grossberg and Cary Nelson, 1992). *How to Have Theory in an Epidemic: Cultural Chronicles of AIDS* is forthcoming from Duke University Press.

CATHERINE A. WARREN is Assistant Professor in the Department of English at North Carolina State University. She is co-editor of *James Carey: A Critical Reader* (University of Minnesota Press, 1997) and has published articles on media activism. She is currently completing a book on silence in medicine, looking at the institution's hidden history of sexual abuse of female patients.

Index

393

Printed in the United States
By Bookmasters